Bone Marrow Transplantation

Editors

BIPIN N. SAVANI
MOHAMAD MOHTY

HEMATOLOGY/ONCOLOGY CLINICS OF NORTH AMERICA

www.hemonc.theclinics.com

Consulting Editors

GEORGE P. CANELLOS
H. FRANKLIN BUNN

December 2014 • Volume 28 • Number 6

ELSEVIER

1600 John F. Kennedy Boulevard • Suite 1800 • Philadelphia, Pennsylvania, 19103-2899

http://www.theclinics.com

HEMATOLOGY/ONCOLOGY CLINICS OF NORTH AMERICA Volume 28, Number 6
December 2014 ISSN 0889-8588, ISBN 13: 978-0-323-35441-7

Editor: Jessica McCool
Developmental Editor: Donald Mumford

Hematology/Oncology Clinics (ISSN 0889-8588) is published bimonthly by Elsevier Inc., 360 Park Avenue South, NewYork, NY10010-1710. Months of issue are February, April, June, August, October, and December. Business and Editorial Offices: 1600 John F. Kennedy Blvd., Ste. 1800, Philadelphia, PA 19103–2899. Customer Service Office: 3251 Riverport Lane, Maryland Heights, MO63043. Periodicals postage paid at New York, NY and at additional mailing offices. Subscription prices are $385.00 per year (domestic individuals), $633.00 per year (domestic institutions), $190.00 per year (domestic students/residents), $440.00 per year (Canadian individuals), $783.00 per year (Canadian institutions) $520.00 per year (international individuals), $783.00 per year (international institutions), and $255.00 per year (international and Canadian students/residents). International air speed delivery is included in all *Clinics* subscription prices. All prices are subject to change without notice. **POSTMASTER:** Send address changes to *Hematology/Oncology Clinics of North America*, Elsevier Health Sciences Division, Subscription Customer Service, 3251 Riverport Lane, Maryland Heights, MO 63043. Customer Service (orders, claims, online, change of address): Elsevier Health Sciences Division, Subscription Customer Service, 3251 Riverport Lane, Maryland Heights, MO 63043. Tel: 1-800-654-2452 (U.S. and Canada); 314-447-8871 (outside U.S. and Canada). Fax: 314-447-8029. E-mail: journalscustomerservice-usa@elsevier.com (for print support); journalsonlinesupport-usa@elsevier.com (for online support).

Reprints. For copies of 100 or more, of articles in this publication, please contact the Commercial Reprints Department, Elsevier Inc., 360 Park Avenue South, New York, New York 10010-1710; Tel.: 212-633-3874, Fax: 212-633-3820, E-mail: reprints@elsevier.com.

Hematology/Oncology Clinics of North America is covered in *MEDLINE/PubMed (Index Medicus), EMBASE/Excerpta Medica, and BIOSIS.*

Contributors

CONSULTING EDITORS

GEORGE P. CANELLOS, MD
William Rosenberg Professor of Medicine; Department of Medical Oncology, Dana-Farber Cancer Institute, Boston, Massachusetts

H. FRANKLIN BUNN, MD
Professor of Medicine; Division of Hematology, Brigham and Women's Hospital, Harvard Medical School, Boston, Massachusetts

EDITORS

BIPIN N. SAVANI, MD
Professor of Medicine, Director, Long Term Transplant Clinic, Division of Hematology/Oncology, Vanderbilt University School of Medicine, Nashville, Tennessee

MOHAMAD MOHTY, MD, PhD
Professor, Head, Clinical Hematology and Cellular Therapy Department, Université Pierre and Marie Curie, Hopital Saint Antoine, INSERM, Paris, France

AUTHORS

ALLISTAIR A. ABRAHAM, MD
Assistant Professor of Pediatrics, George Washington University School of Medicine and Health Sciences, Washington, DC

LAURA ALONSO, LMS
Specialist in Paediatrics, Adult BMT Unit, University Hospitals Bristol National Health Service Foundation Trust, Bristol, United Kingdom

JANE F. APPERLEY, MD, FRCP, FRCPath
Professor of Hematology, Centre for Haematology, Faculty of Medicine, Imperial College London, Hammersmith Hospital; Department of Clinical Haematology, Imperial College Healthcare National Health Service Trust, Hammersmith Hospital, London, United Kingdom

ANDREA BACIGALUPO, MD
Division of Hematology and Bone Marrow Transplant Unit, IRCCS San Martino, Genova, Italy

VIJAYA RAJ BHATT, MBBS
Division of Hematology-Oncology, Department of Internal Medicine, University of Nebraska Medical Center, Omaha, Nebraska

MAMMEN CHANDY, MD, FRACP, FRCPA
Department of Haematology and Bone Marrow Transplant, Tata Medical Center, Rajarhat, Kolkata, India

H. JOACHIM DEEG, MD
Member, Fred Hutchinson Cancer Center; Professor, University of Washington Medical Center, Seattle, Washington

COURTNEY D. FITZHUGH, MD
Assistant Clinical Investigator, National Heart, Lung, and Blood Institute/National Institutes of Health, Bethesda, Maryland

ANDREW GENNERY, MD
Paediatric Immunology Department, Institute of Cellular Medicine, Great North Children's Hospital, Newcastle upon Tyne, United Kingdom

JOHN GRIBBEN, MD, DSc, FRCP, FRCPath, FMedSci
Centre for Haemato-Oncology, Barts Cancer Institute, Queen Mary University of London, London, United Kingdom

SARAH A. HOLSTEIN, MD, PhD
Assistant Professor of Oncology, Department of Medicine, Roswell Park Cancer Institute, Buffalo, New York

MATTHEW M. HSIEH, MD
Staff Clinician, National Heart, Lung, and Blood Institute/National Institutes of Health, Bethesda, Maryland

ANDREW J. INNES, MBChB, MRCP, FRCPath
Clinical Research Fellow, Centre for Haematology, Faculty of Medicine, Imperial College London, Hammersmith Hospital, London, United Kingdom

MADAN JAGASIA, MBBS, MS
Division of Hematology-Oncology, Vanderbilt University Medical Center, Nashville, Tennessee

ELIZABETH KANG, MD
Head, Hematotherapeutics Unit, Laboratory of Host Defenses, National Institute of Allergy and Infectious Diseases, National Institutes of Health, Bethesda, Maryland

HONG LIU, MD, PhD
Assistant Professor of Oncology, Department of Medicine, Roswell Park Cancer Institute, Buffalo, New York

NAVNEET S. MAJHAIL, MD, MS
Blood and Marrow Transplant Program, Cleveland Clinic Taussig Cancer Institute, Cleveland, Ohio

DAVID I. MARKS, MB BS, PhD, FRACP, FRCPath
Professor, Adult BMT Unit, University Hospitals Bristol National Health Service Foundation Trust, Bristol, United Kingdom

VIKRAM MATHEWS, MD, DM
Department of Haematology, Christian Medical College, Vellore, India

PHILIP L. McCARTHY, MD
Professor of Oncology, Department of Medicine, Roswell Park Cancer Institute, Buffalo, New York

FABIENNE McCLANAHAN, MD
Centre for Haemato-Oncology, Barts Cancer Institute, Queen Mary University of London, London, United Kingdom; Division of Molecular Genetics, German Cancer Research Center (DKFZ), Heidelberg, Germany

MIGUEL-ANGEL PERALES, MD
Deputy Chief, Adult Bone Marrow Transplantation Service; Director, Adult Stem Cell Transplantation; Fellowship Associate Member, Memorial Sloan Kettering Cancer Center; Associate Professor of Medicine, Weill Cornell Medical College, New York, New York

UWE PLATZBECKER, MD
Professor, Medical Clinic 1, University Hospital "Carl-Gustav-Carus" at TUD, Dresden, Germany

ROHINI RADIA, MB ChB, MRCP, FRCPath
Adult BMT Unit, University Hospitals Bristol National Health Service Foundation Trust, Bristol, United Kingdom

NISHITHA M. REDDY, MD, MSCI
Associate Professor of Medicine; Clinical director, Lymphoma, Division of Hematology/Oncology, Vanderbilt University Medical Center, Nashville, Tennessee

JACOB M. ROWE, MD
Department of Hematology and Bone Marrow Transplantation, Rambam Health Care Campus, Haifa, Israel; Department of Hematology, Shaare Zedek Medical Center, Jerusalem, Israel; Bruce Rappaport Faculty of Medicine, Technion, Israel Institute of Technology, Haifa, Israel

RACHEL B. SALIT, MD
Assistant Member, Clinical Research Division, Cord Blood Transplant Research Program, Fred Hutchinson Cancer Research Center; Assistant Professor, University of Washington Medical Center, Seattle, Washington

VAISHALI SANCHORAWALA, MD
Stem Cell Transplantation Program, Section of Hematology and Oncology, Amyloidosis Center, Boston Medical Center, Boston, Massachusetts

ALOK SRIVASTAVA, MD, FRACP, FRCPA
Department of Haematology, Christian Medical College, Vellore, India

JOHN F. TISDALE, MD
Senior Investigator, National Heart, Lung, and Blood Institute/National Institutes of Health, Bethesda, Maryland

JULIE M. VOSE, MD, MBA
Division of Hematology-Oncology, Department of Internal Medicine, University of Nebraska Medical Center, Omaha, Nebraska

KATRIN WETZKO, MD
Medical Clinic 1, University Hospital "Carl-Gustav-Carus" at TUD, Dresden, Germany

TSILA ZUCKERMAN, MD
Clinical Assistant Professor, Department of Hematology and Bone Marrow Transplantation, Rambam Health Care Campus; Bruce Rappaport Faculty of Medicine, Technion, Israel Institute of Technology, Haifa, Israel

Contents

Preface: Bone Marrow Transplantation xiii

Bipin N. Savani and Mohamad Mohty

Transplantation in Acute Myeloid Leukemia 983

Tsila Zuckerman and Jacob M. Rowe

Acute myeloid leukemia (AML) is associated with poor outcome mainly because of relapse. The best antileukemic treatment is allogeneic stem cell transplantation. However, the associated significant nonrelapse mortality limits both the application and outcome of the procedure. Recent advances in understanding the genetic landscape of the disease enable educated selection of patients. Improved treatment protocols, supportive therapy, patient selection, and posttransplant manipulations all contribute to a better outcome.

Allogeneic Hematopoietic Cell Transplantation in Adult Patients with Acute Lymphoblastic Leukemia 995

David I. Marks, Laura Alonso, and Rohini Radia

This review discusses the use of prognostic factors, patient and donor selection, choice of conditioning regimens, and timing of transplant. It also describes the management of Philadelphia-positive acute lymphocytic leukemia (ALL) and central nervous system disease. All aggressively treated adults with ALL should be considered for allogeneic transplantation and tissue typed at diagnosis. We further suggest that eligible patients be entered into clinical trials (that incorporate transplantation); these unselected prospective outcome data are essential to evaluate the true value of allogeneic transplantation in adults with ALL.

Transplants in Myelodysplastic Syndromes 1011

Katrin Wetzko and Uwe Platzbecker

Myelodysplastic syndromes are one of the most common hematological disorders in the elderly. Therefore, an increase in the prevalence of de novo but also of secondary forms after prior chemotherapy or radiotherapy, respectively, is anticipated within the next years. Allogeneic stem cell transplantation is considered the only potentially curable therapy, but many patients are not eligible because of age or comorbidities. Reduced-intensity conditioning regimens have improved early tolerability of the procedure, although late effects remain a challenge in the care of these patients. However, hypomethylating agents have become available as alternative therapeutic approaches with a moderate toxicity profile.

Role of Hematopoietic Stem Cell Transplantation in Patients with Myeloproliferative Disease 1023

Rachel B. Salit and H. Joachim Deeg

Myeloproliferative neoplasms (MPN) are clonal hematopoietic stem cell disorders. While some MPN patients have an indolent course, all are at

risk of progressing to severe marrow failure or transforming into acute leukemia. Allogeneic hematopoietic cell transplantation (allo-HCT) is the only potential curative therapy. Major pre-transplant risk factors are disease stage of the MPN, the presence of comorbid conditions and the use of HLA non-identical donors. The development of reduced-intensity conditioning regimens has allowed for successful allo-HCT even for older patients and patients with comorbid conditions. The pre-transplant use of JAK2 inhibitors, which may be effective in down staging a patient's disease, may improve the outcomes following allo-HCT.

Chronic Myeloid Leukemia–Transplantation in the Tyrosine Kinase Era **1037**

Andrew J. Innes and Jane F. Apperley

Allogeneic hematopoietic stem cell transplantation (HSCT) revolutionized the outlook for many patients with chronic myeloid leukemia (CML) in the 1980s. The introduction of the tyrosine kinase inhibitors (TKIs) nearly 15 years ago displaced HSCT as the first-line treatment for most CML patients. However, in the twenty-first century HSCT remains a viable treatment option for many patients with CML. This review focuses on the role of HSCT for CML in the TKI era, paying particular attention to patient selection and transplant outcome.

Transplantation in Chronic Lymphocytic Leukemia: Does It Still Matter in the Era of Novel Targeted Therapies? **1055**

Fabienne McClanahan and John Gribben

Allogeneic stem cell transplantation (HSCT) offers the only potentially curative approach in chronic lymphocytic leukemia (CLL). However, this applies only to a minority of patients, and is associated with significant treatment-related mortality and morbidity. HSCT must therefore always be considered in view of other, potentially less toxic therapies. Several new agents demonstrate impressive and durable responses in high-risk patients who might be candidates for HSCT. Therefore the choice of HSCT versus a novel agent is one that must be gauged on a patient-by-patient basis; this will change as data mature on the use of these novel agents in CLL.

Hematopoietic Stem Cell Transplantation for Non-Hodgkin Lymphoma **1073**

Vijaya Raj Bhatt and Julie M. Vose

Up-front rituximab-based chemotherapy has improved outcomes in non-Hodgkin lymphoma (NHL); refractory or relapsed NHL still accounts for approximately 18,000 deaths in the United States. Autologous hematopoietic stem cell transplantation (SCT) can improve survival in primary refractory or relapsed aggressive NHL and mantle cell lymphoma and in relapsed follicular or peripheral T-cell lymphoma. Autologous SCT as a consolidation therapy after first complete or partial remission in high-risk aggressive NHL, mantle cell lymphoma, and peripheral T-cell lymphoma may improve progression-free survival. Allogeneic SCT offers a lower relapse rate but a higher nonrelapse mortality resulting in overall survival similar to autologous SCT.

center outcomes and accreditation, patient health insurance coverage, geographic location and accessibility, availability of ancillary and support services, and coordination of care after discharge from the transplant center. Ongoing evaluation and research is needed to advise optimal care models for timely referral to a transplant center and transition of care from the transplant center back to the referring physician.

Index **1215**

HEMATOLOGY/ONCOLOGY CLINICS OF NORTH AMERICA

FORTHCOMING ISSUES

February 2015
Colorectal Cancer
Leonard B. Saltz, *Editor*

April 2015
Bladder Cancer
Joaquim Bellmunt, *Editor*

June 2015
Complement-mediated Hemolytic Anemias
Robert A. Brodsky, *Editor*

RECENT ISSUES

October 2014
Multiple Myeloma
Kenneth C. Anderson, *Editor*

August 2014
Iron Disorders
Matthew M. Heeney and Alan R. Cohen, *Editors*

June 2014
Melanoma
F. Stephen Hodi, *Editor*

Preface

Bone Marrow Transplantation

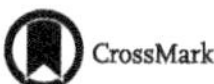

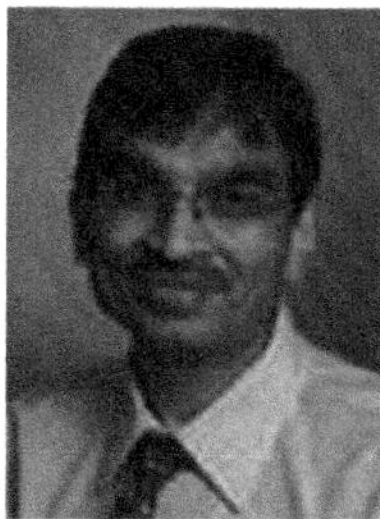

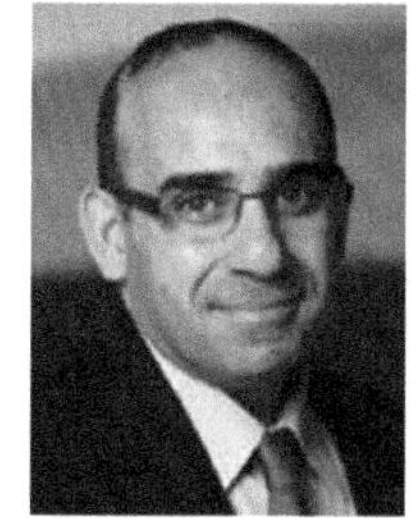

Bipin N. Savani, MD   Mohamad Mohty, MD, PhD
Editors

Since the first 3 cases of successful allogeneic hematopoietic stem cell transplantation (HSCT) in 1968, the number of HSCTs performed annually has increased steadily over the past 3 decades. It is estimated that by 2015 more than 100,000 patients will receive HSCT (combined allogeneic and autologous) annually throughout the world, and numbers are increasing rapidly. We celebrated the one millionth transplant in 2013! With continued improvement in HSCT outcome, the indications for HSCT continue to grow. Hematopoietic cell transplantation provides curative therapy for a variety of diseases. Over the past several decades, significant advances have been made in the field of HSCT, and now HSCT has become an integral part of the treatment modality for a variety of benign and malignant disorders.

Thanks to the advent of reduced-intensity conditioning regimens and improvements in supportive care, we now have the ability to safely perform transplantations for older patients and those with comorbid illnesses. In some centers, it is not uncommon to perform autologous or even allogeneic stem cell transplants in patients as old as age 75 years. Long-term studies suggest that average health-related quality of life and functional status among survivors, including older patients, recover within a couple of years to pretransplant levels.

A major obstacle to success with allogeneic bone marrow transplant has been the frequent lack of suitable matched donors. Only one-quarter of siblings will be an HLA match, and there is only a 50% chance overall, and much lower for African Americans and ethnic minorities, of finding a matched unrelated donor. Time is also a factor; it can take months to coordinate an unrelated transplant. New findings show that HSCTs are more accessible for patients previously not considered good candidates. Since 2007, more allo-HSCT procedures have been performed using alternative donor stem cell sources, such as volunteer unrelated donors or cord blood, than related donors. RIC haploidentical-related donor or cord blood transplantations have emerged as alternatives to fill the gap for those patients who do not have matched related donor or unrelated donor. Recent data support that haploidentical HSCT can be performed

Hematol Oncol Clin N Am 28 (2014) xiii–xv
http://dx.doi.org/10.1016/j.hoc.2014.09.001
0889-8588/14/$ – see front matter Published by Elsevier Inc.

safely, yield good outcomes, and greatly expand the number of patients who can be treated with stem cell transplant. In this era, a stem cell source can be found for virtually all patients who have an indication to receive allogeneic HSCT. Between the cord blood and haploidentical transplant, unrelated donor transplant, and matched sibling donor, there is nobody who needs a transplant who should not get it in this day and age, as long as they are healthy enough to undergo the transplant.

Due to the availability of novel substances and treatment strategies, the standards of care in many malignancies have changed dramatically. These new approaches include new monoclonal antibodies, immune modulatory agents, substances interfering with the BCR signaling pathway, and novel cellular therapies. The choice of HSCT versus a novel agent is one that must be gauged on a patient-by-patient basis.

A very exciting new active immunotherapy strategy is chimeric antigen receptor (CAR) T-cell therapy. CAR technology has recently emerged as a novel and promising perspective to specifically target malignant cells with precisely engineered T cells. Several clinical trials have reported impressive results with anti-CD19 CARs, in both chronic lymphocytic leukemia and acute lymphoblastic leukemia, and therapy has been investigated in other malignancies.

As there are no direct comparisons between HSCT and novel agents, general evidence-based recommendations are very difficult to make at this point. Instead, we need to understand the limitations of each approach and carefully weigh the chances and risks of each procedure on a case-by-case basis. In general, the availability of treatments, their expected benefit and side effects, and individual treatment histories and pretransplant characteristics as determined by the variety of risk score system, need to be taken into consideration. As the success of HSCT is, however, highly dependent on the remission state of the time of HSCT, it seems very desirable to focus on achieving disease control first. This can be facilitated by novel substances. As they are also well tolerated and show only moderate toxicities, they seem a good option to bridge the time until HSCT, and maybe even to postpone HSCT to a later point in the disease. How these substances should be best combined, if there is the option to completely eliminate the chemotherapy backbone from induction or second-line treatment, and whether they will have an effect on graft-versus-tumor and immunomodulation are the major focus of ongoing preclinical and clinical studies.

Indeed, the use of HSCT continues to grow each year in the United States, Europe, and around the world. In parallel with advances in other cancer treatments, HSCT has evolved rapidly in the past 2 decades in ways that may be unfamiliar to those who learned about transplant earlier in their careers. Nevertheless, continued underutilization of transplantation in patients who might otherwise benefit suggests that many of the improvements in the field may not be well-known among referring providers.

In this issue of *Hematology/Oncology Clinics of North America*, a multidisciplinary team has compiled an issue that details the state-of-the-art of HSCT management for commonly indicated benign and malignant hematological disease. The issue is therefore timely and at the same time unique. The contributions from acknowledged experts in the field from around the globe are covering the organizational aspects of transplant patients. This issue presents the most current knowledge about how to integrate transplantation and novel therapies in patients with benign and malignant diseases.

Bipin N. Savani, MD
Long Term Transplant Clinic
Division of Hematology/Oncology
Vanderbilt University School of Medicine
Nashville, TN, USA

Mohamad Mohty, MD, PhD
Clinical Hematology and Cellular Therapy Department
Université Pierre and Marie Curie
Hopital Saint Antoine
INSERM, U938
Paris, France

E-mail addresses:
bipin.savani@Vanderbilt.edu (B.N. Savani)
mohamad.mohty@inserm.fr (M. Mohty)

Transplantation in Acute Myeloid Leukemia

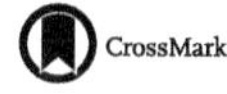

Tsila Zuckerman, MD[a,b,*], Jacob M. Rowe, MD[a,b,c]

KEYWORDS

- Acute myeloid leukemia • Allogeneic stem cell transplantation
- Autologous stem cell transplantation • Complete remission • Genetic alterations

KEY POINTS

- Allogeneic stem cell transplantation (allo-SCT) is recommended for patients with intermediate and unfavorable genetic risk.
- Allo-SCT is best performed in CR1. The chance of achieving CR2 is only 50%.
- Matched unrelated donor is increasingly used with no difference in the outcome compared with matched related donor (MRD).
- Alternative donors such as cord blood (CB) and haploidentical are being used, with encouraging data. There is no recommendation regarding the preferable stem cell source.
- Autologous SCT has a potent antileukemic effect mainly in favorable and intermediate-risk cytogenetic groups with reduced relapse and better leukemia-free survival compared with chemotherapy.
- Allo-SCT can safely be administered to fit older adults (aged 60–75 years), with results similar to those of younger adults.
- Further improvement in allo-SCT outcome includes assessment of minimal residual disease, graft engineering and incorporation of novel approaches (vaccines, adoptive T-cell transfer, and targeted therapy).

INTRODUCTION

Acute myeloid leukemia (AML) is a heterogeneous disease characterized by somatic acquisition of genetic and epigenetic alterations in hematopoietic myeloid progenitors that perturb normal mechanisms of self-renewal, proliferation, and differentiation through accumulation of multistep cooperating mutations. Advance in molecular

[a] Department of Hematology and Bone Marrow Transplantation, Rambam Health Care Campus, 8 Haalia Hshnia Street, Bat Galim, Haifa 3525408, Israel; [b] The Bruce Rappaport Faculty of Medicine, Technion, Israel Institute of Technology, Efron Street, P.O.B. 9649, Bat Galim, Haifa 31096, Israel; [c] Department of Hematology, Shaare Zedek Medical Center, 12 Shmuel Bait Street, Jerusalem 9102102, Israel

* Corresponding author. Department of Hematology and Bone Marrow Transplantation, Rambam Health Care Campus, Bruce Rappaport Faculty of Medicine, Technion, Israel Institute of Technology, PO Box 9602, Haifa 31096, Israel.

E-mail address: t_zuckerman@rambam.health.gov.il

Hematol Oncol Clin N Am 28 (2014) 983–994
http://dx.doi.org/10.1016/j.hoc.2014.08.016 hemonc.theclinics.com

methods showed 23 commonly mutated genes and an average of 13 mutations per patient.[1] The heterogeneity is not only interpatient but also intrapatient, with concomitant presence of genetically different leukemic subclones. This intraclonal genetic diversity reflects natural selection, leading to clonal evolution, disease progression, and relapse.[2] In addition, it was recently shown that the disease may originate from a preleukemic hematopoietic progenitor harboring the DNMT3 or IDH2 mutations, which confers clonal expansion and with additional mutations can transform into AML.[3] The importance of these findings is that to cure leukemia, we need to address not only the dominant clone at disease onset but also minor subclones that can lead to relapse. Until we better define the disease at the genetic level and its origin, AML treatment is intended to achieve complete remission (CR) with induction followed by postremission consolidation with either intensive chemotherapy, autologous stem cell transplantation (ASCT) or allogeneic stem cell transplantation (allo-SCT). This review focuses on the current role of transplantation in AML.

INDICATIONS FOR STEM CELL TRANSPLANTATION IN THE GENOMIC ERA

Evaluation of AML prognosis shifted over the last 2 decades from clinical (or patient related) to a more powerful biological one, based on cytogenetic and molecular alterations present in DNA blasts at diagnosis (disease related). Although under constant revision, biological prognosis is subdivided into 3 main categories of favorable, intermediate, and poor risk.[4] Integrated AML-related prognostic parameters are presented in **Table 1**.

The recommended LeukemiaNet reporting on AML prognosis was developed based on large retrospective studies, such as the Medical Research Council

Table 1
AML-related prognostic parameters

Cytogenetic Markers	Molecular Markers	Clinical Factors
t (8;21)	Mutated *CEBPA* (double)	Minimal residual disease negative
inv(16)/t (16;16)	Mutated *NPM1* (without *FLT3*–ITD mutation)	
t (15;17)		
Adverse prognostic factors		
inv(3)/t (3;3)	Enhanced *Evi-1* expression	Increased age
t (9;22)	*MLL* rearrangements	Increased WBC count
t (9;11)	*FLT3*–ITD mutation	Extramedullary disease
t (6;9)	*DNMT3A* mutation	No early CR
−5 or del (5q)	*BAALC* expression	Persistent minimal residual disease
−7	*ERG* expression	CD34$^+$ blasts
abn (17p)	*MN1* expression	Treatment-related AML
Complex karyotype	*WT1* polymorphism	
Monosomal karyotype	*BCR–ABL*-positive	

Abbreviations: AML, acute myeloid leukemia; *BAALC*, gene encoding brain and acute leukemia cytoplasmic protein; *CEBPA*, gene encoding CCAAT/enhancer-binding protein; *DNMT3A*, gene encoding DNA (cytosine-5)-methyltransferase 3A; *ERG*, gene encoding transcriptional regulator ERG; Evi-1, MDS1 and EVI1 complex locus protein EVI1 (also known as ecotropic viral integration site 1); *FLT3*, fms-like tyrosine kinase receptor-3; ITD, internal tandem duplication; *MLL*, gene encoding histone-lysine *N*-methyltransferase MLL; *MN1*, gene encoding probable tumor suppressor protein MN1; *NPM1*, gene encoding nucleophosmin; WBC, white blood cell; *WT1*, gene encoding Wilms tumor protein.

From Cornelissen JJ, Gratwohl A, Schlenk RF, et al. The European LeukemiaNet AML Working Party consensus statement on allogeneic HSCT for patients with AML in remission: an integrated-risk adapted approach. Nat Rev Clin Oncol 2012;9:581; with permission.

(MRC).[5] However, the postremission treatment was not stratified. The prognostic significance of these genetic alterations was recently evaluated in a large cohort of non–transplant treated patients. The classification clearly separates different genetic groups by outcome and hence can be used for stratification into different treatment groups in clinical trials.[6]

Integrated genetic profiling is a step forward in AML risk assessment. Using mutational analysis of 18 genes known to be involved in AML, Patel and colleagues[7] managed to further refine the large intermediate-risk cytogenetic group into 3 significantly different prognostic subgroups based on molecular alterations, thus emphasizing the significance of coexistence and cooperation of different mutations in AML (**Figs. 1–3**).

Without diminishing the importance of prognostic scores, the predictive value of postremission therapy should be cautiously interpreted, because it has not been prospectively tested in relation to postinduction treatment assignment. In addition, rapidly evolving knowledge and complexity of cooperating genetic alterations dissect patient populations into small cohorts, making analysis more complicated.

Yet, available data, mainly from retrospective subanalyses of patients in large study groups that were genetically randomized to donor versus no donor, can aid in decision making. Patients with the FLT3-ITD mutation have a CR rate similar to that observed in patients with the wild-type after induction therapy; however, they have a higher relapse rate (RR). Most studies, although retrospective, reported that patients harboring the mutation had a better disease-free survival (DFS) and overall survival (OS) after allo-SCT compared with chemotherapy only.[8,9] The beneficial effect of allo-SCT was restricted in some of the studies to patients having a low allelic ratio of mutated to wild-type FLT3 less than 0.8 or less than 0.5.[10] In contrast, other studies failed to show an improved outcome after allo-SCT,[11] whereas a large registry European Group For Blood and Marrow Transplantation (EBMT) study reported inferior outcome after allo-SCT in FLT3-positive versus FLT3-negative patients.[12]

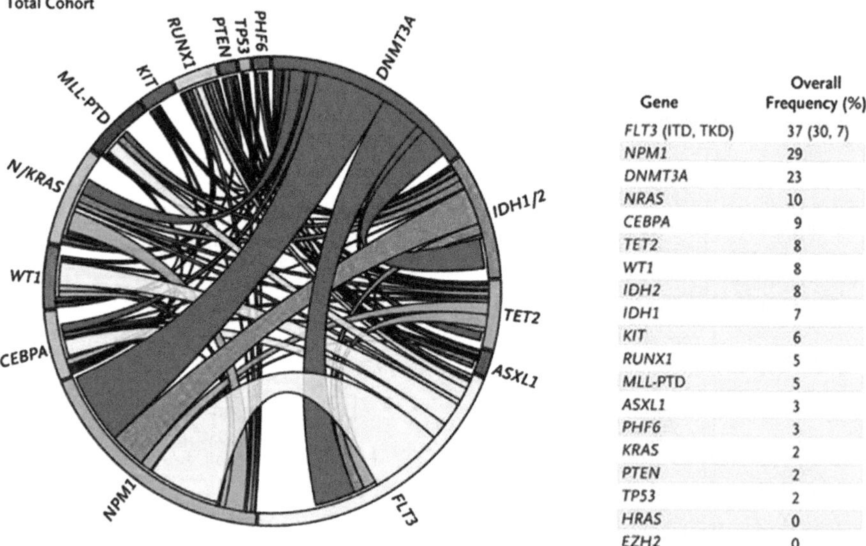

Gene	Overall Frequency (%)
FLT3 (ITD, TKD)	37 (30, 7)
NPM1	29
DNMT3A	23
NRAS	10
CEBPA	9
TET2	8
WT1	8
IDH2	8
IDH1	7
KIT	6
RUNX1	5
MLL-PTD	5
ASXL1	3
PHF6	3
KRAS	2
PTEN	2
TP53	2
HRAS	0
EZH2	0

Fig. 1. Mutational complexity of AML. (*From* Patel JP, Gonen M, Figueroa ME, et al. Prognostic relevance of integrated genetic profiling in acute myeloid leukemia. N Engl J Med 2012;366:1082; with permission.)

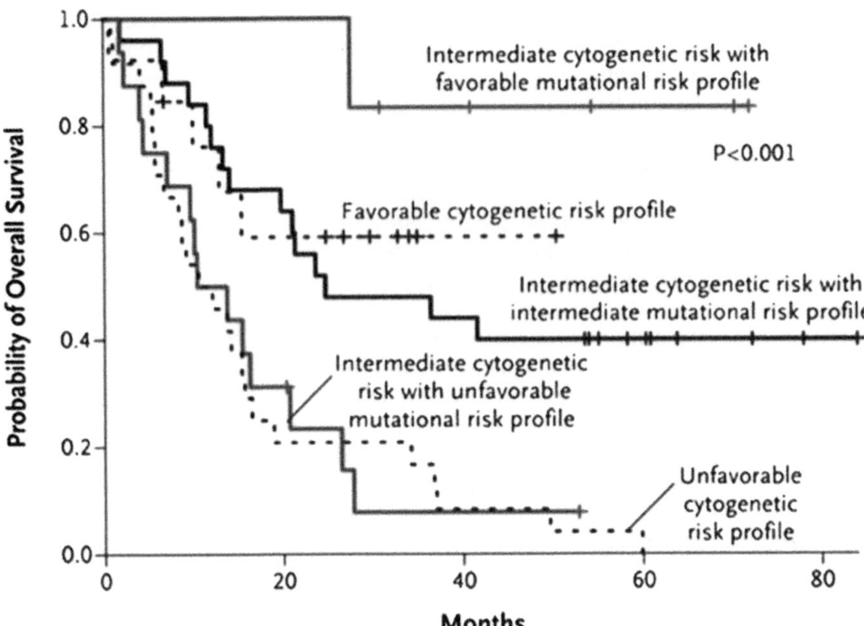

Fig. 2. AML: revised risk classification: integrated genetic analysis. (*From* Patel JP, Gonen M, Figueroa ME, et al. Prognostic relevance of integrated genetic profiling in acute myeloid leukemia. N Engl J Med 2012;366:1085; with permission.)

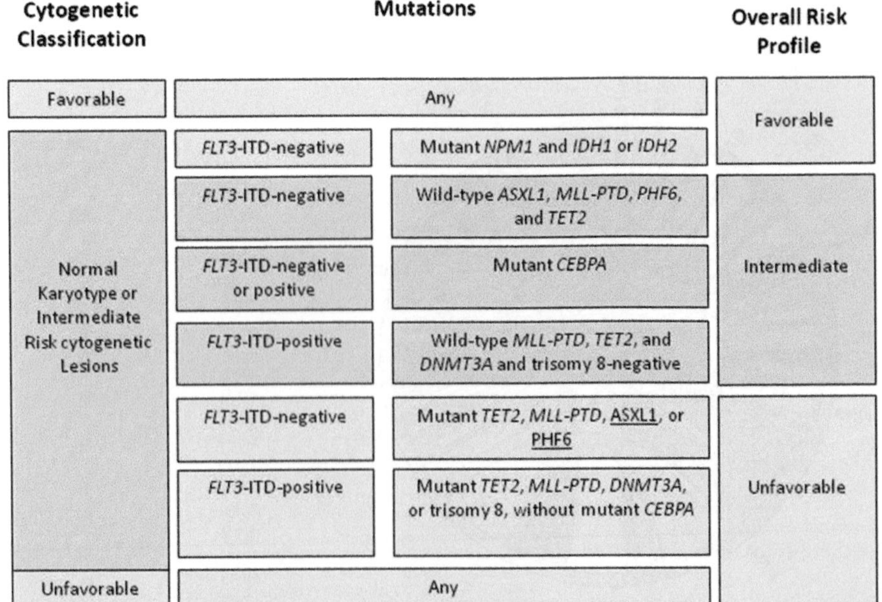

Cytogenetic Classification
Mutations
Overall Risk Profile
Favorable
Any
Favorable
FLT3-ITD-negative
Mutant NPM1 and IDH1 or IDH2
FLT3-ITD-negative
Wild-type ASXL1, MLL-PTD, PHF6, and TET2
Intermediate
Normal Karyotype or Intermediate Risk cytogenetic Lesions
FLT3-ITD-negative or positive
Mutant CEBPA
FLT3-ITD-positive
Wild-type MLL-PTD, TET2, and DNMT3A and trisomy 8-negative
FLT3-ITD-negative
Mutant TET2, MLL-PTD, ASXL1, or PHF6
FLT3-ITD-positive
Mutant TET2, MLL-PTD, DNMT3A, or trisomy 8, without mutant CEBPA
Unfavorable
Unfavorable
Any

Fig. 3. Revised risk stratification. (*From* Patel JP, Gonen M, Figueroa ME, et al. Prognostic relevance of integrated genetic profiling in acute myeloid leukemia. N Engl J Med 2012;366:1085; with permission.)

Monosomal karyotype is known to be associated with a poor outcome in AML. Whether it retains its prognostic effect after allo-SCT is not clear. Although some studies reported an improved outcome, especially when the disease was not associated with complex karyotype,[13,14] others reported no or limited beneficial effect from a transplant.[15]

In the absence of prospective studies, a matched-pair analysis of prospectively treated patients can better clarify the role of allo-SCT in different cytogenetic groups. In a study by the German AML Cooperative Group (AMLCG99), allo-SCT (both from related and unrelated donors) had a significantly superior OS and decrease in RR compared with chemotherapy in both intermediate and unfavorable groups.[16]

Meta-analysis of the role of allo-SCT in AML can aid in decision making, because of the attainment of significant statistical power when data on many patients are combined. Studies by Koreth and colleagues[17] including 6007 patients with AML in CR1 and by Cornelissen and colleagues[18] with 1033 patients from 4 large intergroup trials showed improved leukemia-free survival (LFS) and OS in both poor-risk and intermediate-risk groups.

When considering allo-SCT in AML, it is imperative to include covariates of the transplant itself, such as patient age, comorbidities, availability of a matched related or unrelated donor, and transplant regimen. These data accumulated in the Leukemia-Net recommendations on allo-SCT in AML patients in CR1 are presented in **Table 2**.

STEM CELL TRANSPLANTATION IN FIRST COMPLETE REMISSION AND BEYOND

Given the risks associated with allo-SCT, it may be tempting to postpone the transplant to CR2. A large retrospective analysis of 667 relapsing patients treated in the AML Dutch-Belgian and the Swiss Groups, reported that only 46% of patients achieved CR2. Patients were stratified by duration of relapse-free interval after CR1, cytogenetic risk, age, and previous SCT, into 3 risk categories for outcome at relapse. Overall, the best outcome was achieved using allo-SCT (5-year OS of 26%–88% depending on the risk group). Yet, only 14% to 30% of relapsing patients received allo-SCT.[19] Similar results were obtained in a large Japanese retrospective survey on the outcome of 1535 patients with AML who were treated with chemotherapy only before relapse. Sixty-six percent of patients relapsed and only half entered CR2. The achievement of CR2, using salvage allo-SCT, and a relapse-free interval of 1 year or longer, were independent prognostic factors for long-term outcome.[20] A recent update from the MRC in the United Kingdom reported an outcome of 1271 patients, aged 16 to 49 years, who were treated with chemotherapy only in the MRC AML10, AML12, and AML15 trials, and subsequently relapsed. Only 55% of patients achieved CR2 and only 67% of them received an allo-SCT. The best long-term outcome was achieved with allo-SCT, with an OS of 42% in the transplanted group versus 16% in the nontransplanted group.[21] A recent review by Forman and Rowe[22] suggested that given the low probability of achieving CR2 and proceeding to allo-SCT at that point as well as the dismal prognosis without allo-SCT, it is best to perform transplantation in CR1 according to previously suggested criteria. Moreover, allo-SCT is the only curative modality in CR2.

TRANSPLANTATION FROM A MATCHED UNRELATED DONOR

Because the best long-term results in patients with intermediate-risk and poor-risk AML are achieved with administration of allo-SCT in CR1 and given that only 25% to 30% of patients have a matched related sibling, the question is whether the beneficial effect of SCT remains also with the use of matched unrelated donor (MUD) in

Table 2
Recommendations for allogeneic HSCT in patients with AML in their first CR based on integrated-risk profiles[a]

		Risk of Relapse After Consolidation Approach		Prognostic Scores for Nonrelapse Mortality that Would Indicate Allogeneic HSCT as Preferred Consolidation		
AML Risk Group[b]	**AML Risk Assessment[c]**	**Chemotherapy or AHSCT (%)**	**Allo-HSCT (%)**	**EBMT Score**	**HCT–CI Score**	**Nonrelapse Mortality Risk (%)**
Good	t (8;21) with WBC $\leq$20 Inv(16)/t (16;16) Mutated *CEBPA* (double allelic) Mutated NPM1 (No *FLT3*–ITD mutation) Early first CR and no minimal residual disease	35–40	15–20	NA ($\leq$1)	NA (<1)	10–15
Intermediate	T (8;21) with WBC >20 Cytogenetically normal (or with loss of X and Y chromosomes), WBC count $\leq$100 and early first CR (after first cycle of chemotherapy)	50–55	20–25	$\leq$2	$\leq$2	<20–25
Poor	Otherwise good or intermediate, but no CR after first cycle of chemotherapy Cytogenetically normal and WBC >100 Cytogenetically abnormal	70–80	30–40	$\leq$3–4	$\leq$3–4	<30
Very poor	Monosomal karyotype Abn3q26 Enhanced Evi-1 expression	>90	40–50	$\leq$5	$\leq$5	<40

Abbreviations: AHSCT, autologous hematopoietic stem cell transplantation; AML, acute myeloid leukemia; *CEBPA*, gene encoding CCAAT enhancer-binding protein α; DFS, disease-free survival; EBMT, European Group For Blood and Marrow Transplantation; Evi-1, ecotropic viral integration site 1; *FLT3*, gene encoding fms-like tyrosine kinase receptor-3; HCT–CI, hematopoietic cell transplantation comorbidity index; HSCT, hematopoietic stem cell transplantation; ITD, internal tandem duplication; NA, not advocated; NPM1, gene encoding nucleophosmin; WBC, white blood cell count.

[a] The proposed patient-specific application of allogeneic HSCT in patients with AML in their first CR integrates the individual risks for relapse and nonrelapse mortality and aims for a DFS benefit of at least 10% for the individual patient compared with consolidation by a nonallogeneic HSCT approach.

[b] The categorization of AML is based on cytogenetic, molecular, and clinical parameters (including WBC) into good, intermediate, and (very) poor subcategories and is subject to continuing study and debate. Here, categories are arbitrarily presented according to the latest policy of the Dutch–Belgian Cooperative Trial Group for Hematology Oncology and Swiss Group for Clinical Cancer Research (HOVON–SAKK) consortium. Relapse percentages were derived from published reports.

[c] Includes response to first induction. Categorization requires one of the parameters indicated.

From Cornelissen JJ, Gratwohl A, Schlenk RF, et al. The European LeukemiaNet AML Working Party consensus statement on allogeneic HSCT for patients with AML in remission: an integrated-risk adapted approach. Nat Rev Clin Oncol 2012;9:585; with permission.

CR1. The advance in HLA typing, availability of a large registry of more than 23 million possible donors, and improvement in different aspects of supportive treatment during and after SCT are likely to have translated into a better outcome after MUD transplant. In a retrospective analysis from the Fred Hutchinson Cancer Research Center[23] comparing results of SCT between 1993 and 1997 and 2003 and 2007, with more than 1000 patients in each group, mainly with acute leukemia, and greater than 50% transplanted from a MUD in the more recent cohort, substantial reduction in the rate of death related to transplant, as well as increased long-term survival over the past decade were reported. The improved outcomes appeared to be related to reductions in organ damage, infection, and severe acute graft-versus-host disease (GVHD). Although no randomized trials have evaluated the use of MUD SCT in CR1, data from registry and retrospective studies are available. The Center for International Blood & Marrow Transplant Research (CIBMTR) analyzed the outcome of 2223 adult patients with AML who underwent allo-SCT between 2002 and 2006 (matched related donor [MRD], n = 624; 8/8 HLA locus matched MUD, n = 1193; 7/8 MUD, n = 406). Although a 100-day cumulative incidence of grades II to IV acute GVHD was significantly lower in MRD SCT recipients than in 8/8 MUD and 7/8 MUD SCT recipients, it did not translate into inferior outcome. In multivariate analysis, 8/8 MUD SCT recipients had a similar survival rate compared with MRD SCT recipients (relative risk, 1.03; $P = .62$). These results suggest that MUD and MRD transplants result in similar survival for patients with AML.[24] In 162 prospectively treated patients with high-risk AML, a head-to-head analysis of MRD to MUD SCT in CR1 performed by the German-Austrian AML Study Group reported a similar 5-year OS of 25% and similar non relapse mortality (NRM).[25] A retrospective comparison of 368 patients with AML older than 50 years (median: 57 years, range 50–73 years) performed by the Cooperative German Transplant Study Group[26] found no difference in patient outcome with regard to donor source. These data are even more encouraging in view of a probable preselection bias associated with application of MUD SCT in higher-risk patients. However, the findings of the CIBMTR analysis show in a large cohort of patients no superior impact of graft-versus-leukemia effect in recipients of MUD compared with a sibling donor transplant.[27] Results of prospective studies in intermediate-risk AML are eagerly awaited.

AUTOLOGOUS STEM CELL TRANSPLANTATION IN ACUTE MYELOID LEUKEMIA

ASCT is considered as a postremission treatment option, especially in patients with favorable and intermediate cytogenetic risk AML. The intensity of the treatment coupled with its low risk of mortality can offer cure to patients without a matched donor. Although ASCT has been studied extensively over the years, the interpretation of data is not clearcut because of different factors such as projection of historical outcome data to the current treatment area with improved supportive care, small subgroups of patients in different treatment arms, and significance of results based on intent-to-treat analysis when many patients did not receive the assigned treatment.[28] In a recent prospective randomized trial conducted by the HOVON-SAKK groups, patients in the ASCT arm had a significantly reduced RR (58% vs 70%) and a better 5-year relapse-free survival (38% vs 29%) compared with the chemotherapy arm. However, this factor did not translate into improved OS, because there were fewer salvage opportunities in the ASCT group compared with the chemotherapy one.[29] ASCT was compared with allo-SCT and chemotherapy in a subgroup of patients with the CEBPA double mutant, which, according to the World Health Organization classification, belongs to the favorable risk group. In this combined study conducted by the HOVON-SAKK and the German-Austrian (AMLSG) groups, relapse-free survival was better in patients transplanted in CR1 versus those receiving chemotherapy, but again it did not translate into a better OS; however, patients relapsing after ASCT were salvageable by allo-SCT in CR2.[30] The issue of performing allo-SCT from MUD after ASCT was addressed by the CIBMTR. MUD allogeneic hematopoietic cell transplantation (allo-HCT) after autologous hematopoietic cell transplantation (auto-HCT) relapse resulted in long-term LFS of 20% in 302 patients, with the best outcome seen in patients with a longer interval to secondary MUD transplantation, with a Karnofsky performance status score 90% or greater, in CR, and using an reduced intensity conditioning (RIC) regimen.[31] Similar results regarding the role of ASCT versus chemotherapy were obtained in a recent meta-analysis.[32] The available data suggest that ASCT has the most potent antileukemic effect after an allo-SCT and it may be beneficial in all patients in CR1 in whom a donor cannot be found. Prospective randomized studies are warranted to evaluate this approach, although it is unlikely that this will ever be done.

ALLOGENEIC STEM CELL TRANSPLANTATION IN OLDER ADULTS

AML is a disease of older adults, with a median age of 70 years. Yet, most studies on SCT exclude patients older than 60 years. Moreover, AML in this age group has an increased probability of poor prognosis, because the cytogenetic profile is more often unfavorable and it is more likely to evolve from previous myelodysplastic syndrome or is therapy related. With the introduction of reduced intensity and reduced toxicity protocols, improvement in the outcome of MUD and integrating the comorbidity scores in refined patient selection, the use of allo-SCT is becoming a feasible option for fit older patients.[33] The outcome of 94 patients aged 60 to 70 years with AML receiving reduced intensity allo-SCT in CR1 (as reported by the CIBMTR) was compared with the outcome in 96 matched patients uniformly treated with chemotherapy protocols of the Cancer and Leukemia Group B. Allo-SCT was associated, at 3 years, with a significantly lower risk of relapse (32% vs 81%; $P<.001$), higher NRM (36% vs 4%; $P<.001$), and longer LFS (32% vs 15% at 3 years; $P = .001$). Although the OS was better for SCT recipients, the difference was not statistically significant (37% vs 25%; $P = .08$).[34] The CIBMTR analyzed the outcome of 545 patients with AML transplanted in CR1 between 1995 and 2005 and found no effect of age on relapse, transplant related mortality (TRM), DFS, or OS.[35] The Eastern Cooperative Oncology Group has incorporated allo-SCT in older adults with AML as part of phase III E2906 study. This study enables prospective evaluation of allo-SCT compared with chemotherapy in this age group.

FUTURE DIRECTIONS

Post–allo-SCT relapse remains a major issue in AML, with an incidence of 25% to 30%. The management of posttransplant relapse is a major challenge to the immune system. A recent EBMT study evaluated the effect of donor lymphocyte infusion (DLI) administration in 399 patients in first relapse: comparison was made between 171 patients who received a single dose of DLI ($>1.10^8$) (most with active disease) and 228 individuals to whom it was not administered. The beneficial effect of DLI was shown in patients in remission, suggesting that the immunologic effect is significantly diminished in active disease.[36] The hypomethylating agent azacitidine, besides its role in the treatment of the aberrant methylation profile in AML, has an immunomodulatory effect, such as increasing functional regulatory T cells and killer cell immunoglobulin-like receptor expression. Combination of graded DLI and azacytidine in a small phase 2 study yielded a modest response, with 23% CR and 17% long-term remission.[37]

Should the focus be moved to preemptive DLI in patients with evidence of minimal residual disease? This theory has yet to be studied.

Assessment of minimal residual disease at different time points is another area of active research. Minimal residual disease can be evaluated either by real-time quantitative polymerase chain reaction for a known mutated marker and or by multiparametric flow cytotometry for the leukemia-associated immunophenotype. In several recent studies, minimal residual disease positivity pre–allo-SCT or post–allo-SCT was found to be unequivocally associated with reduced LFS and increased relapse risk.[38] With the recent discovery of a preleukemic clone, the meaning of minimal residual disease is probably about to be redefined.

Integration of targeted therapy with allo-SCT is another venue of research. Many new targeted therapies for AML are continuously developed, such as FLT3 inhibitors.[39]

Various immunologic strategies to modulate the immune system after transplant using either monoclonal antibodies or adoptive cellular therapies are being studied.[40]

The enormous advance over the last 2 decades in cytogenetic risk profiling, supportive care, HLA typing, and transplant protocols, increased availability of donors and data from large registries and phase 3 studies have contributed to better transplant outcomes. Future targeted therapies and immunologic manipulations are under way, with initial promising data.

REFERENCES

1. Cancer Genome Atlas Research Network. Genomic and epigenomic landscapes of adult de novo acute myeloid leukemia. N Engl J Med 2013;368:2059–74.
2. Ding L, Saunders TL, Enikolopov G, et al. Endothelial and perivascular cells maintain haematopoietic stem cells. Nature 2012;481:457–62.
3. Shlush LI, Zandi S, Mitchell A, et al. Identification of pre-leukaemic haematopoietic stem cells in acute leukaemia. Nature 2014;506:328–33.
4. Dohner H, Estey EH, Amadori S, et al. Diagnosis and management of acute myeloid leukemia in adults: recommendations from an international expert panel, on behalf of the European LeukemiaNet. Blood 2010;115:453–74.
5. Grimwade D, Hills RK, Moorman AV, et al. Refinement of cytogenetic classification in acute myeloid leukemia: determination of prognostic significance of rare recurring chromosomal abnormalities among 5876 younger adult patients treated in the United Kingdom Medical Research Council trials. Blood 2010; 116:354–65.
6. Mrozek K, Marcucci G, Nicolet D, et al. Prognostic significance of the European LeukemiaNet standardized system for reporting cytogenetic and molecular alterations in adults with acute myeloid leukemia. J Clin Oncol 2012;30:4515–23.
7. Patel JP, Gonen M, Figueroa ME, et al. Prognostic relevance of integrated genetic profiling in acute myeloid leukemia. N Engl J Med 2012;366:1079–89.
8. Bornhauser M, Illmer T, Schaich M, et al. Improved outcome after stem-cell transplantation in FLT3/ITD-positive AML. Blood 2007;109:2264–5 [author reply: 2265].
9. Schlenk RF, Dohner K, Krauter J, et al. Mutations and treatment outcome in cytogenetically normal acute myeloid leukemia. N Engl J Med 2008;358:1909–18.
10. Pfirrmann M, Ehninger G, Thiede C, et al. Prediction of post-remission survival in acute myeloid leukaemia: a post-hoc analysis of the AML96 trial. Lancet Oncol 2012;13:207–14.
11. Gale RE, Hills R, Kottaridis PD, et al. No evidence that FLT3 status should be considered as an indicator for transplantation in acute myeloid leukemia

(AML): an analysis of 1135 patients, excluding acute promyelocytic leukemia, from the UK MRC AML10 and 12 trials. Blood 2005;106:3658–65.
12. Brunet S, Labopin M, Esteve J, et al. Impact of FLT3 internal tandem duplication on the outcome of related and unrelated hematopoietic transplantation for adult acute myeloid leukemia in first remission: a retrospective analysis. J Clin Oncol 2012;30:735–41.
13. Fang M, Storer B, Estey E, et al. Outcome of patients with acute myeloid leukemia with monosomal karyotype who undergo hematopoietic cell transplantation. Blood 2011;118:1490–4.
14. Cornelissen JJ, Breems D, van Putten WL, et al. Comparative analysis of the value of allogeneic hematopoietic stem-cell transplantation in acute myeloid leukemia with monosomal karyotype versus other cytogenetic risk categories. J Clin Oncol 2012;30:2140–6.
15. Kayser S, Zucknick M, Dohner K, et al. Monosomal karyotype in adult acute myeloid leukemia: prognostic impact and outcome after different treatment strategies. Blood 2012;119:551–8.
16. Stelljes M, Krug U, Beelen DW, et al. Allogeneic transplantation versus chemotherapy as postremission therapy for acute myeloid leukemia: a prospective matched pairs analysis. J Clin Oncol 2014;32:288–96.
17. Koreth J, Schlenk R, Kopecky KJ, et al. Allogeneic stem cell transplantation for acute myeloid leukemia in first complete remission: systematic review and meta-analysis of prospective clinical trials. JAMA 2009;301:2349–61.
18. Cornelissen JJ, van Putten WL, Verdonck LF, et al. Results of a HOVON/SAKK donor versus no-donor analysis of myeloablative HLA-identical sibling stem cell transplantation in first remission acute myeloid leukemia in young and middle-aged adults: benefits for whom? Blood 2007;109:3658–66.
19. Breems DA, Van Putten WL, Huijgens PC, et al. Prognostic index for adult patients with acute myeloid leukemia in first relapse. J Clin Oncol 2005;23:1969–78.
20. Kurosawa S, Yamaguchi T, Miyawaki S, et al. Prognostic factors and outcomes of adult patients with acute myeloid leukemia after first relapse. Haematologica 2010;95:1857–64.
21. Burnett AK, Goldstone A, Hills RK, et al. Curability of patients with acute myeloid leukemia who did not undergo transplantation in first remission. J Clin Oncol 2013;31:1293–301.
22. Forman SJ, Rowe JM. The myth of the second remission of acute leukemia in the adult. Blood 2013;121:1077–82.
23. Gooley TA, Chien JW, Pergam SA, et al. Reduced mortality after allogeneic hematopoietic-cell transplantation. N Engl J Med 2010;363:2091–101.
24. Saber W, Opie S, Rizzo JD, et al. Outcomes after matched unrelated donor versus identical sibling hematopoietic cell transplantation in adults with acute myelogenous leukemia. Blood 2012;119:3908–16.
25. Schlenk RF, Dohner K, Mack S, et al. Prospective evaluation of allogeneic hematopoietic stem-cell transplantation from matched related and matched unrelated donors in younger adults with high-risk acute myeloid leukemia: German-Austrian trial AMLHD98A. J Clin Oncol 2010;28:4642–8.
26. Schetelig J, Bornhauser M, Schmid C, et al. Matched unrelated or matched sibling donors result in comparable survival after allogeneic stem-cell transplantation in elderly patients with acute myeloid leukemia: a report from the cooperative German Transplant Study Group. J Clin Oncol 2008;26:5183–91.

27. Ringden O, Pavletic SZ, Anasetti C, et al. The graft-versus-leukemia effect using matched unrelated donors is not superior to HLA-identical siblings for hematopoietic stem cell transplantation. Blood 2009;113:3110–8.
28. Rowe JM. Optimal induction and post-remission therapy for AML in first remission. Hematology Am Soc Hematol Educ Program 2009;396–405.
29. Vellenga E, van Putten W, Ossenkoppele GJ, et al. Autologous peripheral blood stem cell transplantation for acute myeloid leukemia. Blood 2011;118:6037–42.
30. Schlenk RF, Taskesen E, van Norden Y, et al. The value of allogeneic and autologous hematopoietic stem cell transplantation in prognostically favorable acute myeloid leukemia with double mutant CEBPA. Blood 2013;122:1576–82.
31. Foran JM, Pavletic SZ, Logan BR, et al. Unrelated donor allogeneic transplantation after failure of autologous transplantation for acute myelogenous leukemia: a study from the center for international blood and marrow transplantation research. Biol Blood Marrow Transplant 2013;19:1102–8.
32. Wang J, Ouyang J, Zhou R, et al. Autologous hematopoietic stem cell transplantation for acute myeloid leukemia in first complete remission: a meta-analysis of randomized trials. Acta Haematol 2010;124:61–71.
33. Hahn T, McCarthy PL Jr, Hassebroek A, et al. Significant improvement in survival after allogeneic hematopoietic cell transplantation during a period of significantly increased use, older recipient age, and use of unrelated donors. J Clin Oncol 2013;31:2437–49.
34. Farag SS, Maharry K, Zhang MJ, et al. Comparison of reduced-intensity hematopoietic cell transplantation with chemotherapy in patients age 60–70 years with acute myelogenous leukemia in first remission. Biol Blood Marrow Transplant 2011;17:1796–803.
35. McClune BL, Weisdorf DJ, Pedersen TL, et al. Effect of age on outcome of reduced-intensity hematopoietic cell transplantation for older patients with acute myeloid leukemia in first complete remission or with myelodysplastic syndrome. J Clin Oncol 2010;28:1878–87.
36. Schmid C, Labopin M, Nagler A, et al. Donor lymphocyte infusion in the treatment of first hematological relapse after allogeneic stem-cell transplantation in adults with acute myeloid leukemia: a retrospective risk factors analysis and comparison with other strategies by the EBMT Acute Leukemia Working Party. J Clin Oncol 2007;25:4938–45.
37. Schroeder T, Czibere A, Platzbecker U, et al. Azacitidine and donor lymphocyte infusions as first salvage therapy for relapse of AML or MDS after allogeneic stem cell transplantation. Leukemia 2013;27:1229–35.
38. Anthias C, Dignan FL, Morilla R, et al. Pre-transplant MRD predicts outcome following reduced-intensity and myeloablative allogeneic hemopoietic SCT in AML. Bone Marrow Transplant 2014;49:679–83.
39. Dinner SN, Giles FJ, Altman JK. New strategies for relapsed acute myeloid leukemia: fertile ground for translational research. Curr Opin Hematol 2014;21:79–86.
40. Tettamanti S, Magnani CF, Biondi A, et al. Acute myeloid leukemia and novel biological treatments: monoclonal antibodies and cell-based gene-modified immune effectors. Immunol Lett 2013;155:43–6.

FURTHER READINGS

Brunet S, Martino R, Sierra J. Hematopoietic transplantation for acute myeloid leukemia with internal tandem duplication of FLT3 gene (FLT3/ITD). Curr Opin Oncol 2013;25:195–204.

Champlin R. Reduced intensity allogeneic hematopoietic transplantation is an established standard of care for treatment of older patients with acute myeloid leukemia. Best Pract Res Clin Haematol 2013;26:297–300.

Copelan EA, Hamilton BK, Avalos B, et al. Better leukemia-free and overall survival in AML in first remission following cyclophosphamide in combination with busulfan compared with TBI. Blood 2013;122:3863–70.

Estey EH. Acute myeloid leukemia: 2012 update on diagnosis, risk stratification, and management. Am J Hematol 2012;87:89–99.

Foran JM. Frontline therapy of AML: should the older patient be treated differently? Curr Hematol Malig Rep 2014;9:100–8.

Gönen M, Sun Z, Figueroa ME, et al. CD25 expression status improves prognostic risk classification in AML independent of established biomarkers: ECOG phase 3 trial, E1900. Blood 2012;120:2297–306.

Liersch R, Müller-Tidow C, Berdel WE, et al. Prognostic factors for acute myeloid leukaemia in adults–biological significance and clinical use. Br J Haematol 2014;165:17–38.

Martelli MF, Di Ianni M, Ruggeri L, et al. HLA-haploidentical transplantation with regulatory and conventional T cell adoptive immunotherapy prevents acute leukemia relapse. Blood 2014;124(4):638–44.

Ofran Y, Rowe JM. Genetic profiling in acute myeloid leukaemia–where are we and what is its role in patient management. Br J Haematol 2013;160:303–20.

Porter DL. Allogeneic immunotherapy to optimize the graft-versus-tumor effect: concepts and controversies. Hematology Am Soc Hematol Educ Program 2011; 2011:292–8.

Rowe JM. Important milestones in acute leukemia in 2013. Best Pract Res Clin Haematol 2013;26:241–4.

Schiller GJ. High-risk acute myelogenous leukemia: treatment today... and tomorrow. Hematology Am Soc Hematol Educ Program 2013;2013:201–8.

Stern M, de Wreede LC, Brand R, et al. Sensitivity of hematological malignancies to graft-versus-host effects: an EBMT megafile analysis. Leukemia 2014. [Epub ahead of print].

Versluis J, Labopin M, Niederwieser D, et al. Prediction of non-relapse mortality in recipients of reduced intensity conditioning allogeneic stem cell transplantation with AML in first complete remission. Leukemia 2014. [Epub ahead of print].

Allogeneic Hematopoietic Cell Transplantation in Adult Patients with Acute Lymphoblastic Leukemia

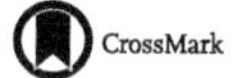

David I. Marks, MB BS, PhD, FRACP, FRCPath*, Laura Alonso, LMS, Rohini Radia, MB ChB, MRCP, FRCPath

KEYWORDS

- Acute lymphoblastic leukemia • Allogeneic hematopoietic cell transplantation
- Timing of transplant • Pretransplant conditioning • Prognostic factors

KEY POINTS

- Pretreatment and posttreatment prognostic factors should be used to guide transplant decisions.
- CR1 allografts remain controversial in standard risk patients.
- Novel conditioning regimens that do not include total body irradiation are being evaluated.
- Posttransplant relapse is a major cause of treatment failure; novel therapies such as blinatumamab for pH-negative disease and tyrosine kinase inhibitors for Ph-positive disease may improve outcome.
- Chimeric antigen receptor T cells directed against CD19 are a potentially exciting advance.

INTRODUCTION

Acute lymphoblastic leukemia (ALL) in adults is a rare, aggressive neoplasm of immature lymphoid cells that involves the blood, marrow, lymphoid organs, liver, testes, and central nervous system. With intensive therapy, greater than 90% of adults achieve complete remission[1] but nearly one half relapse.

Treatment outcomes in ALL in adult patients remain unsatisfactory, but recent developments suggest that there will be significant improvements over the next 10 years.[2] The optimal use of high-dose chemo(radio)therapy and hematopoietic cell transplantation (HCT) from allogeneic donors will be a major part of this progress.

Conflict of Interest Disclosure: D.I. Marks has performed advisory work for Amgen and Pfizer.
Adult BMT Unit, University Hospitals Bristol NHS Foundation Trust, Upper Mandlin Street, Bristol BS2 8BJ, UK
* Corresponding author.
E-mail address: David.Marks@UHBristol.nhs.uk

Hematol Oncol Clin N Am 28 (2014) 995–1009
http://dx.doi.org/10.1016/j.hoc.2014.08.008 hemonc.theclinics.com
0889-8588/14/$ – see front matter

Allogeneic HCT, despite its limitations and toxicities, is an accepted therapy for adults with this disease. A number of prospective studies and a meta-analyses support the use of sibling allografts for adults with ALL in first remission.[1,3–5] Nonetheless, there are greatly differing views about its role in adult ALL. Chemotherapy and HCT have complementary roles in ALL management and leukemia physicians should acknowledge that chemotherapy fails in many adults and that in some patients early transplant is a better option. Transplantation should be considered from the day of diagnosis.

PATIENT EVALUATION AND SELECTION OVERVIEW: USING PROGNOSTIC FACTORS

Many simple clinical parameters affect the outcome of chemotherapy and should be used to guide management of patients in CR1.[6,7] These include age greater than 40 years, a high white blood cell count (WBC) at diagnosis, greater than 4 weeks to achievement of CR1, and certain cytogenetic abnormalities.[8] Having more than 1 adverse factor has a cumulative impact on prognosis.[7] Some factors are not independently predictive of outcome. For example, a high WBC is more commonly seen in patients with t(4;11) disease. In adult acute myeloid leukemia patients, known risk factors have been statistically manipulated to calculate risk scores that guide chemotherapy and transplant decisions.[9] This has been harder to do in ALL, because patient numbers are much smaller but this will be required to individualize therapy. At present we do not know how much weight to give each risk factor, especially when they interact.

Adverse prognostic factors predict failure of chemotherapy, but it cannot be assumed that allogeneic transplant will be better therapy. However, it is reasonable to design clinical trials to test this hypothesis.[10,11] Entering patients on trials that examine the role of transplantation may answer these questions, but we accept that many patients and physicians will not have access to such trials and will require recommendations based on available evidence.

Does transplantation improve the outcome of patients with adverse risk factors? In a Center of International BMT research (CIBMTR) study of 169 patients with ALL who received unrelated donor stem cell transplantation in CR1, 157 patients had at least 1 risk factor and 97 had more than 1 risk factor.[12] One quarter had a WBC of greater than 100×10^9/L at diagnosis, 28% were greater than 40 years, and 25% had adverse cytogenetics; these risk factors were associated with 5-year survivals of 21%, 26%, and 22% to 28%, respectively, in the UKALL XII/ECOG 2993 study. Therefore, the answer is that transplantation probably did improve survival; 39% of the 169 patients survived and most had multiple risk factors. However, these are selected historical data and only prospective studies can provide clear answers. Notably, there is evidence from a prospective French study that allograft improves the outcome of patients with t(4;11).[13] In the UKALL XIV study, high-risk patients are assigned to sibling or unrelated donor stem cell transplantation if they have an 8/8 donor enabling their outcome to be compared with patients without a donor.

A high WBC at diagnosis implies greater tumor bulk to eradicate. In B-cell disease, a count of greater than 30 and in T-cell disease a count of greater than 100×10^9/L confer a worse prognosis, although that effect is modest with still 40% being cured.[14] Advancing age (>40–50 years) is the hardest risk factor to address (**Fig. 1**). Older patients with ALL are less easily cured because of a variety of biologic (patient-related) and disease-related factors.[11] The outcome of older patients with chemotherapy is poor, but myeloablative stem cell transplantation has not been shown to improve survival because of the 36% 2-year treatment-related mortality (TRM) seen in this age group.[1] The UKALL XIV trial prospectively tests whether reduced intensity allografts

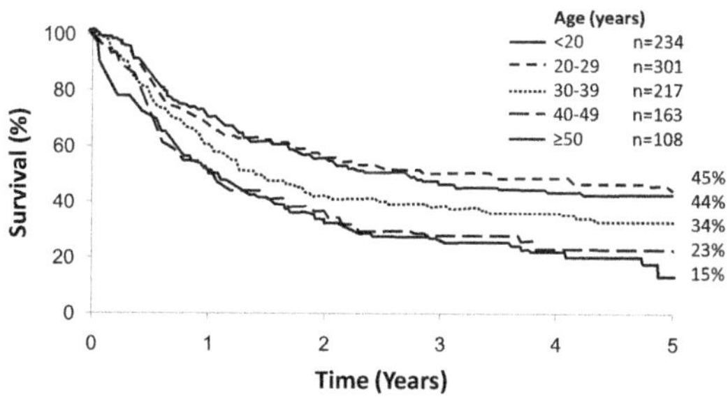

Fig. 1. The probability of survival (%) with age (years) in the UKALL XII/ECOG 2993 trial. (*From* Rowe JM, Buck G, Burnett AK, et al. ECOG; MRC/NCRI Adult Leukemia Working Party. Induction therapy for adults with acute lymphoblastic leukemia: results of more than 1500 patients from the international ALL trial: MRC UKALL XII/ECOG 2993. Blood 2005;106:3760–7.)

(sibling and unrelated donor) can reduce TRM and improve survival. At present, there are no data supporting this strategy, so I enter my patients in our national clinical trial. Older patients without access to clinical trials should be considered for allografting if they are fit and have a well-matched donor, but this has not been shown to improve survival.

Response to therapy may trump all risk factors. For example, patients with a high diagnostic WBC may have a good outcome if they become minimum residual disease (MRD) negative and it may be unnecessary to regard them as high risk and therefore an allograft candidate. However, this is being examined further in prospective trials.

MRD data in adult ALL are protocol specific, but it is clear that patients who are MRD positive 10 weeks from diagnosis have a low chance of cure with continued chemotherapy and are candidates for allogeneic transplantation.[15] In the UKALL XII protocol, there was 85% survival of patients who were MRD positive after phase II induction if sibling allograft was performed.[16] MRD status did not the affect outcome in patients who had a sibling allograft in CR1, suggesting that allografting may mitigate the adverse effect of a suboptimal response to chemotherapy. Larger numbers are required to confirm this encouraging finding.

Evaluation of prognostic factors is essential for decision making. We offer fit high-risk patients with appropriate donors an allograft in CR1. For standard-risk patients with a sibling donor who are MRD negative, the decision is difficult. After discussion of the options, some patients decide to continue with chemotherapy.

SPECIFIC DISEASE SUBTYPES

Philadelphia-Positive Acute Lymphocytic Leukemia

One quarter of adults have this adverse chromosomal abnormality. Older patients have an increased incidence, but this plateaus at 50 years.[17] Patients with additional chromosomal abnormalities (deletion 9p) have a worse prognosis.

Treatment of this disease has been recently reviewed.[18] Although response rates and survival have undoubtedly improved with concomitant tyrosine kinase inhibitor therapy,[19] we assume that all fit intensively treated adults will require an allogeneic transplant if they have a suitable donor. Pediatric data showing excellent medium-term survival without allograft[20] cannot be extrapolated to adults currently. Tissue typing should be performed at diagnosis and the transplant center notified.

The results of myeloablative allografting in CR1 are modest: 44% and 36% 5-year survivals in sibling and unrelated donor transplant patients.[21] About 30% of patients will not have these donor options. Our view is that, although some centers specializing in cord blood transplantation achieve outstanding results,[22] there are now data indicating that this stem cell source is equivalent to mismatched unrelated donors[23] and therefore this approach is reasonable in selected patients in CR1. Haplo-identical HCT should be performed in centers with a specific interest. Posttransplant cyclophosphamide graft-versus-host disease (GVHD) prophylaxis is a promising advance that may promote immune recovery but requires further data.

There is considerable interest in the use of posttransplant tyrosine kinase inhibitor and whether they can prevent relapse or treat it effectively if it occurs. The German ALL group and the CIBMTR are studying this issue.[24]

t(4;11) Acute Lymphocytic Leukemia

Marks and colleagues[25] reported the outcome of 85 patients with t(4;11) ALL treated on the UKALLXII protocol. On multivariate analysis, allografting in CR1 was not associated with improved survival, but this may be related to small numbers. However, in the group less than 25 years, the strategy of allografting with sibling or unrelated donor stem cells was associated with 70% survival.

THE PROBLEM OF RELAPSE

Relapse of ALL occurs in more than 50% of adults treated with chemotherapy and is not curable with chemotherapy.[26] Only 40% to 60% of adults who relapse will achieve CR2.[27] Patients achieving CR2 may be cured by allogeneic transplantation, but unselected prospective results are not as good as selected single-center series with a large study showing 23% survival with sibling allograft and 16% with unrelated donor transplantation.[26] In this study, only 7% of patients were salvaged. Many patients died within 2 weeks of relapse.

The goal at relapse is to achieve CR2 without undue toxicity then proceed to allograft rapidly. There is no standard-of-care regimen, but FLAG is well tolerated and efficacious. If CR1 duration is greater than 2 years we may recommend a 4-drug reinduction, but this may be toxic. Careful assessment of cardiac function should be made in patients with high cumulative anthracycline doses. If there is no sibling donor available, a timely allograft is only possible if tissue typing and donor identification have been undergone previously. Cord blood and haplo-identical stem cell transplantation should be considered.

Efforts are being made to improve the outcome of relapse with trials of B-cell antibodies[28] and nelarabine.[29] However, currently the results are poor and patients at high risk of relapse should be considered for transplantation in CR1.

ALLOGRAFTING IN YOUNG ADULTS

Adolescents aged 15 to 19 years achieve better results when treated on pediatric-inspired protocols.[2] Adults aged 20 to 25 years (or perhaps older) also benefit from this approach, but this idea requires further study. In these protocols transplant has a smaller role. Our experience is that chemotherapy-associated toxicity is more common than in children[30] and that allografting retains a role in high-risk young adults and those in whom chemotherapy cannot be effectively delivered.

ALLOGRAFTS FOR PATIENTS NOT IN REMISSION

We do not recommend allogeneic HCT for patients with ALL not in remission; their outcome is dismal. All reasonable efforts are made to achieve remission, but we do not proceed if it cannot be achieved. However, some patients can be cured with active disease. Duval and colleagues[31] reported the outcome of allografts in 582 adults and children with ALL not in remission. Fourteen percent of patients survived 5 years with better results if the marrow blasts were less than 20% and performance status (PS) good. This showed that cure is possible but patients were selected. Similar results (10% survival) were reported by Doney and associates from Seattle in 95 patients.[32] Current patients who are refractory to all therapies may constitute a worse prognosis group than those previously reported. There is little place for allografting patients with refractory high blast count disease and poor PS.

DONOR ISSUES AND STEM CELL SOURCE

Finding a donor at the right time is critical. Timing is discussed further, but additional therapy can be toxic and affect transplant outcome or even eligibility. In CR1 patients, we prefer to perform the allograft after 1 cycle of consolidative post-remission therapy; this allows time for neurologic prophylaxis. In relapsed patients, we perform the allograft about 6 weeks after starting therapy provided remission is achieved. To do this, patients must have had a donor search at initial diagnosis. Some patients do not remain in CR2 long enough for a donor to be identified.

Matched sibling donors are preferred for patients with ALL undergoing an allograft on the grounds of practicability, availability, and cost. Only 25% to 30% of patients will have a fit matched sibling willing to donate.[33,34] There is increasing evidence that 8/8 molecularly matched unrelated donors achieve similar outcomes.[12,35] However, TRM may be higher (42% at 5 years in the CIBMTR series). Some of this excess mortality may be mitigated by a lower relapse rate (20% in high-risk patients). Less well-matched donors using CIBMTR definitions[36] achieve poorer outcomes (RR of treatment failure, 2.09; $P = .003$). It is our experience that 7/8 matched unrelated donor transplants (full or reduced intensity) in adults with ALL are problematic with a high incidence of infection, poor immune reconstitution and refractory GVHD, resulting in a greater impact on survival than that seen in Lee's landmark study.[37] This may be related to prior therapy of ALL including steroid exposure. These outcomes often tip the balance in favor of chemotherapy, except in the patients at greatest risk of conventional treatment failure.

The Use of Cord Blood

In a CIBMTR 3-way comparison of cord blood with 8/8 and 7/8 unrelated donor stem cells, the adjusted probability of survival was very similar in all 3 groups.[25] The cord blood group was younger, had a better PS, and was more likely to be from ethnic minorities and in CR2. This group experienced more graft failure (usually a fatal complication), more grade II to IV acute GVHD but no difference in relapse, non-relapse mortality (NRM), or GVHD.

The Minneapolis group have published encouraging data, but this requires large-scale confirmation as more units gain experience of using this graft source.[22,38] Cord stem cells are underutilized for patients in CR2. Almost all patients have suitable units available within the desired time frame.

An alternative rapidly available graft source is stem cells from haplo-identical donors.[39] The major issue has been that aggressive T-cell depletion results in poor immune reconstitution and high infection rates. However, the Beijing group using pretransplant antithymocyte globulin and no in vivo T-cell depletion, report excellent results in standard risk ALL.[40] The newer strategy of posttransplant cyclophosphamide to prevent GVHD (with more rapid immune recovery) is likely to make requires further evaluation.[41]

ISSUES OF CONDITIONING

Unfortunately, no large study has compared myeloablative allograft regimens. Some of the best long-term survival data are from the Stanford/City of Hope group using etoposide (60 mg/kg) and 13.2 Gy of total body irradiation (TBI) in 9 fractions.[42] CIBMTR compared this regimen with standard cyclophosphamide and TBI.[43] Cyclophosphamide and 12 Gy TBI produced markedly inferior survival compared with etoposide-containing or higher dose TBI regimens. However, if more than 13 Gy TBI was given, etoposide/TBI was not superior to cyclophosphamide/TBI. Transplant-related mortality was not higher in the etoposide/TBI arm, although this is undoubtedly more toxic. Etoposide plus TBI was superior in CR2 patients. We recommend etoposide and TBI in fit patients less than 40 years, but are concerned about its mucosal toxicity especially when mini-dose methotrexate is used as GVHD prophylaxis. Palifermin may reduce mucosal toxicity but needs formal testing.

Non–TBI-containing regimens seem to be well tolerated and achieve disease control. Santarone and associates[44] used fludarabine and pharmacologically targeted busulfan in 44 adults with ALL, reporting a 2 year TRM of 18% and leukemia free survival (LFS) of 63% in patients in CR1. Kebriaei and coworkers[45] used pharmacokinetic (PK)-targeted IV busulfan and clofarabine in 51 patients. The 1-year overall survival, disease-free survival and nonrelapse mortality rates were 67%, 54%, and 32%. Kebriaei and colleagues[46] have also investigated IV busulfan combined with melphalan, but NRM was high in patients greater than 40 years. Intravenous busulfan, therapeutic monitoring, and targeted dose adjustments has reduced toxicity and may allow for myeloablative or intermediate-intensity conditioning transplant regimens in older patients and those with comorbidities.

Reduced Intensity Conditioning

Full intensity allografting causes excessive TRM in patients greater than 40 years; this negates its antileukemic effect so that allograft does not improve outcome in this patient group.[1] Patients in the 40- to 45-year-old age group who have no comorbidities can receive full intensity allografts.

Reduced intensity conditioning (RIC) allografting has been tested less in ALL. The graft-versus-leukemia effect is only curative if the leukemia can be reduced to a minimal residual disease state. There is evidence that the intensity of conditioning may influence outcome in full intensity transplant[43] and data for chemotherapy-only conditioning are limited.

RIC allografting in ALL has not been subjected to prospective study, so first it was necessary to analyze data from international registries (**Fig. 2**). The initial EBMT study[47] found that patients not in remission had a dismal outcome; subsequent studies have focused on patients in CR1/2. Two studies require detailed description. Marks and colleagues[48] compared patients who received full intensity transplants for ALL with 92 patients who had a variety of RIC regimens using sibling or unrelated donors. The RIC group was 17 years older. Adjusted survival was similar in the 2 groups and TRM not significantly different. This finding was disappointing (reducing TRM was the reason to use RIC); it reflects outcomes in older patients who have significant comorbidities. Relapse was slightly higher in the RIC group (35% vs 26%), but this was not significant ($P = .08$).

The EBMT study had a different methodology.[49] It compared outcomes of full and reduced intensity allografts in 576 patients greater than 45 years using only sibling donors. This is a 'fairer' test of the difference between conditioning regimen intensities. Findings were different. TRM was lower in the RIC group (21% vs 29%) and

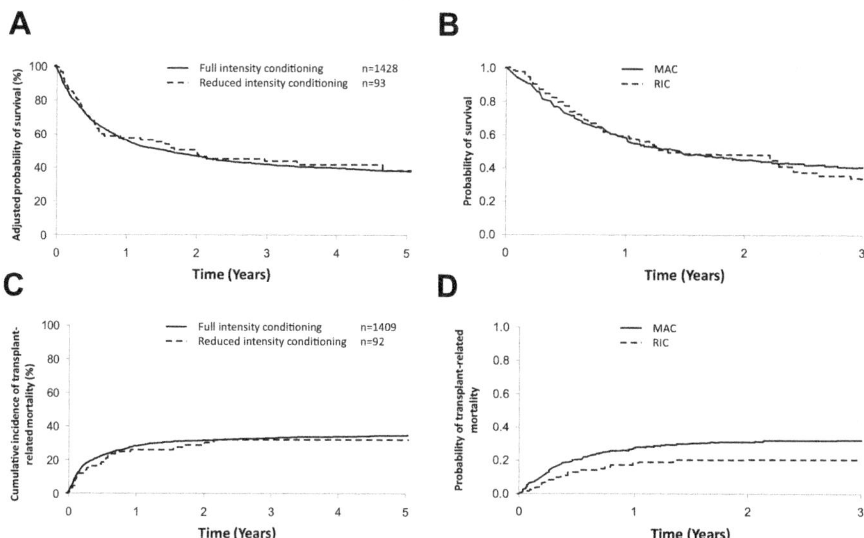

Fig. 2. Comparison of outcomes between full and reduced intensity allografts for adults with acute lymphoblastic leukemia. (*A*) Center of International BMT Research (CIBMTR) study: Comparison of adjusted overall survival between the full and reduced intensity conditioning arms. (*B*) European Blood and Marrow Transplant Group (EBMT) study: Comparison of overall survival between the 2 conditioning intensity arms in sibling transplant patients greater than 45 years. MAC, myeloablative conditioning; RIC, reduced intensity conditioning. (*C*) CIBMTR study: Comparison of transplant-related mortality between the 2 arms. (*D*) EBMT study: Comparison of transplant-related mortality between the 2 conditioning intensity arms in sibling transplant patients greater than 45 years. (*Data from* [*A, C*] Marks DI, Wang T, Pérez WS, et al. The outcome of full-intensity and reduced-intensity conditioning matched sibling or unrelated donor transplantation in adults with Philadelphia chromosome-negative acute lymphoblastic leukemia in first and second complete remission. Blood 2010;116:366–74; and [*B, D*] Mohty M, Labopin M, Volin L, et al. Acute Leukemia Working Party of EBMT. Reduced-intensity versus conventional myeloablative conditioning allogeneic stem cell transplantation for patients with acute lymphoblastic leukemia: a retrospective study from the European Group for Blood and Marrow Transplantation. Blood 2010;116:4439–43.)

counterbalancing this, relapse was more common (47% vs 31%). However, the 6% higher survival in the full intensity group compared with the RIC group was not significant (P = .07).

There were other important findings. In an EBMT study, chronic GVHD was associated with better survival.[47] This is a problematic but unsurprising finding. Severe chronic GVHD may not be well tolerated by the older subgroup and certainly affects quality of life. Patients with a poor PS (karnofsky score [KS] <80) did very poorly; they do not benefit from RIC allografting. Finally, using less well-matched unrelated donors resulted in poor outcomes. There was a suggestion of a worse outcome in patients who did not receive TBI (RR of treatment failure, 1.4; P = .02), but this finding was in a small numbers of patients who received various TBI regimens.[49] Fludarabine and TBI conditioning in 51 patients (25 Ph positive) resulted in 34% survival, 20% relapse, and 20% TRM.[50]

What should we recommend to our patients? If a patient can tolerate full intensity conditioning this is preferred, because there are more data with longer follow-up. It is possible that RIC survival curves will worsen with further follow-up owing to late relapse. But what about patients older than 40? Will RIC allografts improve their survival? The data are inconclusive and only prospective studies will answer this. Entering these patients into a clinical trial is advised. It is reasonable to recommend a RIC allograft (with a sibling or well-matched unrelated donor) if the patient cannot tolerate chemotherapy, although there is no evidence to support transplanting older patients routinely. Reduced neurologic-directed therapy is a theoretic issue with RIC allografts.

EXPLOITING THE GRAFT-VERSUS-LEUKEMIA EFFECT

Some transplant physicians describe the graft-versus-leukemia effect in ALL as 'weak.' The graft-versus-leukemia effect was first described in this disease[51] and there are multiple lines of evidence for its existence and importance. In a large study, Passweg and colleagues[52] showed that grade II or IV acute GVHD and/or chronic GVHD reduced the risk of relapse after allografts for ALL 2.5-fold or that, if there was GVHD, the relative risk of relapse was 0.40 compared with those without GVHD. This effect should be exploited and it is our goal in most patients that they experience some GVHD. Spontaneous GVHD is common after T-replete sibling and unrelated donor allografts but in the absence of GVHD at 3 months we rapidly withdraw immune suppression in patients at high risk of relapse.

The importance of a graft-versus-leukemia effect would argue against T-cell depletion of grafts. However, there are some provocative data from a UK group who report excellent (60%) survival in alemtuzumab in-vivo T-cell–depleted unrelated donor transplant patients with ALL in CR1.[53] A significant minority of these partially T-cell–depleted patients experienced GVHD and the alemtuzumab may have had some direct antileukemic activity countering the possible reduction in the graft-versus-leukemia effect.

TIMING OF TRANSPLANT

There is little evidence concerning timing of allograft in adults with ALL in CR1. 'Deeper' remissions (MRD <0.01%, achieved with additional chemotherapy) before transplant may result in better outcomes. However, intensive chemotherapy may result in infection (including fungal infection) and organ dysfunction; this should be weighed against the potential advantages. Data in children with Philadelphia-negative ALL in CR1 shows that achieving a low level MRD status improves transplant outcome.[30,54]

Allograft is powerful antileukemic therapy. In patients with acute myeloid leukemia, post-remission therapy does not improve outcome.[55] Of course, ALL may be different. In the UKALL XII/ECOG 2993 study the median time from diagnosis to transplant was 7 months[1]; this may have been associated with a high TRM. For sibling donors transplant can be performed after consolidation chemotherapy when neurologic prophylaxis has been given.

Unrelated donors take longer to identify and procure stem cells from but with 'fit' panels most transplants should be able to be performed less than 4 months from diagnosis if searching occurs at the first opportunity. The highest risk patients may not remain in remission if transplant is delayed.

In children in CR2 achieving a molecular remission or low level MRD improves outcome[56,57] but not in all studies.[58] This cannot necessarily be extrapolated to adults where second remissions are brief and post relapse therapy commonly very toxic. We are content with 1 course of reinduction therapy in these patients if flow cytometry shows less than 1% leukemic cells. A second course is sometimes needed to provide time to identify a donor.

CENTRAL NERVOUS SYSTEM INVOLVEMENT

Central nervous system involvement at diagnosis is increased in patients with T-cell disease, a high presenting WBC, and mediastinal involvement.[14,59] Prognosis is slightly worse[59] but not all studies demonstrate this.[14] Some patients relapse in the central nervous system; this may be associated with systemic relapse. The evidence base for managing these patients is extrapolated from pediatric experience. Eradication of leukemic cells is achieved by chemoradiotherapy because the graft-versus-leukemia effect is less within the central nervous system. In these patients, we perform a transplant with cyclophosphamide and TBI (14.4 Gy) and a cranial 'boost,' commonly 6 Gy in 4 fractions. This is well tolerated, but oral mucositis is more marked and we occasionally see acute cerebral toxicity that is usually reversible. An alternative strategy is posttransplant intrathecal therapy. Relapse in the central nervous system is a major cause of treatment failure.

RELAPSE POSTTRANSPLANT AND MONITORING

Until recently, most patients who relapsed after stem cell transplantation were palliated with few achieving remission. A retrospective analysis of 465 adults patients with relapsed ALL postallograft reported 5-year survival of 8% and median survival of 5.5 months.[60] Among 93 patients who underwent second allograft, only 6 remained alive. Early results with blinatumamab suggest this may be a less toxic but effective way of achieving CR, which may mean the role of a second RIC allograft may require reevaluation in selected fit patients particularly if graft-versus-leukemia effects can be exploited (Gokbuget EBMT 2013).[60] Another strategy would be to monitor patients post allografting and use immunotherapy or novel agents in patients with high-risk disease, MRD relapse or mixed T-cell chimerism before overt relapse. However, these interventions have not been shown to be effective.

ASSESSMENT OF THE PATIENT AND COMMUNICATION

Organ function, past complications, and estimation of TRM are the focus of pretransplant assessment.[61,62] We see the patient when there is sufficient information required to make a recommendation. Knowledge of risk factors, remission status (including MRD data) and progress with the donor search are needed to describe accurately the risks and benefits of the proposed allograft. Explaining the short- and long-term risks of transplant and comparison with nontransplant therapy are the major components of the transplant consultation (**Box 1**).

NOVEL THERAPIES AND INTEGRATION INTO TRANSPLANTATION

Achieving optimal outcomes in adult ALL is a moving target (**Table 1**). Randomized trials will establish the role of rituximab and nelarabine in upfront therapy (see **Table 1**).[28,63] Novel antibodies are being tested in phase III relapse studies and prospective studies will evaluate novel transplant strategies.[64,65] Larger scale results of pediatric-inspired protocols will also affect which patients are offered allografts. There is evidence that the outcome of younger adults with ALL is continually improving.[66] Similarly, transplant methodology is changing and in particular reduced intensity and radioimmunotherapy-based transplant regimens require testing prospectively.[67]

Box 1
Assessment of the patient and communication

Is the patient fit for myeloablative conditioning?

Microbiological assessment of past bacterial/fungal infections and targeted prophylaxis

Assessment of hepatic dysfunction, cessation of hepatotoxic drugs

Calculation of hematopoietic cell transplantation—comorbidity index: Assessment of renal and pulmonary function

The transplant consultation

- Timing: When risk factors, disease response, donor status known
- Calculation of transplant-related mortality and relapse risk
- Comparison with nontransplant chemotherapy
- Description of long-term risks (chronic graft-versus-host disease, infertility, secondary malignancy)

Recently T cells genetically engineered to express chimeric antigen receptors targeting CD19 (and other surface antigens) have resulted in clinical and molecular responses in small numbers of patients with B-ALL with minimal toxicity.[68–70] These T cells dramatically expand and may penetrate the central nervous system. Further work will focus on optimizing platforms for chimeric antigen receptors and determining whether remissions are durable. Relapse with CD19-negative disease may be an issue.

Table 1
Novel therapies and integration into transplantation

Novel Therapies/Approaches	Likely Applications/Advantages	Limitations/Caveats
Rituximab	CD20-positive disease up front[a]	2 randomized, controlled trials currently investigating
Nelarabine[63]	Upfront for T-cell ALL	
Blinatumamab[64]	Persistent minimum residual disease, post stem cell transplantation relapse	Neurotoxicity
Inotuzamab[65]	Relapse, possibly upfront therapy	Hepatotoxicity and veno-occlusive disease
Pediatric-inspired protocols[66]	Upper age limit remains undefined	Data in >30 y old group lacking, toxic if >45 y
Radioimmunotherapy[67]	Enhance cell kill of transplant by increasing marrow radiation dose	Not readily available
CD19 chimeric antigen receptor directed T cells (chimeric antigen receptors)[68–70]	Relapse including post stem cell transplantation, possibly in patients unfit for stem cell transplantation, may penetrate central nervous system	? are remissions durable, potential relapse of CD19 negative disease

[a] Upfront means part of initial 6 months of therapy.

REFERENCES

1. Goldstone AH, Richards SM, Lazarus HM, et al. In adults with standard-risk acute lymphoblastic leukemia, the greatest benefit is achieved from a matched sibling allogeneic transplantation in first complete remission, and an autologous transplantation is less effective than conventional consolidation/maintenance chemotherapy in all patients: final results of the International ALL Trial (MRC UKALL XII/ECOG E2993). Blood 2008;111:1827–33.
2. Marks DI. Treating the older patient with ALL. 'Hematology 2010'. 30th edition. American Society of Hematology Education Program Book; 2010. p. 13–20.
3. Yanada M, Matsuo K, Suzuki T, et al. Allogeneic hematopoietic stem cell transplantation as part of postremission therapy improves survival for adult patients with high-risk acute lymphoblastic leukemia: a metaanalysis. Cancer 2006;106: 2657–63.
4. Attal M, Blaise D, Marit G, et al. Consolidation treatment of adult acute lymphoblastic leukemia: a prospective, randomized trial comparing allogeneic versus autologous bone marrow transplantation and testing the impact of recombinant interleukin-2 after autologous bone marrow transplantation. BGMT Group. Blood 1995;86:1619–28.
5. Hunault M, Harousseau JL, Delain M, et al, GOELAMS (Groupe Ouest-Est des Leucémies Airguës et Maladies du Sang) Group. Better outcome of adult acute lymphoblastic leukemia after early genoidentical allogeneic bone marrow transplantation (BMT) than after late high-dose therapy and autologous BMT: a GOELAMS trial. Blood 2004;104:3028–37.
6. Marks DI. Allogeneic stem cell transplantation for acute lymphoblastic leukaemia in adults. In: Advani AS, Lazarus HM, editors. Adult ALL. Biology and treatment. New York: Humana Press, Springer Science; 2011. p. 297–304.
7. Hoelzer D, Thiel H, Loffler H, et al. Prognostic factors in a multicenter study for treatment of acute lymphoblastic leukemia in adults. Blood 1988;71: 123–31.
8. Moorman AV, Harrison CJ, Buck GAN, et al, Adult Leukaemia Working Party, Medical Research Council/National Cancer Research Institute. Karyotype is an independent prognostic factor in acute lymphoblastic leukaemia: analysis of cytogenetic data from patients treated on the MRC UKALL XII/ECOG 2993 trial. Blood 2007;109:3189–97.
9. Burnett A, Wetzler M, Löwenberg B. Therapeutic advances in acute myeloid leukemia. J Clin Oncol 2011;29:487–94.
10. Rowe JM. Prognostic factors in adult acute lymphoblastic leukaemia. Br J Haematol 2010;150:389–405.
11. Rowe JM, Buck G, Burnett AK, et al, ECOG, MRC/NCRI Adult Leukemia Working Party. Induction therapy for adults with acute lymphoblastic leukaemia: results of more than 1500 patients from the international ALL trial: MRC UKALL XII/ECOG 2993. Blood 2005;106:3760–7.
12. Marks DI, Pérez WS, He W, et al. Unrelated donor transplants in adults with Philadelphia-negative acute lymphoblastic leukemia in first complete remission. Blood 2008;112:426–34.
13. Vey N, Thomas X, Picard C, et al, GET-LALA Group the Swiss Group for Clinical Cancer Research (SAKK). Allogeneic stem cell transplantation improves the outcome of adults with t(1;19)/E2A-PBX1 and t(4;11)/MLL-AF4 positive B-cell acute lymphoblastic leukemia: results of the prospective multicenter LALA-94 study. Leukemia 2006;20:2155–61.

14. Marks DI, Paietta EM, Moorman AV, et al. T-cell acute lymphoblastic leukemia in adults: clinical features, immunophenotype, cytogenetics and outcome from the large randomised prospective trial (UKALL XII/ECOG 2993). Blood 2009;114: 5136–45.
15. Bruggeman M, Raff T, Flohr T, et al, German Multicenter Study Group for Adult Acute Lymphoblastic Leukemia. Clinical significance of minimal residual disease quantification in adult patients with standard risk acute lymphoblastic leukemia. Blood 2006;107:1116–23.
16. Patel B, Rai L, Buck G, et al. Minimal residual disease is a significant predictor of treatment failure in non T-lineage adult acute lymphoblastic leukaemia: final results of the international trial UKALL XII/ECOG2993. Br J Haematol 2010;148:80–9.
17. Moorman AV, Chilton L, Wilkinson J, et al. A population-based cytogenetic study of adults with acute lymphoblastic leukemia. Blood 2010;115:206–14.
18. Fielding AK. How I treat Philadelphia chromosome-positive acute lymphoblastic leukemia. Blood 2010;116:3409–17.
19. Ravandi F, O'Brien S, Thomas D, et al. First report of phase 2 study of dasatinib with hyper-CVAD for the frontline treatment of patients with Philadelphia chromosome-positive (Ph+) acute lymphoblastic leukemia. Blood 2010;116: 2070–7.
20. Schultz KR, Bowman WP, Aledo A, et al. Improved early event-free survival with imatinib in Philadelphia chromosome-positive acute lymphoblastic leukemia: a children's oncology group study. J Clin Oncol 2009;27:5175–81.
21. Fielding AK, Rowe JM, Richards SM, et al. Prospective outcome data on 267 unselected adult patients with Philadelphia chromosome-positive acute lymphoblastic leukemia confirms superiority of allogeneic transplantation over chemotherapy in the pre-imatinib era: results from the International ALL Trial MRC UKALLXII/ECOG 2993. Blood 2009;113:4489–96.
22. Bachanova V, Verneris MR, DeFor T, et al. Prolonged survival in adults with acute lymphoblastic leukemia after reduced-intensity conditioning with cord blood or sibling donor transplantation. Blood 2009;113:2902–5.
23. Laughlin MJ, Eapen M, Rubinstein P, et al. Outcomes after transplantation of cord blood or bone marrow from unrelated donors in adults with leukemia. N Engl J Med 2004;351:2265–75.
24. Bachanova V, Marks DI, Zhang MJ, et al. Ph+ ALL patients in first complete remission have similar survival after reduced intensity and myeloablative allogeneic transplantation: impact of tyrosine kinase inhibitor and minimal residual disease. Leukemia 2014;28(3):658–65.
25. Marks DI, Woo KA, Zhong X, et al. Unrelated umbilical cord blood transplant for adult acute lymphoblastic leukemia in first and second complete remission: a comparison with allografts from adult unrelated donors. Haematologica 2014; 99(2):322–8.
26. Fielding AK, Richards SM, Chopra R, et al, Medical Research Council of the United Kingdom Adult ALL Working Party, Eastern Cooperative Oncology Group. Outcome of 609 adults after relapse of acute lymphoblastic leukaemia (ALL); an MRC UKALL XII/ECOG 2993 study. Blood 2007;109:944–50.
27. Tavernier E, Boiron JM, Huguet F, et al, GET-LALA Group, Swiss Group for Clinical Cancer Research SAKK, Australasian Leukaemia and Lymphoma Group. Outcome of treatment after first relapse in adults with acute lymphoblastic leukemia initially treated by the LALA-94 trial. Leukemia 2007;21:1907–14.
28. Hoelzer D, Huettmann A, Kaul F, et al. Immunochemotherapy with rituximab improves molecular CR rate and outcome in CD20+ B-lineage standard and high

risk patients; results of 263 CD20+ patients studied prospectively in GMALL study 07/2003 ASH Annual Meeting Abstracts 2010 116:170. Orlando (FL), December, 2010.

29. DeAngelo DJ. Nelarabine for the treatment of patients with relapsed or refractory T-cell acute lymphoblastic leukemia or lymphoblastic lymphoma. Hematol Oncol Clin North Am 2009;23:1121–35.
30. Huguet F, Leguay T, Raffoux E, et al. Pediatric inspired therapy in adults with Philadelphia chromosome negative acute lymphoblastic leukemia: the GRAALL 2003 study. J Clin Oncol 2009;27:911–8.
31. Duval M, Klein JP, He W, et al. Hematopoietic stem-cell transplantation for acute leukemia in relapse or primary induction failure. J Clin Oncol 2010;28:3730–8.
32. Doney K, Hägglund H, Leisenring W, et al. Predictive factors for outcome of allogeneic hematopoietic cell transplantation for adult acute lymphoblastic leukemia. Biol Blood Marrow Transplant 2003;9:472–81.
33. Goldstone AH, Rowe J. How I treat acute lymphocytic leukaemia. Blood 2007; 110:2268–75.
34. Marks DI, Aversa F, Lazarus HM. Alternative donor transplants for adult acute lymphoblastic leukaemia: a comparison of the three major options. Bone Marrow Transplant 2006;38:467–75.
35. Kako S, Morita S, Sakamaki H, et al. Decision analysis of unrelated hematopoietic stem cell transplantation for adult patients with Philadelphia Chromosome-Negative Acute Lymphoblastic Leukemia In First Remission Who Lack An HLA-Matched Sibling ASH Annual Meeting Abstracts 2010 116:3527. Orlando (FL), December, 2010.
36. Weisdorf D, Spellman S, Haagenson M, et al. Classification of HLA-matching for retrospective analysis of unrelated donor transplantation: revised definitions to predict survival. Biol Blood Marrow Transplant 2008;14:748–58.
37. Lee SJ, Klein J, Haagenson M, et al. High-resolution donor-recipient HLA matching contributes to the success of unrelated donor marrow transplantation. Blood 2007;110:4576–83.
38. Tomblyn MB, Arora M, Baker KS, et al. Myeloablative hematopoietic cell transplantation for acute lymphoblastic leukemia: analysis of graft sources and long-term outcome. J Clin Oncol 2009;27:3634–41.
39. Aversa F, Tabilio A, Velardi A, et al. Treatment of high-risk acute leukemia with T-cell-depleted stem cells from related donors with one fully mismatched HLA haplotype. N Engl J Med 1998;339:1186–93.
40. Lu DP, Dong L, Wu T, et al. Conditioning including antithymocyte globulin followed by unmanipulated HLA-mismatched/haploidentical blood and marrow transplantation can achieve comparable outcomes with HLA-identical sibling transplantation. Blood 2006;107:3065–73.
41. Luznik L, Bolaños-Meade J, Zahurak M, et al. High-dose cyclophosphamide as single-agent, short-course prophylaxis of graft-versus-host disease. Blood 2010;115:3224–30.
42. Laport GG, Alvarnas JC, Palmer JM, et al. Long-term remission of Philadelphia chromosome-positive acute lymphoblastic leukemia after allogeneic hematopoietic cell transplantation from matched sibling donors: a 20-year experience with the fractionated total body irradiation-etoposide regimen. Blood 2008;112: 903–9.
43. Marks DI, Forman SJ, Blume KG, et al. A comparison of cyclophosphamide and total body irradiation with etoposide and total body irradiation as conditioning regimens for patients undergoing sibling allografting for acute lymphoblastic

leukaemia in first or second complete remission. Biol Blood Marrow Transplant 2006;12:438–53.

44. Santarone S, Pidala J, Di Nicola M, et al. Fludarabine and pharmacokinetic-targeted busulfan before allografting for adults with acute lymphoid leukemia. Biol Blood Marrow Transplant 2011;17(10):1505–11.
45. Kebriaei P, Basset R, Ledesma C, et al. Clofarabine combined with busulfan provides excellent disease control in adult patients with acute lymphoblastic leukemia undergoing allogeneic hematopoietic stem cell transplantation. Biol Blood Marrow Transplant 2012;18(12):1819–26.
46. Kebriaei P, Madden T, Wang X, et al. Intravenous BU plus Mel: an effective, chemotherapy-only transplant conditioning regimen in patients with ALL. Bone Marrow Transplant 2013;48(1):26–31. http://dx.doi.org/10.1038/bmt.2012.114.
47. Mohty M, Labopin M, Tabrizzi R, et al, Acute Leukemia Working Party, European Group for Blood and Marrow Transplantation. Reduced intensity conditioning allogeneic stem cell transplantation for adult patients with acute lymphoblastic leukemia: a retrospective study from the European Group for Blood and Marrow Transplantation. Haematologica 2008;93:303–6.
48. Marks DI, Wang T, Pérez WS, et al. The outcome of full-intensity and reduced-intensity conditioning matched sibling or unrelated donor transplantation in adults with Philadelphia chromosome-negative acute lymphoblastic leukemia in first and second complete remission. Blood 2010;116:366–74.
49. Mohty M, Labopin M, Volin L, et al, Acute Leukemia Working Party of EBMT. Reduced-intensity versus conventional myeloablative conditioning allogeneic stem cell transplantation for patients with acute lymphoblastic leukemia: a retrospective study from the European Group for Blood and Marrow Transplantation. Blood 2010;116:4439–43.
50. Ram R, Storb R, Sandmaier BM, et al. Non-myeloablative conditioning with allogeneic hematopoietic cell transplantation for the treatment of high-risk acute lymphoblastic leukemia. Haematologica 2011;96(8):1113–20.
51. Weiden PL, Flournoy N, Thomas ED, et al. Antileukemic effect of graft-versus-host disease in human recipients of allogeneic-marrow grafts. N Engl J Med 1979;300:1068–73.
52. Passweg JR, Cahn JY, Tiberghien P, et al. Graft versus leukaemia effect in T-lineage and cALLa+ (B-lineage) acute lymphoblastic leukaemia. Bone Marrow Transplant 1998;21:153–8.
53. Patel B, Kirkland KE, Szydlo R, et al. Favorable outcomes with alemtuzumab-conditioned unrelated donor stem cell transplantation in adults with high-risk Philadelphia chromosome-negative acute lymphoblastic leukemia in first complete remission. Haematologica 2009;94:1399–406.
54. Schrauder A, Stanulla M, Flohr T, et al. Prospective evaluation of MRD-kinetics in 274 children with high-risk ALL treated in trial ALL-BFM 2000: insights into development of resistance and impact on further refinement of treatment stratification strategies. Blood (ASH Annual Meeting Abstracts) 2007 110: Abstract 585. Atlanta (GA), December, 2007.
55. Tallman MS, Rowlings PA, Milone G, et al. Effect of postremission chemotherapy before human leukocyte antigen-identical sibling transplantation for acute myelogenous leukemia in first complete remission. Blood 2000;96:1254–8.
56. Eckert C, Biondi A, Seeger K, et al. Prognostic value of minimal residual disease in relapsed childhood acute lymphoblastic leukaemia. Lancet 2001;358:1239–41.
57. Knechtli CJ, Goulden NJ, Hancock JP, et al. Minimal residual disease status before allogeneic bone marrow transplantation is an important determinant of

successful outcome for children and adolescents with acute lymphoblastic leukemia. Blood 1998;92:4072–9.
58. Leung W, Pui CH, Coustan-Smith E, et al. Detectable minimal residual disease before hematopoietic cell transplantation is prognostic but does not preclude cure for children with very-high-risk leukemia. Blood 2012;120:468–72.
59. Lazarus HM, Richards SM, Chopra R, et al, Medical Research Council (MRC)/ National Cancer Research Institute (NCRI), Adult Leukaemia Working Party of the United Kingdom and the Eastern Cooperative Oncology Group. Central nervous system involvement in adult acute lymphoblastic leukemia at diagnosis: results from the international ALL trial MRC UKALL XII/ECOG E2993. Blood 2006; 108:465–72.
60. Spyridonidis A, Labopin M, Schmid C, et al, Immunotherapy Subcommittee of Acute Leukemia Working Party of European Blood and Marrow Transplant Group. Outcomes and prognostic factors of adults with acute lymphoblastic leukemia who relapse after allogeneic hematopoietic cell transplantation. An analysis on behalf of the Acute Leukemia Working Party of EBMT. Leukemia 2012;26: 1211–7.
61. Blume KG, Krance RA. The evaluation and counselling of candidates for hematopoietic cell transplantation. In: Appelbaum FR, Forman SJ, Negrin RS, et al, editors. Thomas' hematopoietic cell transplantation 4th edition. Oxford (United Kingdom): Wiley-Blackwell; 2007. p. 445–60.
62. Sorror ML, Giralt S, Sandmaier BM, et al. Hematopoietic cell transplantation specific comorbidity index as an outcome predictor for patients with acute myeloid leukemia in first remission: combined FHCRC and MDACC experiences. Blood 2007;110:4606–13.
63. Gokbuget N, Basara B, Baurmann H, et al. High single drug activity of nelarabine in relapsed T-lymphoblastic leukemia/lymphoma offers curative option with subsequent stem cell transplantation. Blood 2011;118(13):3504–11.
64. Topp MS, Kufer P, Gökbuget N, et al. Targeted therapy with the T-cell-engaging antibody blinatumomab of chemotherapy-refractory minimal residual disease in B-lineage acute lymphoblastic leukemia patients results in high response rate and prolonged leukemia-free survival. J Clin Oncol 2011;29(18):2493–8.
65. Kantarjian H, Thomas D, Jorgensen J, et al. Results of inotuzumab ozogamicin, a CD22 monoclonal antibody, in refractory and relapsed acute lymphocytic leukemia. Cancer 2013;1(119):2728–36.
66. Pulte D, Gondos A, Brenner H. Improvement in survival in younger patients with acute lymphoblastic leukemia from the 1980s to the early 21st century. Blood 2009;113:1408–11.
67. Matthews DC, Appelbaum FR, Eary JF, et al. Phase I study of (131)I-anti-CD45 antibody plus cyclophosphamide and total body irradiation for advanced acute leukemia and myelodysplastic syndrome. Blood 1999;94:1237–47.
68. Fry TJ, Mackall CL. T cell adoptive immunotherapy for ALL. Hematology Am Soc Hematol Educ Program 2013;2013:348–53.
69. Advani AS. New immune strategies for the treatment of acute lymphoblastic leukemia: antibodies and chimeric antigen receptors. Hematology Am Soc Hematol Educ Program 2013;2013:131–7.
70. Brentjens RJ, Davila ML, Riviere I, et al. CD19-targeted T cells rapidly induce molecular remissions in adults with chemotherapy-refractory acute lymphoblastic leukemia. Sci Transl Med 2013;5(177):177ra138.

Transplants in Myelodysplastic Syndromes

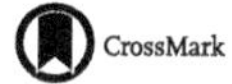

Katrin Wetzko, MD, Uwe Platzbecker, MD*

KEYWORDS

- MDS • Allogeneic HSCT • Relapse • Conditioning • Azacitidine

KEY POINTS

- Transplantation can be a potential curative option in elderly patients with myelodysplastic syndromes within prospective trials investigating the success of allogeneic stem cell transplantation (SCT) compared with other treatment options.
- In the absence of prospective trials, a careful individual selection should be done and patients should be stratified according to comorbidities, performance status, and disease risk.
- Chronic graft-versus-host disease (GVHD) and relapse are still the major challenges after SCT.
- Special attention should be paid to posttransplant care in terms of GVHD management, minimal residual disease (MRD) monitoring, and prevention of relapse.

INTRODUCTION

Because of the great variability of biology and presentation of the disease, the therapeutic management of patients with myelodysplastic syndromes (MDS) is challenging. Over the last decade, there has been a remarkable increase in scientific research on the pathogenesis and therapeutic approaches in MDS. However, despite a rapidly expanding therapeutic drug arsenal, allogeneic hematopoietic stem cell transplantation (SCT) remains the only potentially curative treatment. Only a minority of patients are considered for this treatment modality because cumulative mortality rates after SCT can exceed 30% and also because graft-versus-host disease (GVHD) as well as relapse remain major clinical challenges following transplantation. Because of the heterogeneous nature of MDS, ranging from low-risk patients with a life expectancy of 10 years with best supportive care only to high-risk patients with MDS with a median survival of 5 months with the very best standard treatment, not every patient

Medical Clinic 1, University Hospital "Carl-Gustav-Carus" at TUD, Fetscherstraße 74, 01307 Dresden, Germany
* Corresponding author.
E-mail address: uwe.platzbecker@uniklinikum-dresden.de

Hematol Oncol Clin N Am 28 (2014) 1011–1022
http://dx.doi.org/10.1016/j.hoc.2014.08.012 hemonc.theclinics.com
0889-8588/14/$ – see front matter

with MDS will benefit from this potential curative but risky treatment procedure. In fact, physicians who treat patients with MDS are faced primarily with an older patient population (median age of 70 years at diagnosis) with significant comorbidities and reduced biological ability to regenerate. In these patients, the potential high treatment-related mortality (TRM) of standard conditioning would limit the benefit of this procedure. With the introduction of reduced-intensity conditioning (RIC), early TRM could be reduced, allowing a potentially curative treatment approach even for patients in the seventh decade of life. On the other hand, the use of RIC is accompanied by a higher risk of relapse, especially in patients with higher-risk disease.[1] Defining patients who should be referred to allogeneic SCT and the best time point within the treatment course of MDS is, therefore, essential. In fact, prospective randomized trials supporting these decisions are still not available. This review highlights the current selection process and therapeutic strategies before and after allogeneic SCT to potentially improve the outcome of patients with MDS undergoing this procedure.

PATIENT EVALUATION OVERVIEW

Diagnostic and Prognosis

According to the recently published guidelines from the European LeukemiaNet (ELN) (**Table 1**), every patient should receive a complete blood count, a peripheral blood (PB) smear with differential leukocyte count, a bone marrow (BM) aspiration for morphologic evaluation, as well as a BM biopsy to assess marrow fibrosis. Furthermore, cytogenetic analysis of BM should be undertaken in all cases of suspected MDS. At least 20 metaphases have to be analyzed; if less than 20 metaphases are

Table 1
Diagnostic tools for MDS in adults, recommendations from the ELN (modified)

Diagnostic Tool	Diagnostic Value	
1. Peripheral blood smear	Evaluation of dysplasia and blast count	Mandatory
2. Bone marrow aspirate	Evaluation of dysplasia and blast count, Quantification of ring sideroblasts	
3. Bone marrow biopsy	Assessment of cellularity, CD34+ count and fibrosis	
4. Cytogenetic analysis	Detection of clonal chromosomal abnormalities for conclusive diagnosis/prognostic assessment	
5. FISH	Detection of targeted chromosomal abnormalities in interphase nuclei following repeated failure of standard G banding	Recommended
6. Immunophenotyping	Detection of abnormalities in erythroid, myeloid, and lymphoid compartment	
7. SNP-array	Detection of chromosomal defects at a high resolution in combination with metaphase cytogenetic	Suggested
8. Mutation analysis of candidates genes	Detection of somatic mutations that can allow a conclusive diagnosis and also reliable for prognostic evaluation	

Abbreviations: FISH, fluorescence in situ hybridization; SNP, single-nucleotide polymorphism.

Adapted from Malcovati L, Hellstrom-Lindberg E, Bowen D, et al. Diagnosis and treatment of primary myelodysplastic syndromes in adults: recommendations from the European LeukemiaNet. Blood 2013;122(17):2943–64; with permission.

scored, then the results should be considered invalid, provided the karyotype appears normal. Fluorescence in situ hybridization analysis, with a validated panel of probes, is recommended in certain instances (eg, to clarify complex aberrations, to detect specific anomalies [eg, monosomy 7 or del (5q)], or when only a low number of metaphases are available for standard G banding).

The cytomorphological assessment of the bone marrow smear is the basic diagnostic when an MDS is suspected. As a result of cytogenetic and epigenetic changes, there will be found more or less pronounced morphologic alterations in at least 1 cell line up to trilinear dysplasia and is associated with a normal or increased blast count.

Many clinical trials use the IPSS[2] for differentiation between lower- versus higher-risk disease. However, some patients classified as lower risk, particularly those in the IPSS intermediate-1 group, may have higher-risk features (eg, patients with red blood cell [RBC] transfusion–dependent [TD] refractory cytopenia with multilineage dysplasia [RCMD] with intermediate karyotype). Consequently, a revised IPSS (IPSS-R)[3] has been proposed, which incorporates several changes, including an updated system for assessing cytogenetic risk and the consideration of the severity of cytopenias (with thresholds of hemoglobin: 10 g/dL; absolute neutrophil count: $0.8 \times 10^9\ L^{-1}$; platelets: $100 \times 10^9\ L^{-1}$). Using this new R-IPSS, 27% of lower-risk patients with MDS per classic IPSS were reclassified as having a higher risk and may potentially require more intensive treatment, whereas 18% of higher-risk patients per classic IPSS were reclassified as low risk, suggesting that IPSS-R can refine the classification of MDS and more individual prognosis estimation is possible. Still, the benefit of IPSS-R for guided therapy decisions is under investigation. Quite recently, Della Porta and colleagues[4] developed an IPSS-R–based score to predict outcome of patients after SCT.

Chromosomal aberrations are present in approximately 50% of patients with MDS. The impact of cytogenetic risk groups on prognosis and the rate of transformation to acute myeloid leukemia (AML) are well known. Moreover, the selection of certain therapeutic options may be driven by the existence of specific chromosomal abnormalities. For example, lenalidomide (Revlimid) is particularly effective in patients with low-risk, TD MDS with a deletion of chromosome 5q.

More frequently, there are somatic mutations, which are, however, not exclusively found in MDS. Mutations (eg, in regulator genes of central pathways in the pathophysiology in MDS) are suitable as prognostic parameters and may also be, in the future, a specific therapeutic target. An extract of recurrent mutations in MDS is listed in **Table 2**.

Accurate diagnostics and subsequent prognostication are crucial in determining the appropriate treatment, including best supportive care, immunomodulatory drugs, chemotherapy, or SCT. Additionally, accompanying diseases, preexisting organ dysfunction, clinical condition and symptoms, as well as the biological age must be considered carefully. The Seattle group developed a hematopoietic cell transplantation specific comorbidity index (CI) to predict the influence of the pretransplant comorbidities on TRM and overall survival (OS) in hematopoietic SCT recipients.[5] In a Web-based available questionnaire (www.HCTci.org), hepatic, pulmonary, cardiac, and renal impairments as well as other pretransplant variables can be translated into a patient-specific score. The predictive value of this score on the posttransplant outcome has been evaluated in different studies worldwide. Furthermore, the predictive relevance of patients' physical condition on outcomes has been shown by Deschler and colleagues[6] with several performance status scores being predictive for post-SCT mortality.

Table 2
Somatic mutations found in MDS according to frequency and clinical impact in patients treated with supportive care only

Function	Mutation	Prognosis	Frequency (%)
Splicing	SF3B1	Good	15–30
	SRSF2	Poor	5–10
	U2AF1	Poor	5–10
	ZRSR2	Neutral	5
Methylation	DNMT3A	Poor	5–10
	TET2	Neutral	15–25
Methylation/histone modifications	IDH1/IDH2	Mixed evidence	4–5
Histone modification	ASXL1	Poor	10–20
	EZH2	Poor	3–7
Transcription factor	RUNX1	Poor	5–10
	TP53	Poor	5–10
	BCOR-L1	Poor	5–6
	ETV6	Poor	3
Signal transduction	NRAS/KRAS	Poor	5–10

INDICATIONS FOR TRANSPLANTATION

First, we have to be aware of the fact that allogeneic SCT is the only potentially curative therapy for MDS; but there is finally no warranty for treatment success. As pointed out earlier, individual risk assessment determined by disease-related as well as patient-related factors is, therefore, absolutely mandatory. Because of the reduction of therapy-associated adverse events, mainly by better supportive therapies and the introduction of reduced RIC, the indication has been extended within the last years even to patients in their seventh decade of life. In contrast, hypomethylating agents (HMAs) (azacitidine, decitabine) have become available and effective drugs, with azacitidine (AZA) being superior compared with conventional care.[7]

Whether patients with advanced MDS actually benefit from an allogeneic SCT has only been studied in retrospective analyses with varying results (**Table 3**). Prospective studies are lacking so far, but several studies have been initiated to compare allogeneic SCT and nontransplant among older patients with MDS.[8]

So far, an early allogeneic SCT is recommended for fit patients, with an available, compatible donor, up to 65 to 70 years of age at intermediate-2 and high-risk MDS

Table 3
Is allogeneic SCT superior to nontransplant treatment? Summary of results of retrospective studies

	n	Age (y)	Conditioning
Yes			
Koreth et al,[9] 2013	184	60–70	RIC
Alessandrino et al,[10] 2013	1109	46–63	RIC/MAC
Platzbecker et al,[11] 2012	178	63–66	RIC/MAC
Cutler et al,[12] 2004	674	39–50	MAC
No			
Jabbour et al,[13] 2013	93	51–54	MAC
Brand et al,[14] 2013	384	55–69	RIC/MAC

according to IPSS, respectively, with very high, high, or intermediate risk referred to IPSS-R.[9] A very poor prognosis, even after transplantation, is apparent in patients with monosomal karyotype (especially in chromosome 7)[15] and advanced disease stage at the time of transplantation mainly because of relapse.[16] TRM is substantially influenced by individual comorbidities and age.[4] Furthermore, a simple score including performance status as well as age and IPSS-R allows for a prediction of outcome after SCT (**Table 4**).[4]

TIMING OF ALLOGENEIC TRANSPLANTATION

In addition to the question of who actually benefits from allogeneic SCT, the question of the proper time point still remains to be determined. Performing allogeneic SCT immediately after diagnosis was shown to be superior in patients with higher-risk MDS, whereas younger patients with lower-risk MDS may benefit from delaying allogeneic SCT until progression of the disease.[12] For patients with less advanced disease, however, an early transplant seems to be an overtreatment and exposes patients to a high risk of TRM.

A low-as-possible tumor burden before SCT minimizes the risk of post-SCT relapse and improves disease-free survival.[17–20] Large retrospective analyses have demonstrated improved outcomes for patients who have underwent a transplant in complete remission compared with those with active disease at the time of SCT.[21] Importantly, these analyses are hampered by a certain selection bias for patients with chemosensitive disease and do not take patients into consideration who did not undergo SCT because of therapy-related toxicity. Therefore, the value of prior induction chemotherapy (IC) is still not clear in the absence of randomized trials[22] and also because IC can be associated with considerable toxicity mainly in the absence of response. Two recent retrospective studies have demonstrated that pre-SCT therapy with AZA compared with IC may allow for similar outcomes after allogeneic SCT.[23,24] Nevertheless, as the rate of complete remissions is generally higher with IC compared with HMA, that strategy might still be the best option in selected, medically fit (younger) patients with a high disease burden. An important prerequisite before the

Table 4
MDS transplantation risk index predicts for outcome after allogeneic SCT

	A	B	C	D	E
Scores	**Age**	**IPSS-R**	**Monosomal Karyotype**	**SCT-CI**	**Refractory to IC**
0	<50	Low	No	Low/intermediate	No
1	≥50	Intermediate	Yes	High	Yes
2	—	High			
3	—	Very high	—	—	—
		$\sum$ = score (A) + (B) + (C) + (D) + (E)			
		0–1 = Low	2–3 = Intermediate	4 = High	>4 = Very high
		↓	↓	↓	↓
	2-y OS (%)	78	55	30	10

Abbreviations: CI, comorbidity index; IC, induction chemotherapy.

From Della Porta MG, Alessandrino EP, Bacigalupo A, et al. Predictive factors for the outcome of allogeneic transplantation in patients with myelodysplastic syndrome stratified according to the revised International Prognostic Scoring System (IPSS-R). Blood 2014;123(15):2333–42; with permission.

initiation of IC may be the availability of a suitable donor mainly to be able to rescue nonresponding patients.[25,26] This factor is especially true for patients with poor-risk cytogenetics and an expected lower response rate compared with other karyotypic abnormalities.

The use of HMA instead of IC for reduction of disease burden has changed potential strategies in preparation for SCT.[27,28] Treatment with HMA is feasible and mostly well tolerated and should be considered mainly for older (>60 years) and comorbid patients and as a bridging strategy to SCT when no donor has been identified. However, the authors disagree with the notion that HMA always allow for a safe bridging to SCT because infectious complications during the first cycles of therapy remain a big challenge in the clinical routine. Several predictive factors for long-term outcomes with HMA have been determined (**Fig. 1**) and might, therefore, guide treatment decisions regarding when to finally proceed to transplant during an HMA-based therapy.[29] In fact, Eastern Cooperative Oncology Group performance status, blasts in PB, RBC transfusion dependency, and IPSS karyotype were proven as independent risk factors and summarized as the AZA prognostic score. The IPSS karyotype allows for an estimation of the survival with AZA mono-therapy (see **Fig. 1**).[29] In fact, the estimated median 2-year OS is 35% (6 months) with a high AZA score, 50% (15 months) with intermediate score, and 85% with a low AZA score.

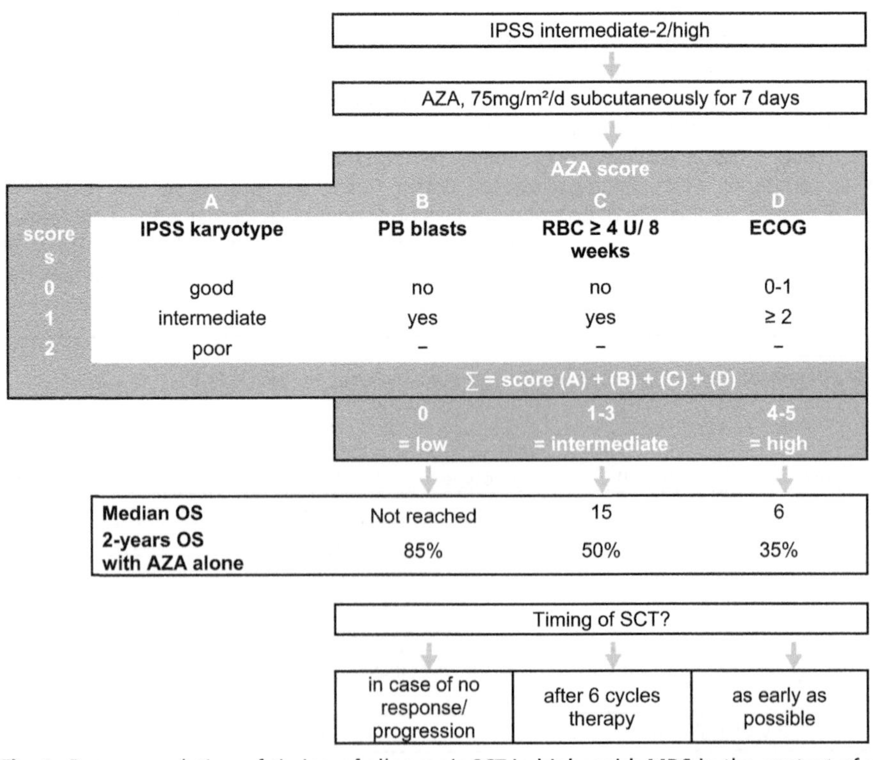

Fig. 1. Recommendation of timing of allogeneic SCT in higher-risk MDS in the context of a planned AZA therapy; based on AZA prognostic score. ECOG, Eastern Cooperative Oncology Group. (*Data from* Itzykson R, Thepot S, Quesnel B, et al. Prognostic factors for response and overall survival in 282 patients with higher-risk myelodysplastic syndromes treated with azacitidine. Blood 2011;117(2):403–11.)

A large body of evidence exists from retrospective studies stating that systemic iron overload (SIO) in patients with MDS (mainly as a result of RBC-TD before SCT) is associated with an increased risk of *early* mortality after allogeneic SCT.[30,31] The reasons for this observation remain, at least in part, not very well defined. Given the limitation of serum ferritin measurements including its association with variables important for transplantation outcomes like comorbidities,[31] noninvasive MRI or the detection of labile plasma iron (LPI) are currently the most promising methods to evaluate SIO and its potential toxic metabolites. In fact, the authors and others[32,33] have presented data demonstrating that MRI-based liver iron concentration rather than ferritin is of prognostic significance after allogeneic SCT. LPI is released as a result of pretransplant conditioning; however, so far, the direct consequences of this observation in vivo and on the posttransplant period are not well described. Nevertheless, treatment approaches to prevent severe iron overload are reasonable and warranted. It is recommended to use iron chelation before SCT in selected patients with SIO, although no definitive cutoff for ferritin or liver iron has been systematically defined. Alternatively, allogeneic SCT should be considered earlier before SIO becomes clinically evident.

PREPARATION OF PATIENTS FOR ALLOGENEIC HEMATOPOIETIC STEM CELL TRANSPLANTATION

Today there are several different concepts in use for patients with MDS undergoing a transplant, and it is recommended to treat patients preferentially within clinical studies only.

Stem Cell Donor

A matched related donor is preferred in general because of the lower incidence of chronic GVHD compared with unrelated or mismatched donors. However, several recent studies showed almost comparable outcomes with a compatible high-resolution matched unrelated donor. Just because of the advanced age of most patients with MDS, available siblings are also mostly of advanced age with accompanying comorbidities; so the question arises about whether a younger unrelated donor should be preferred. Two studies investigated that question with opposing results.[34,35] As a result, no general recommendation can be drawn.

Source of Stem Cells

Bone marrow from HLA-identical siblings had been the only source of stem cells for decades. Today, granulocyte colony-stimulating factor (G-CSF)–stimulated blood stem cells (PB stem cells [PBSCs]) are preferred and predominantly used because they are associated with a faster engraftment and a lower relapse rate through the graft-versus-leukemia (GVL) effect caused by the higher amount of T cells in the apheresis products.[36] However, PBSCs are associated with a higher incidence of chronic GVHD compared with bone marrow.[37] According to a recent randomized study in patients with hematological malignancies (including MDS) undergoing bone marrow transplantation, the rate of severe chronic GVHD was significantly reduced compared with PBSCs.[38] Therefore, this approach might be an option, especially in older patients.

Conditioning Regimes

Myeloablative conditioning (MAC) (eg, busulfan/cyclophosphamide containing or total body irradiation [TBI] based) regimens are considered the standard of care mainly in younger patients with MDS, younger than 60 years. Additionally, the addition of ATG is recommended in case of a matched unrelated donor and MAC according to a randomized study.[39]

The introduction of RIC has broadened the use of allogeneic SCT for patients with MDS with advanced age and comorbidities through reduced tissue damage, toxicity, and the risk of acute GVHD. However, RIC is associated with a less effective reduction of MDS burden resulting in an increased rate of relapse.[1,40–42] It is hoped that the results of a randomized study comparing RIC versus MAC will be available shortly (ClinicalTrials.gov, NCT01339910, NCT01203228).

MANAGEMENT OF RELAPSE AFTER TRANSPLANTATION

Despite all of the improvements in allogeneic SCT, about 30% of patients who have undergone a transplant do relapse, mostly within 6 to 12 month after the procedure.[43–45] Thus, relapse remains the most frequent cause of treatment failure and is mostly associated with a very poor prognosis. There is still no standard salvage treatment defined today. According to the patients' clinical status, the available therapy options range from palliative care, HMA, and conventional chemotherapy to second SCT and donor lymphocyte infusion (DLI), respectively.

Recently, AZA has been investigated in the treatment of patients with relapsed MDS or AML after allogeneic SCT.[44] This study demonstrated an overall response rate of 30% with durable responses in 5 out of 30 patients. Apart from the direct antiproliferative and cytotoxic effects on leukemic cells, AZA might also influence the donor immune system, thereby enhancing the GVL effect.[46] Therefore, the combination of HMA and DLI seems to be an interesting treatment approach in relapsed patients.

NOVEL THERAPIES AND THEIR INTEGRATION IN TRANSPLANTATION

Considering the limited treatment opportunities in patients with MDS relapsing after SCT, prevention of disease recurrence should be one of the major goals for future clinical research.[47] Because relapse occurs predominantly within the first year after SCT, a potential maintenance therapy should start as early as possible. Because of its tolerability, AZA can be administered on an outpatient basis, which is an ideal prerequisite for this kind of approach. In fact, a recent study confirmed that early posttransplant maintenance therapy with AZA is feasible without serious side effects and without an increased rate of GVHD,[48] which has been the backbone for a randomized trial comparing AZA versus the current standard of care after allogeneic SCT (NCT00887068). Another potentially appealing drug for maintenance therapy is lenalidomide mainly in case of del (5q) disease. However, the results of a recent study in patients with MDS and AML[47] as well as in patients with multiple myeloma have shown an increased risk of GVHD.

In general, during maintenance therapy to prevent relapse, there will be a subset of patients with MDS who will never relapse after SCT and will, thus, unjustifiably be exposed to the potential risks and adverse events of drug treatment. The optimal strategy to circumvent this situation is an MRD-guided therapy, which offers treatment to patients with detectable MRD only after SCT. Until recently, most patients with MDS often lacked a disease-specific molecular marker for MRD detection. In these patients, chimerism analyses have remained an important diagnostic tool to monitor the success of SCT. The authors' group has recently reported the first trial evaluating the efficacy of a preemptive treatment with AZA for MRD defined by a decreasing $CD34^+$ donor chimerism to prevent or delay hematologic relapse in patients with $CD34^+$ MDS or AML after allogeneic SCT.[49] Flow cytometry–based detection of

MRD represents an additional tool for interventions.[50] In the near future, it can be anticipated that mutational analyses will increasingly be used for MRD-guided approaches.

AUTOLOGOUS HEMATOPOIETIC STEM CELL TRANSPLANTATION

Currently, there is no evidence for the use of autologous SCT in MDS, even when no suitable allogeneic donor is available.

SUMMARY/DISCUSSION

Finally, should transplantation be a potential curative option in elderly patients with MDS? Yes it should be, but within prospective trials investigating the success of allogeneic SCT compared with other treatment options. In the absence of prospective trials, a careful individual selection should be done; patients should be stratified according to comorbidities, performance status, and disease risk. Chronic GVHD and relapse are still the major challenges after SCT. Therefore, special attention should be paid to posttransplant care in terms of GVHD management, MRD monitoring, and prevention of relapse.

REFERENCES

1. Martino R, de Wreede L, Fiocco M, et al. Comparison of conditioning regimens of various intensities for allogeneic hematopoietic SCT using HLA-identical sibling donors in AML and MDS with <10% BM blasts: a report from EBMT. Bone Marrow Transplant 2013;48(6):761–70.
2. Greenberg P, Cox C, LeBeau MM, et al. International scoring system for evaluating prognosis in myelodysplastic syndromes. Blood 1997;89(6):2079–88.
3. Greenberg PL, Tuechler H, Schanz J, et al. Revised international prognostic scoring system for myelodysplastic syndromes. Blood 2012;120(12):2454–65.
4. Della Porta MG, Alessandrino EP, Bacigalupo A, et al. Predictive factors for the outcome of allogeneic transplantation in patients with myelodysplastic syndrome stratified according to the revised International Prognostic Scoring System (IPSS-R). Blood 2014;123(15):2333–42.
5. Sorror ML, Maris MB, Storb R, et al. Hematopoietic cell transplantation (SCT)-specific comorbidity index: a new tool for risk assessment before allogeneic SCT. Blood 2005;106(8):2912–9.
6. Deschler B, Ihorst G, Platzbecker U, et al. Parameters detected by geriatric and quality of life assessment in 195 older patients with myelodysplastic syndromes and acute myeloid leukemia are highly predictive for outcome. Haematologica 2013;98(2):208–16.
7. Gore SD, Fenaux P, Santini V, et al. A multivariate analysis of the relationship between response and survival among patients with higher-risk myelodysplastic syndromes treated within azacitidine or conventional care regimens in the randomized AZA-001 trial. Haematologica 2013;98(7):1067–72.
8. Saber W, Le Rademacher J, Sekeres M, et al. Multi-center biologic assignment trial comparing reduced intensity allogeneic hematopoietic cell transplant to hypomethylating therapy or best supportive care in patients aged 50-75 with intermediate-2 and high risk myelodysplastic syndrome: Blood and Marrow Transplant Clinical Trials Network #1102 study rationale, design and methods. Biol Blood Marrow Transplant 2014;20(10):1566–72.

9. Koreth J, Pidala J, Perez WS, et al. Role of reduced-intensity conditioning allogeneic hematopoietic stem-cell transplantation in older patients with de novo myelodysplastic syndromes: an international collaborative decision analysis. J Clin Oncol 2013;31(21):2662–70.
10. Alessandrino EP, Porta MG, Malcovati L, et al. Optimal timing of allogeneic hematopoietic stem cell transplantation in patients with myelodysplastic syndrome. Am J Hematol 2013;88(7):581–8.
11. Platzbecker U, Schetelig J, Finke J, et al. Allogeneic hematopoietic cell transplantation in patients age 60-70 years with de novo high-risk myelodysplastic syndrome or secondary acute myelogenous leukemia: comparison with patients lacking donors who received azacitidine. Biol Blood Marrow Transplant 2012; 18(9):1415–21.
12. Cutler CS, Lee SJ, Greenberg P, et al. A decision analysis of allogeneic bone marrow transplantation for the myelodysplastic syndromes: delayed transplantation for low-risk myelodysplasia is associated with improved outcome. Blood 2004;104(2):579–85.
13. Jabbour E, Mathisen MS, Garcia-Manero G, et al. Allogeneic hematopoietic stem cell transplantation versus hypomethylating agents in patients with myelodysplastic syndrome: a retrospective case-control study. Am J Hematol 2013; 88(3):198–200.
14. Brand R, Putter H, van Biezen A, et al. Comparison of allogeneic stem cell transplantation and non-transplant approaches in elderly patients with advanced myelodysplastic syndrome: optimal statistical approaches and a critical appraisal of clinical results using non-randomized data. PLoS One 2013;8(10):e74368.
15. van Gelder M, de Wreede LC, Schetelig J, et al. Monosomal karyotype predicts poor survival after allogeneic stem cell transplantation in chromosome 7 abnormal myelodysplastic syndrome and secondary acute myeloid leukemia. Leukemia 2013;27(4):879–88.
16. Deeg HJ, Scott BL, Fang M, et al. Five-group cytogenetic risk classification, monosomal karyotype, and outcome after hematopoietic cell transplantation for MDS or acute leukemia evolving from MDS. Blood 2012;120(7):1398–408.
17. Sierra J, Perez WS, Rozman C, et al. Bone marrow transplantation from HLA-identical siblings as treatment for myelodysplasia. Blood 2002;100(6): 1997–2004.
18. Warlick ED, Cioc A, Defor T, et al. Allogeneic stem cell transplantation for adults with myelodysplastic syndromes: importance of pretransplant disease burden. Biol Blood Marrow Transplant 2009;15(1):30–8.
19. Lim Z, Brand R, Martino R, et al. Allogeneic hematopoietic stem-cell transplantation for patients 50 years or older with myelodysplastic syndromes or secondary acute myeloid leukemia. J Clin Oncol 2010;28(3):405–11.
20. Alessandrino EP, Della Porta MG, Bacigalupo A, et al. WHO classification and WPSS predict posttransplantation outcome in patients with myelodysplastic syndrome: a study from the Gruppo Italiano Trapianto di Midollo Osseo (GITMO). Blood 2008;112(3):895–902.
21. de Witte T, Suciu S, Verhoef G, et al. Intensive chemotherapy followed by allogeneic or autologous stem cell transplantation for patients with myelodysplastic syndromes (MDSs) and acute myeloid leukemia following MDS. Blood 2001;98(8):2326–31.
22. Scott BL, Storer B, Loken MR, et al. Pretransplantation induction chemotherapy and posttransplantation relapse in patients with advanced myelodysplastic syndrome. Biol Blood Marrow Transplant 2005;11(1):65–73.

23. Gerds AT, Gooley TA, Estey EH, et al. Pretransplantation therapy with azacitidine vs induction chemotherapy and posttransplantation outcome in patients with MDS. Biol Blood Marrow Transplant 2012;18(8):1211–8.
24. Damaj G, Duhamel A, Robin M, et al. Impact of azacitidine before allogeneic stem-cell transplantation for myelodysplastic syndromes: a study by the Societe Francaise de Greffe de Moelle et de Therapie-Cellulaire and the Groupe-Francophone des Myelodysplasies. J Clin Oncol 2012;30(36):4533–40.
25. Platzbecker U, Thiede C, Fussel M, et al. Reduced intensity conditioning allows for up-front allogeneic hematopoietic stem cell transplantation after cytoreductive induction therapy in newly-diagnosed high-risk acute myeloid leukemia. Leukemia 2006;20(4):707–14.
26. Schmid C, Schleuning M, Ledderose G, et al. Sequential regimen of chemotherapy, reduced-intensity conditioning for allogeneic stem-cell transplantation, and prophylactic donor lymphocyte transfusion in high-risk acute myeloid leukemia and myelodysplastic syndrome. J Clin Oncol 2005;23(24): 5675–87.
27. Lubbert M, Bertz H, Ruter B, et al. Non-intensive treatment with low-dose 5-aza-2'-deoxycytidine (DAC) prior to allogeneic blood SCT of older MDS/AML patients. Bone Marrow Transplant 2009;44(9):585–8.
28. Field T, Perkins J, Huang Y, et al. 5-Azacitidine for myelodysplasia before allogeneic hematopoietic cell transplantation. Bone Marrow Transplant 2010; 45(2):255–60.
29. Itzykson R, Thepot S, Quesnel B, et al. Prognostic factors for response and overall survival in 282 patients with higher-risk myelodysplastic syndromes treated with azacitidine. Blood 2011;117(2):403–11.
30. Armand P, Kim HT, Cutler CS, et al. Prognostic impact of elevated pretransplantation serum ferritin in patients undergoing myeloablative stem cell transplantation. Blood 2007;109(10):4586–8.
31. Platzbecker U, Bornhauser M, Germing U, et al. Red blood cell transfusion dependence and outcome after allogeneic peripheral blood stem cell transplantation in patients with de novo myelodysplastic syndrome (MDS). Biol Blood Marrow Transplant 2008;14(11):1217–25.
32. Armand P, Sainvil MM, Kim HT, et al. Does iron overload really matter in stem cell transplantation? Am J Hematol 2012;87(6):569–72.
33. Wermke M, Schmidt A, Middeke JM, et al. MRI-based liver iron content predicts for nonrelapse mortality in MDS and AML patients undergoing allogeneic stem cell transplantation. Clin Cancer Res 2012;18(23):6460–8.
34. Kroger N, Zabelina T, de Wreede L, et al. Allogeneic stem cell transplantation for older advanced MDS patients: improved survival with young unrelated donor in comparison with HLA-identical siblings. Leukemia 2013;27(3):604–9.
35. Alousi AM, Le-Rademacher J, Saliba RM, et al. Who is the better donor for older hematopoietic transplant recipients: an older-aged sibling or a young, matched unrelated volunteer? Blood 2013;121(13):2567–73.
36. Anasetti C, Logan BR, Lee SJ, et al. Peripheral-blood stem cells versus bone marrow from unrelated donors. N Engl J Med 2012;367(16):1487–96.
37. Guardiola P, Runde V, Bacigalupo A, et al. Retrospective comparison of bone marrow and granulocyte colony-stimulating factor-mobilized peripheral blood progenitor cells for allogeneic stem cell transplantation using HLA identical sibling donors in myelodysplastic syndromes. Blood 2002;99(12):4370–8.
38. Anasetti C, Logan BR, Confer DL, et al. Peripheral-blood versus bone marrow stem cells. N Engl J Med 2013;368(3):288.

39. Finke J, Bethge WA, Schmoor C, et al. Standard graft-versus-host disease prophylaxis with or without anti-T-cell globulin in haematopoietic cell transplantation from matched unrelated donors: a randomised, open-label, multicentre phase 3 trial. Lancet Oncol 2009;10(9):855–64.
40. Scott BL, Sandmaier BM, Storer B, et al. Myeloablative vs nonmyeloablative allogeneic transplantation for patients with myelodysplastic syndrome or acute myelogenous leukemia with multilineage dysplasia: a retrospective analysis. Leukemia 2006;20(1):128–35.
41. Martino R, Valcarcel D, Brunet S, et al. Comparable non-relapse mortality and survival after HLA-identical sibling blood stem cell transplantation with reduced or conventional-intensity preparative regimens for high-risk myelodysplasia or acute myeloid leukemia in first remission. Bone Marrow Transplant 2008;41(1):33–8.
42. Chen YB, Coughlin E, Kennedy KF, et al. Busulfan dose intensity and outcomes in reduced-intensity allogeneic peripheral blood stem cell transplantation for myelodysplastic syndrome or acute myeloid leukemia. Biol Blood Marrow Transplant 2013;19(6):981–7.
43. Pollyea DA, Artz AS, Stock W, et al. Outcomes of patients with AML and MDS who relapse or progress after reduced intensity allogeneic hematopoietic cell transplantation. Bone Marrow Transplant 2007;40(11):1027–32.
44. Schroeder T, Czibere A, Platzbecker U, et al. Azacitidine and donor lymphocyte infusions as first salvage therapy for relapse of AML or MDS after allogeneic stem cell transplantation. Leukemia 2013;27(6):1229–35.
45. Warren EH, Fujii N, Akatsuka Y, et al. Therapy of relapsed leukemia after allogeneic hematopoietic cell transplantation with T cells specific for minor histocompatibility antigens. Blood 2010;115(19):3869–78.
46. Goodyear O, Agathanggelou A, Novitzky-Basso I, et al. Induction of a CD8+ T-cell response to the MAGE cancer testis antigen by combined treatment with azacitidine and sodium valproate in patients with acute myeloid leukemia and myelodysplasia. Blood 2010;116(11):1908–18.
47. Sockel K, Bornhaeuser M, Mischak-Weissinger E, et al. Lenalidomide maintenance after allogeneic HSCT seems to trigger acute graft-versus-host disease in patients with high-risk myelodysplastic syndromes or acute myeloid leukemia and del(5q): results of the LENAMAINT trial. Haematologica 2012;97(9):e34–5.
48. de Lima M, Giralt S, Thall PF, et al. Maintenance therapy with low-dose azacitidine after allogeneic hematopoietic stem cell transplantation for recurrent acute myelogenous leukemia or myelodysplastic syndrome: a dose and schedule finding study. Cancer 2010;116(23):5420–31.
49. Platzbecker U, Wermke M, Radke J, et al. Azacitidine for treatment of imminent relapse in MDS or AML patients after allogeneic HSCT: results of the RELAZA trial. Leukemia 2012;26(3):381–9.
50. Scott BL, Wells DA, Loken MR, et al. Validation of a flow cytometric scoring system as a prognostic indicator for posttransplantation outcome in patients with myelodysplastic syndrome. Blood 2008;112(7):2681–6.

Role of Hematopoietic Stem Cell Transplantation in Patients with Myeloproliferative Disease

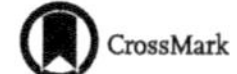

Rachel B. Salit, MD[a,b], H. Joachim Deeg, MD[a,b,*]

KEYWORDS

- Myeloproliferative neoplasms (MPN) • Myelofibrosis • Polycythemia vera
- Essential thrombocythemia • Hematopoietic stem cell transplantation • Ruxolitinib

KEY POINTS

- Allogeneic stem cell transplantation remains the only curative therapy for Myeloproliferative neoplasms.
- Transplantation following reduced-intensity conditioning provides survival equivalent to that with high-intensity (myeloablative) regimens.
- Alternative stem cell sources, including umbilical cord blood, are acceptable for patients without HLA-matched siblings.
- Janus kinase 2 inhibitors (ruxolitinib) may provide beneficial adjuvant therapy in patients undergoing allogeneic hematopoietic cell transplantation.

INTRODUCTION

Myelofibrosis (MF) can present as de novo primary MF (PMF) or evolve from other myeloproliferative neoplasms (MPN), such as polycythemia vera (PV) or essential thrombocythemia (ET).[1,2] Regardless of the cause, MF is characterized as a clonal stem cell disorder associated with dysregulated Janus kinase (JAK)/signal transducers and activators of transcription signaling and elevated levels of proinflammatory and proangiogenic cytokines, such as tumor necrosis factor alpha, interleukin 6, and interferon gamma, resulting in a bone marrow stromal reaction that includes varying degrees of reticulin and collagen fibrosis and osteosclerosis.[3–5] Clinically, MF is typified by progressive anemia, leukopenia or leukocytosis, thrombocytopenia or thrombocythemia, and multi-organ extramedullary hematopoiesis. It frequently involves the

Funding: Funded by National Institutes of Health grant number HL036444.
[a] Clinical Research Division, Cord Blood Transplant Research Program, Fred Hutchinson Cancer Research Center, Seattle, WA 98109, USA; [b] University of Washington Medical Center, Seattle, WA 98195, USA
* Corresponding author. Clinical Research Division, Cord Blood Transplant Research Program, Fred Hutchinson Cancer Research Center, Seattle, WA 98109.
E-mail address: jdeeg@fhcrc.org

Hematol Oncol Clin N Am 28 (2014) 1023–1035
http://dx.doi.org/10.1016/j.hoc.2014.08.003
0889-8588/14/$ – see front matter Published by Elsevier Inc.
hemonc.theclinics.com

spleen, resulting in massive splenomegaly, severe constitutional symptoms, a hypermetabolic state, and cachexia.[6,7] The median age at diagnosis is 60 to 65 years.[8] The clinical course is heterogeneous, ranging from indolent disease and survival for decades to aggressive disease in other cases, with survival measured in months.[9] The most common causes of death are progressive marrow failure leading to infection or hemorrhage, transformation to acute myelogenous leukemia, and complications of portal hypertension.

PATIENT EVALUATION OVERVIEW

Prognosis of MF varies with the presence or absence of specific risk factors. Historical prognostic scoring systems, such as the Lille or Dupriez classification, focused primarily on blood cell counts as the major prognostic factor.[10] In 2009, Cervantes and colleagues[6] published a multicenter analysis of risk factors and their impact on prognosis in patients with MF. Age greater than 65 years; presence of constitutional symptoms, including weight loss, fever, or night sweats, anemia (hemoglobin [Hb] <10 g/dL), leukocytosis (white blood cells [WBC] greater than 25 × 109/L); and a circulating blast percentage of 1% or greater were identified as most predictive of outcome. Median survival among patients with no risk factors (low-risk group) was 135 months, compared with 95 months among patients with one risk factor (intermediate 1 risk), 48 months among those with 2 risk factors (intermediate 2 risk), and 27 months among those with 3 or more risk factors (high risk).[6] This risk stratification is referred to as the international prognostic scoring system (IPSS) (**Table 1**).

The *Dynamic* IPSS (DIPSS), which was subsequently developed, uses the same 5 variables but can be used at any time in the disease course. However, unlike the IPSS, Hb less than 10 g/L receives a score of 2 points. The risk groups are scored as follows: low risk (score = 0), intermediate 1 (score = 1), intermediate 2 (score = 2 or 3), or high risk (score = 4–6) with corresponding median survivals of 185, 78, 35, and 16 months, respectively.[11] The DIPSS *plus* scoring system includes an additional 3 risk factors: transfusion dependence, unfavorable cytogenetics (+8, -7/7q-, i [17q], inversion [inv] [3], -5, 5q-, 12p-, 11q23, and complex karyotype), and platelet count less than 100 × 10^9/L.[12]

INDICATIONS FOR TRANSPLANTATION

IPSS, DIPPS, or DIPPS-plus risk classifications, comorbidities, and donor availability should be used to identify patients who are candidates for allogeneic stem cell

Table 1
Prognostic score systems developed for patients with PMF

Variable	IPSS	DIPSS	DIPSS-Plus
Age >65 y	X	X	X
Constitutional symptoms	X	X	X
Hb <100 g/L	X	X	X
WBC >25 × 10^9/L	X	X	X
Circulating blasts >1%	X	X	X
Platelets <100 × 10^9/L	—	—	X
RBC transfusion need	—	—	X
Unfavorable karyotype	—	—	X
	1 Point each	1 Point each but Hb = 2	1 Point each

Abbreviations: DIPSS, *Dynamic* IPSS; RBC, red blood cell.

transplantation (allo-SCT).[13] Current recommendations imply that the potential risk of transplant-related complications is justified in transplant-eligible patients with less than 5 years expected survival if not transplanted.[14] Based on DIPSS data, this would include patients in the intermediate 2– and high-risk groups. Those patients are, indeed, the patients included in most clinical transplant trials; however, lower-risk patients actually have a better outcome following allogeneic hematopoietic cell transplantation (allo-HCT), raising questions as to the most appropriate selection of patients and timing for allo-HCT.[15] Published data from the Fred Hutchinson Cancer Research Center (FHCRC) on 170 patients, with a median age of 51.5 years, with MF showed that the 6-year post–allo-HCT survival for low, intermediate 1–, intermediate 2–, and high-risk patients was 80%, 67%, 54%, and 38%, respectively, validating the DIPSS as an accurate prognosticator for post–allo-HCT outcomes in MF.[16]

Tefferi and colleagues[17] recently completed an analysis of 884 patients aimed at identifying risk factors associated with a greater than 80% 2-year mortality. Poor prognostic features included monosomal karyotype, inv (3)/i (17q) abnormalities, or any 2 of the following factors: peripheral blast percentage greater than 9%, WBC greater than 40×10^9/L, or other unfavorable karyotypes. Those patients meeting the performance status and donor criteria for allo-HCT should be referred directly to allo-HCT rather than undergo conventional treatment. In another study, which characterized 793 patients with PMF using DIPSS-plus criteria, the only 2 risk factors for leukemic transformation were unfavorable karyotype and platelet count less than 100×10^9/L; the 10-year risk of leukemic transformation was 12% in the absence of these 2 risk factors and 31% in the presence of one or both risk factors.[12] As is becoming evident for overall survival (OS), leukemia-free survival is also significantly compromised in patients carrying certain mutations, including ASXL1, *IDH1/2*, *EZH2*, and *SRSF2*.[18–20]

Transformation into acute leukemia occurs in 10% to 20% of patients and is associated with a median 5-month survival.[21,22] Previous studies have shown that postponing transplantation in MF until patients are at a more advanced stage of disease resulted in worse outcome.[16,23] In a study performed by the MPN subcommittee of the Chronic Myeloid Leukemia Working Party of the European Bone Marrow Transplant (EBMT) group looking at 46 patients with leukemic transformation of PMF or post–ET/PV MF, 3-year OS, and progression-free survival (PFS) were 33% and 26%, respectively.[24] Only remission status was significantly predictive for OS and PFS (69% vs 22%; $P = .0008$). However, the survival benefit of patients transplanted in complete remission (CR) was caused by significantly lower treatment-related mortality (TRM) while relapse incidence was identical. The consensus by the EBMT/european leukemia net (ELN) working committee in 2014 is that patients with leukemic transformation should receive cytoreductive therapy and be considered for transplantation only after achieving a partial or CR of leukemia.[25]

TIMING OF AND PREPARING PATIENTS FOR TRANSPLANT

Although allo-HCT remains the only known curative therapy for MF, any treatment that improves the patients' performance status and reduces the individual transplant-specific risk should be considered in the pretransplant phase.[25] In the past, drug therapies, including hydroxyurea, busulfan, 6-mercaptopurine, anagrelide, thalidomide, lenalidomide, interferon, corticosteroids, androgens, and erythropoiesis-stimulating agents or other growth factors, were used as the first-line treatment of MF.[26,27] These treatments may be helpful for palliation of symptoms; but responses are typically of short duration, usually less than 1 year. The Food and Drug Administration (FDA) recently approved ruxolitinib, a selective JAK-1/2 inhibitor, for the treatment of primary and secondary MF. JAK2 inhibitor therapy (ruxolitinib or others) is indicated in patients with a spleen extending more than 5 cm from the left costal margin and patients with constitutional symptoms. The drug should be administered for a minimum of 1 month but tapered off before transplant conditioning.[25] Impressive symptom control in patients with MF on ruxolitinib treatment is predominantly mediated by profound suppression of proinflammatory and proangiogenic cytokines.[28] Reduction of cytokine levels is typically accompanied by a substantial decrease in spleen size. Patients should be treated to best response.

The potential benefits of (surgical) splenectomy are a matter of debate. Data from Mayo Clinic on 314 patients with MF undergoing splenectomy showed significant perioperative complications in 28% of patients and a mortality of 6.7%.[29] The report by Ballen and colleagues[30] in 2010 on 289 patients with MF failed to show a significant effect of prior splenectomy on graft failure or PFS. Ciurea in 2008 noted that successful engraftment still was achieved even with massive splenomegaly.[31] Michallet and colleagues[32] showed in 2009 greater severity of graft-versus-host disease (GVHD) in splenectomized patients. A recent report from the MD Anderson Cancer Center demonstrated improvement in symptoms, such as anemia and thrombocytopenia, as well as abdominal discomfort at the cost of increased TRM.[33] However, there are also proponents for pre–allo-HCT splenectomy in patients with MF. Li and colleagues[34] showed in 2001 that splenectomized patients had faster neutrophil recovery and decreased transfusion requirements. Robin and colleagues,[35] in a multivariate analysis of results in patients receiving peripheral blood stem cells, showed faster engraftment in patients without splenomegaly and those who had undergone splenectomy pretransplant. Kroger and colleagues[36] demonstrated a trend toward more rapid neutrophil engraftment in splenectomized versus nonsplenectomized patients with reduced-intensity conditioning (RIC) allo-HCT. However, in that study a higher rate of relapse at 3 years was seen in splenectomized patients. On the other hand, the retrospective analysis by Scott and colleagues[16] in 170 patients transplanted at the FHCRC, suggests that splenectomized patients had superior post–allo-HCT survival (P = .05). Bacigalupo and colleagues[37] suggested that a spleen size greater than 22 cm was an independent risk factor for survival.

In summary, for patients with refractory, symptomatic splenomegaly, the evidence in support of splenectomy to improve transplant outcome is not sufficient to recommend splenectomy as a standard pretransplant procedure.[25] Pretransplant splenectomy in patients with refractory splenomegaly should be decided on an individual basis. If this procedure is performed, it should be in the setting of a clinical trial and at a center that performs many procedures per year and has a proven track record of success.

Autologous Stem Cell Transplant

Data on autologous SCT for MPN are sparse. In a multicenter study, 27 patients with MF in the setting of PMF, PV, or ET underwent autologous hematopoietic cell collection and 21 underwent conditioning with busulfan only, followed by autologous HCT.[38] The median time to platelet and neutrophil recovery was 21 days (for both), with clinically significant responses seen in 10 of 17 patients with anemia, 4 of 8 patients with thrombocytopenia, and 7 of 10 patients with symptomatic splenomegaly. However, the study was closed because of graft failure or incomplete hematopoietic recovery in 5 patients (27%). The high graft failure rate was attributed to the fact that autologous hematopoietic cells had been collected late in the disease course, and the investigators speculated that engraftment might be improved if autologous cells had been harvested earlier. The benefit achieved with autologous cells was thought to be caused by the faster growth of normal stem cells than that of clonal malignant cells. To carry out autologous HCT for MPN with curative intent, purging of clonal hematopoietic cells from the harvested cells would be necessary; currently, no effective method to achieve this objective is available.[39]

Allogeneic Stem Cell Transplant

Allo-HCT remains the only curative therapy for MF. Initial trials at the FHCRC showed that patients with *severe* marrow fibrosis were prone to experience engraftment failure (33% in a cohort of 15 patients), whereas engraftment was prompt in patients with mild or moderate fibrosis (6% failure in a cohort of 32 patients).[40] However, subsequently patients with severe MF or even osteosclerosis were shown to achieve sustained engraftment and regression or even complete resolution of marrow fibrosis with normalization of the marrow architecture following allo-HCT.[39]

Myeloablative Conditioning

Although a broad range of conditioning regimens of different intensities has been developed, the initial studies of allo-HCT for MF used high-intensity myeloablative conditioning (MAC) regimens, usually including total body irradiation (TBI) or busulfan. For MAC regimens, graft failure rates of less than 5% to 30% have been reported, reflecting the heterogeneity in patient populations and specific conditioning regimens.[41,42] Published TRM rates of 10% to 35% at 1 year and OS from 30% to 67% at 5 years have been reported (**Table 2**).[41,43–48]

One of the first studies reported by the EBMT included 55 patients with a median age of 42 years and showed a 5-year OS of 47%. Anemia was a predictive factor for poor

Table 2
Selected transplant studies in patients with PMF and secondary MF

Study	N	Conditioning	Age (y)	1-y TRM (%)	5-y OS (%)	5-y PFS (%)
Ballen et al,[30] 2010	229	MAC	47	27 (Sib) 43 (URD)	37 (Sib) 30 (URD)	33 (Sib) 27 (URD)
Patriarca et al,[50] 2008	100	MAC	49	35	31	28
Kerbauy et al,[41] 2007	104	MAC	49	27	61 (7 y)	—
Deeg et al,[47] 2003	56	MAC	43	35	58	—
Guardiola et al,[43] 1999	55	MAC	42	27	47	—
Abelsson et al,[58] 2012	40 52	MAC RIC	46 55	—	49 59	—
Robin et al,[35] 2011	46 101	MAC RIC	53	29 (4 y)	39 (4 y)	32 (4 y)
Stewart et al,[59] 2010	27 24	MAC RIC	38 54	41 (3 y) 32 (3 y)	44 (3 y) 31 (3 y)	44 (3 y) 24 (3 y)
Kroger et al,[36] 2009	103	RIC	53	16	67	51
Ballen et al,[30] 2010	60	RIC	—	15	—	39
Bacigalupo et al,[37] 2010	46	RIC	51	24	45	43
Alchaby et al,[23] 2012	150	RIC	57	—	60	—
Rondelli et al,[53] 2005	21	RIC	54	10	85 (2.5 y)	—
Gupta et al,[56] 2014	233	RIC	55	24 (5 y)	47	27

Abbreviations: Sib, sibling; URD, unrelated donor.

survival.[43] The largest study to date was reported from the Center for International Blood and Marrow Transplant Research (CIBMTR), analyzing data in 289 patients with PMF.[30] Patients underwent a transplant between 1989 and 2002 at 118 centers, with a variety of conditioning regimens. A total of 162 patients received an HLA-matched sibling transplant, 101 received HLA-matched unrelated donor (URD) transplants, and 26 received transplants from HLA nonidentical related donors. Most of the patients received bone marrow as the stem cell source, and 83% were conditioned with an MAC regimen. The 100-day TRM was 18% for HLA-matched sibling patients and 33% for the URD patients. The graft failure rate was 9% for HLA-matched sibling transplants and 20% for URD transplants. Splenomegaly did not impact the graft failure rate. GVHD grades II to IV occurred in 43% of sibling patients and 40% of the URD patients. The OS at 5 years was 37% for sibling transplants and 30% for URD transplants. Relapse-free survival (RFS) at 5 years was 33% for recipients of an HLA-identical sibling allografts and 27% for recipients of URD transplants. Positive predictors for survival included HLA-identical sibling donors, performance status greater than 90%, and absence of peripheral blood blasts at the time of transplantation.[30] Patients who had a poor Karnofsky score, peripheral blood blasts, or received a transplant from a URD had a 15% probability of 3-year survival.[49]

Other reports of allo-HCT for MF have confirmed the findings of the CIBMTR study. The Italian group analyzed results in patients from 26 centers; 48% received a MAC regimen.[50] The risk of graft failure was 13%, and the 1-year TRM was 35%. The 5-year OS and PFS rates were 31% and 28%, respectively. Positive predictors for survival included an HLA-matched sibling donor, transplantation after 1995, and a short interval between diagnosis and transplantation.[49]

A French group reported results in 147 patients with primary or secondary MF who received an allo-HCT, 31% with MAC regimens, with similar results.[35] Sixty percent of patients received transplants from HLA-identical sibling donors. The 4-year rates were 39% OS, 32% PFS, and 39% nonrelapse mortality. In a multivariate analysis, neither the Lille nor the IPSS score predicted survival. Positive predictors for survival included prior splenectomy, female sex, and transplantation from an HLA-identical sibling donor.

The authors' group at the FHCRC reported on 104 patients with MF, either PMF or after PV or ET.[41] The survival at 7 years was 61% in patients conditioned with targeted intravenous busulfan and cyclophosphamide. The use of a targeted busulfan-based chemotherapy regimen, younger patient age, and a lower comorbidity score predicted for better survival. This finding was consistent with a prior report by Deeg and colleagues[47] in 2003 that demonstrated that patients conditioned with cyclophosphamide plus targeted busulfan had a higher probability of survival at 3 years (76%). A more recent study demonstrated that administering cyclophosphamide, 120 mg/kg over 2 days *before* targeted busulfan for 4 days, conferred significantly less liver toxicity than busulfan *followed* by cyclophosphamide,[51] which translated into decreased early TRM.

Reduced-Intensity Conditioning

TRM has generally been high in older patients and those with comorbidities. To improve outcomes in those patient groups, several small studies of older patients with MF who underwent a transplant after RIC have reported encouraging results with decreased TRM. Early RIC studies for MF included reports by Devine and colleagues[52] and Rondelli and colleagues[53]; Kroger and colleagues[54] (2005) treated 21 patients with PMF or MF after PV or ET with RIC regimens consisting of fludarabine (180 mg/m^2) and busulfan (10 mg/kg) plus antithymocyte globulin followed by related-donor or URD allo-HCT and observed no graft failures and no day-100 TRM. The 1-year TRM was 16%. At 3 years, the PFS was 84%; 78% of patients became JAK2 mutation polymerase chain reaction (PCR) negative. A follow-up report included 103 patients, median age of 55 years. Among these, 33 had HLA-matched sibling donors and 60 had URD of which 30% were mismatched.[36] Engraftment occurred in 98%, and acute GVHD grades II to IV occurred in 27% of patients. The incidence of relapse at 3 years was 22%; patients with a low Lille score had a lower incidence of relapse, 14% versus 34%, suggesting that patients who underwent a transplant earlier in the course of their disease fared better. The 5-year PFS was 51%. Younger patients and those with HLA-matched donors did better. Thus, these results are comparable with those obtained with MAC regimens.[49]

The CIBMTR study by Ballen and colleagues[30] (described earlier) included 60 patients who received RIC (or nonmyeloablative) regimens. Graft failure occurred in 7 patients, none of whom survived. The TRM rate at 1 year was 15% for HLA-matched sibling transplants and 49% among those transplanted from URD. The RFS at 3 years was 39% for matched sibling allo-HCT and 17% with URD.[55] A more recent retrospective analysis by the CIBMTR included 233 patients undergoing RIC HCT for PMF. In this study, 12% of patients were low risk, 49% of patients were intermediate 1, 37% were intermediate 2, and 1% were high risk by DIPSS. Probability of OS at 5 years was 47%. In a multivariate analysis, donor type was the only factor associated with survival.[56]

With the use of RIC regimens, older patients with higher comorbidities have been transplanted successfully. However, results from these small, retrospective studies must be interpreted with great caution because of selection bias.

A comparison of outcomes by the Nordic MPD study group in 2009 revealed that when adjustments were made for age, survival after RIC versus MAC was significantly better ($P = .0003$).[57] A follow-up study by the same group published the results of 92 patients undergoing MAC versus RIC in 2012.[58] Patients in the RIC arm had an estimated 5 year OS of 78% compared with 52% in the MAC arm for patients younger than 53 years and a 5-year OS of 44% compared with 38% for patients aged 53 years and older. Within the RIC group, the outcomes were significantly better for patients younger than 60 years, with an estimated 5-year OS of 75% as compared with 20% for older patients. However, the poor outcome in the older population was worse than in prior publications comparing the two strategies. Discordantly, in a study by Stewart and colleagues[59] in which 27 patients were treated with MAC and 24 patients with RIC, there was no difference in nonrelapse mortality, OS, or PFS between the two intensity groups.

Donor Selection and Stem Cell Source

Only 30% of patients have HLA-matched sibling donors, and it is often difficult for African Americans and other minorities to find suitably matched URDs. Alternative stem cell sources for these patients include umbilical cord blood (UCB) or HLA-haploidentical donors: child, parent, or HLA half-matched sibling. Because of the delayed engraftment often seen after UCB transplantation (UCBT), transplant physicians have been reluctant to extend UCBT to patients with MF. However, a recent report by Takagi and colleagues[60] suggests that successful engraftment can be achieved after RIC with UCBT in patients with MF. Fourteen patients with MF, including several whose disease had transformed to acute myelogenous leukemia, underwent UCBT following RIC, mostly consisting of fludarabine 125 mg/m^2, melphalan 80 mg/m^2, and TBI 4 Gy. Neutrophil engraftment occurred in 92% of patients (n = 13) at a median of 23 days, and platelet engraftment occurred in 43% of patients at a median of 56 days. Complete donor chimerism was achieved in all evaluable patients. The estimated 4-year survival was 28.6%. Preliminary data by a French group presented as an abstract at ASH 2013 looking at MAC and RIC followed by UCBT for PMF, ET, and PV (12 patients had transformed to acute myelogenous leukemia) demonstrated only 64% engraftment but 44% 2-year survival.[61]

Alternative donor sources, such as HLA-mismatched URD, UCB, or HLA-haploidentical donors, may be effective; but the actual success rates and the incidence of complications, such as graft failure and GVHD, remain to be determined. The ELN/EBMT International Working Group concluded that patients with DIPSS intermediate 2–risk or high-risk disease lacking HLA-matched sibling or URD should be enrolled in prospective clinical trials using HLA-nonidentical donors.[25] The working group also agreed on considering peripheral blood as the most appropriate source of hematopoietic stem cells for HLA-matched sibling and URD transplants.[25]

Posttransplant Monitoring

In patients undergoing a transplant in the presence of splenomegaly, monitoring of spleen size with ultrasound after allo-SCT is recommended.[25] Persistence of splenomegaly in the early posttransplant phase should be considered the normal process of disease clearance and does not need specific management, unless there is pancytopenia. If patients have persistent splenomegaly (and complete donor cell chimerism), splenectomy may be a therapeutic option. JAK2 inhibition in this setting has not been tested so far and may contribute to cytopenias. Persistence of splenomegaly late after transplantation, when associated with incomplete donor chimerism, is typically a sign of disease persistence or recurrence.[25] Treatment may consist of reduction of immunosuppression, donor lymphocyte infusion (DLI), or both. JAK2 inhibitors alone may reduce the spleen size and persistent constitutional symptoms but will not increase donor cell chimerism or clear minimal residual disease. Splenomegaly appearing after allo-SCT should raise the suspicion of hepatic venoocclusive disease, posttransplant lymphoproliferative disorders, infections, or relapse.[25]

In the presence of poor graft function, bone marrow assessment by biopsy to assess cellularity and persistence of fibrosis and osteosclerosis as well as chimerism determination should be performed.[25] Chimerism studies on peripheral blood CD3+ cells and unfractionated bone marrow cells are necessary to establish the degree of donor cell engraftment and may assist in the decision regarding withdrawal of immunosuppression. In patients with poor graft function, use of growth factors may be useful. In patients with a late decline in graft function who have full donor chimerism and no evidence of active GVHD, an infusion of additional donor hemopoietic stem cells is recommended.[25] In patients with graft failure and no autologous reconstitution, the only available option is a second transplant.

MANAGEMENT OF RELAPSES AFTER TRANSPLANTATION

Disease-specific markers, such as JAK2V617, CALR, and myeloproliferative leukemia (MPL) mutations, have been shown to be beneficial in detecting minimal residual disease after allo-SCT.[62] Those molecular markers can be monitored by PCR or by direct sequencing. In patients who relapse after allo-SCT and do not have severe GVHD, reduction of immunosuppressive drugs or DLI are currently considered the treatment strategies of choice. In patients who fail to achieve complete remission despite these measures, a second allo-HCT may be considered. Patients relapsing with constitutional symptoms or splenomegaly may benefit from treatment with a JAK2 inhibitor.

NOVEL THERAPIES AND THEIR INTEGRATION IN TRANSPLANTATION

Presently, ruxolitinib is the only FDA-approved JAK2 inhibitor for MF and the only non-HCT therapy to date associated with a survival benefit. In a phase I/II study of ruxolitinib therapy at the MD Anderson Cancer Center, OS was significantly superior in ruxolitinib-treated patients compared with a historical cohort in an analysis adjusted for IPSS.[63] Spleen volume reduction alone was associated with a survival advantage in ruxolitinib-treated patients; 63% of patients achieved greater than 50% reduction in spleen volume with a median duration of approximately 2 years. Patients with greater than 50% reduction in splenomegaly had superior survival when compared with patients with less than 25% spleen size reduction ($P<.0001$). Furthermore, the finding of superimposable survival curves for high-risk and intermediate 2–risk patients treated with ruxolitinib suggested that ruxolitinib therapy may downgrade an individual's prognostic score category and improve predicted survival.[63]

Using JAK2 inhibitors to reduce spleen size before HCT may be useful in improving engraftment. In a study by a German group, 14 patients received allo-HCT following a median of 6.5 months treatment with ruxolitinib.[64] Under ruxolitinib therapy, spleen size was reduced in 64% of patients and engraftment was achieved in 93% of patients. TRM was 7% and survival 79%, but the median follow-up was only 9 months. Another German group reported a retrospective analysis of results in 22 patients with PMF or after ET/PV MF who had received a median of 97 days of ruxolitinib before allo-HCT.[65] At the time of transplant, 86% had improvement in constitutional symptoms and 41% had a major response in spleen size. With a median follow-up of 12 months, the 1-year OS was 81% and PFS was 76%. Whether JAK2 inhibitor treatment before HCT can consistently improve patient performance status and the degree of splenomegaly and lead to more favorable outcomes is an important area of ongoing investigation. A prospective study (JAK-ALLO) is ongoing in France on behalf of French Society of Bone Marrow Transplantation and Cell Therapies (SFGM-TC) to evaluate the role of ruxolitinib before allo-HCT, and a similar trial is under way at the FHCRC.

SUMMARY/DISCUSSION

Considering the lack of long-term effective drug therapies for patients with MF, the potential risk of transplant-related complications seems justified in patients with DIPSS plus high- or intermediate 2–risk disease as well as those with either unfavorable karyotype or a platelet count of less than 100×10^9/L. Currently, TRM is too high to justify pursuing allo-HCT systematically in lower-risk patient populations, even though the data indicate that those patients have a much higher probability to benefit from HCT. As we modify our treatment regimens and enhance peri-transplant strategies for supportive care, transplant results are improving. Increasing success rates are being reported with RIC as well as with regimens historically designated as MAC. The JAK2 inhibitor era provides a unique opportunity to begin to incorporate novel agents into the transplant algorithm for high-risk patients. Clinical trials, which examine the best way to use these agents in concert with allo-HCT and the optimal timing, will be the key to providing the best therapy for patients.

REFERENCES

1. Barosi G, Mesa RA, Thiele J, et al. Proposed criteria for the diagnosis of post-polycythemia vera and post-essential thrombocythemia myelofibrosis: a consensus statement from the International Working Group for Myelofibrosis Research and Treatment. Leukemia 2008;22:437–8.

2. Tefferi A. How I treat myelofibrosis. Blood 2011;117:3494–504.
3. Vannucchi AM. Management of myelofibrosis. Hematology Am Soc Hematol Educ Program 2011;2011:222–30.
4. Vainchenker W, Delhommeau F, Constantinescu SN, et al. New mutations and pathogenesis of myeloproliferative neoplasms. Blood 2011;118:1723–35.
5. Tefferi A, Vaidya R, Caramazza D, et al. Circulating interleukin (IL)-8, IL-2R, IL-12, and IL-15 levels are independently prognostic in primary myelofibrosis: a comprehensive cytokine profiling study. J Clin Oncol 2011;29:1356–63.
6. Cervantes F, Dupriez B, Pereira A, et al. New prognostic scoring system for primary myelofibrosis based on a study of the International Working Group for Myelofibrosis Research and Treatment. Blood 2009;113:2895–901.
7. Mesa RA, Niblack J, Wadleigh M, et al. The burden of fatigue and quality of life in myeloproliferative disorders (MPDs): an international Internet-based survey of 1179 MPD patients. Cancer 2007;109:68–76.
8. Barosi G, Berzuini C, Liberato LN, et al. A prognostic classification of myelofibrosis with myeloid metaplasia. Br J Haematol 1988;70:397–401.
9. Tefferi A. Myelofibrosis with myeloid metaplasia. N Engl J Med 2000;342: 1255–65.
10. Dupriez B, Morel P, Demory JL, et al. Prognostic factors in agnogenic myeloid metaplasia: a report on 195 cases with a new scoring system. Blood 1996;88: 1013–8.
11. Passamonti F, Cervantes F, Vannucchi AM, et al. Dynamic International Prognostic Scoring System (DIPSS) predicts progression to acute myeloid leukemia in primary myelofibrosis. Blood 2010;116:2857–8.
12. Gangat N, Caramazza D, Vaidya R, et al. DIPSS plus: a refined Dynamic International Prognostic Scoring System for primary myelofibrosis that incorporates prognostic information from karyotype, platelet count, and transfusion status. J Clin Oncol 2011;29:392–7.
13. Sorror ML, Maris MB, Storb R, et al. Hematopoietic cell transplantation (HCT)-specific comorbidity index: a new tool for risk assessment before allogeneic HCT. Blood 2005;106:2912–9.
14. Barbui T, Barosi G, Birgegard G, et al. Philadelphia-negative classical myeloproliferative neoplasms: critical concepts and management recommendations from European LeukemiaNet. J Clin Oncol 2011;29:761–70.
15. Deeg HJ, Appelbaum FR. Indications for and current results with allogeneic hematopoietic cell transplantation in patients with myelofibrosis. Blood 2011;117: 7185.
16. Scott BL, Gooley TA, Sorror ML, et al. The Dynamic International Prognostic Scoring System for myelofibrosis predicts outcomes after hematopoietic cell transplantation. Blood 2012;119:2657–64.
17. Tefferi A, Jimma T, Gangat N, et al. Predictors of greater than 80% 2-year mortality in primary myelofibrosis: a Mayo Clinic study of 884 karyotypically annotated patients. Blood 2011;118:4595–8.
18. Lasho TL, Jimma T, Finke CM, et al. SRSF2 mutations in primary myelofibrosis: significant clustering with IDH mutations and independent association with inferior overall and leukemia-free survival. Blood 2012;120:4168–71.
19. Tefferi A, Lasho TL, Abdel-Wahab O, et al. IDH1 and IDH2 mutation studies in 1473 patients with chronic-, fibrotic- or blast-phase essential thrombocythemia, polycythemia vera or myelofibrosis. Leukemia 2010;24:1302–9.
20. Vannucchi AM, Lasho TL, Guglielmelli P, et al. Mutations and prognosis in primary myelofibrosis. Leukemia 2013;27:1861–9.

21. Cervantes F, Tassies D, Salgado C, et al. Acute transformation in nonleukemic chronic myeloproliferative disorders: actuarial probability and main characteristics in a series of 218 patients. Acta Haematol 1991;85:124–7.
22. Mesa RA, Li CY, Ketterling RP, et al. Leukemic transformation in myelofibrosis with myeloid metaplasia: a single-institution experience with 91 cases. Blood 2005;105:973–7.
23. Alchalby H, Yunus DR, Zabelina T, et al. Risk models predicting survival after reduced-intensity transplantation for myelofibrosis. Br J Haematol 2012;157: 75–85.
24. Alchalby H, Zabelina T, Stubig T, et al. Allogeneic stem cell transplantation for myelofibrosis with leukemic transformation: a study from the Myeloproliferative Neoplasm Subcommittee of the CMWP of the European Group for Blood and Marrow Transplantation. Biol Blood Marrow Transplant 2014;20:279–81.
25. Group EEIW. Indication and management of allogeneic stem cell transplantation in myelofibrosis: a consensus process by a EBMT/ELN international working group. March 6, 2014.
26. Cervantes F, Alvarez-Larran A, Hernandez-Boluda JC, et al. Erythropoietin treatment of the anaemia of myelofibrosis with myeloid metaplasia: results in 20 patients and review of the literature. Br J Haematol 2004;127:399–403.
27. Tefferi A, Cortes J, Verstovsek S, et al. Lenalidomide therapy in myelofibrosis with myeloid metaplasia. Blood 2006;108:1158–64.
28. Verstovsek S, Kantarjian H, Mesa RA, et al. Safety and efficacy of INCB018424, a JAK1 and JAK2 inhibitor, in myelofibrosis. N Engl J Med 2010;363:1117–27.
29. Mesa RA, Nagorney DS, Schwager S, et al. Palliative goals, patient selection, and perioperative platelet management: outcomes and lessons from 3 decades of splenectomy for myelofibrosis with myeloid metaplasia at the Mayo Clinic. Cancer 2006;107:361–70.
30. Ballen KK, Shrestha S, Sobocinski KA, et al. Outcome of transplantation for myelofibrosis. Biol Blood Marrow Transplant 2010;16:358–67.
31. Ciurea SO, Sadegi B, Wilbur A, et al. Effects of extensive splenomegaly in patients with myelofibrosis undergoing a reduced intensity allogeneic stem cell transplantation. Br J Haematol 2008;141:80–3.
32. Michallet M, Corront B, Bosson JL, et al. Role of splenectomy in incidence and severity of acute graft-versus-host disease: a multicenter study of 157 patients. Bone Marrow Transplant 1991;8:13–7.
33. Santos FP, Tam CS, Kantarjian H, et al. Splenectomy in patients with myeloproliferative neoplasms: efficacy, complications and impact on survival and transformation. Leuk Lymphoma 2014;55:121–7.
34. Li Z, Gooley T, Applebaum FR, et al. Splenectomy and hemopoietic stem cell transplantation for myelofibrosis. Blood 2001;97:2180–1.
35. Robin M, Tabrizi R, Mohty M, et al. Allogeneic haematopoietic stem cell transplantation for myelofibrosis: a report of the Societe Francaise de Greffe de Moelle et de Therapie Cellulaire (SFGM-TC). Br J Haematol 2011;152:331–9.
36. Kroger N, Holler E, Kobbe G, et al. Allogeneic stem cell transplantation after reduced-intensity conditioning in patients with myelofibrosis: a prospective, multicenter study of the Chronic Leukemia Working Party of the European Group for Blood and Marrow Transplantation. Blood 2009;114:5264–70.
37. Bacigalupo A, Soraru M, Dominietto A, et al. Allogeneic hemopoietic SCT for patients with primary myelofibrosis: a predictive transplant score based on transfusion requirement, spleen size and donor type. Bone Marrow Transplant 2010; 45:458–63.

38. Anderson JE, Tefferi A, Craig F, et al. Myeloablation and autologous peripheral blood stem cell rescue results in hematologic and clinical responses in patients with myeloid metaplasia with myelofibrosis. Blood 2001;98:586–93.
39. Tse W, Deeg HJ. Hematopoietic cell transplantation for chronic myeloproliferative disorders. Arch Immunol Ther Exp (Warsz) 2006;54:375–80.
40. Rajantie J, Sale GE, Deeg HJ, et al. Adverse effect of severe marrow fibrosis on hematologic recovery after chemoradiotherapy and allogeneic bone marrow transplantation. Blood 1986;67:1693–7.
41. Kerbauy DM, Gooley TA, Sale GE, et al. Hematopoietic cell transplantation as curative therapy for idiopathic myelofibrosis, advanced polycythemia vera, and essential thrombocythemia. Biol Blood Marrow Transplant 2007;13:355–65.
42. Gupta V, Kroger N, Aschan J, et al. A retrospective comparison of conventional intensity conditioning and reduced-intensity conditioning for allogeneic hematopoietic cell transplantation in myelofibrosis. Bone Marrow Transplant 2009;44:317–20.
43. Guardiola P, Anderson JE, Bandini G, et al. Allogeneic stem cell transplantation for agnogenic myeloid metaplasia: a European Group for Blood and Marrow Transplantation, Societe Francaise de Greffe de Moelle, Gruppo Italiano per il Trapianto del Midollo Osseo, and Fred Hutchinson Cancer Research Center Collaborative Study. Blood 1999;93:2831–8.
44. Ditschkowski M, Beelen DW, Trenschel R, et al. Outcome of allogeneic stem cell transplantation in patients with myelofibrosis. Bone Marrow Transplant 2004;34:807–13.
45. Ditschkowski M, Elmaagacli AH, Trenschel R, et al. Dynamic International Prognostic Scoring System scores, pre-transplant therapy and chronic graft-versus-host disease determine outcome after allogeneic hematopoietic stem cell transplantation for myelofibrosis. Haematologica 2012;97:1574–81.
46. Mittal P, Saliba RM, Giralt SA, et al. Allogeneic transplantation: a therapeutic option for myelofibrosis, chronic myelomonocytic leukemia and Philadelphia-negative/BCR-ABL-negative chronic myelogenous leukemia. Bone Marrow Transplant 2004;33:1005–9.
47. Deeg HJ, Gooley TA, Flowers ME, et al. Allogeneic hematopoietic stem cell transplantation for myelofibrosis. Blood 2003;102:3912–8.
48. Daly A, Song K, Nevill T, et al. Stem cell transplantation for myelofibrosis: a report from two Canadian centers. Bone Marrow Transplant 2003;32:35–40.
49. Ballen K. How to manage the transplant question in myelofibrosis. Blood Cancer J 2012;2:e59.
50. Patriarca F, Bacigalupo A, Sperotto A, et al. Allogeneic hematopoietic stem cell transplantation in myelofibrosis: the 20-year experience of the Gruppo Italiano Trapianto di Midollo Osseo (GITMO). Haematologica 2008;93:1514–22.
51. Rezvani AR, McCune JS, Storer BE, et al. Cyclophosphamide followed by intravenous targeted busulfan for allogeneic hematopoietic cell transplantation: pharmacokinetics and clinical outcomes. Biol Blood Marrow Transplant 2013;19:1033–9.
52. Devine SM, Hoffman R, Verma A, et al. Allogeneic blood cell transplantation following reduced-intensity conditioning is effective therapy for older patients with myelofibrosis with myeloid metaplasia. Blood 2002;99:2255–8.
53. Rondelli D, Barosi G, Bacigalupo A, et al. Allogeneic hematopoietic stem-cell transplantation with reduced-intensity conditioning in intermediate- or high-risk patients with myelofibrosis with myeloid metaplasia. Blood 2005;105:4115–9.

54. Kroger N, Zabelina T, Schieder H, et al. Pilot study of reduced-intensity conditioning followed by allogeneic stem cell transplantation from related and unrelated donors in patients with myelofibrosis. Br J Haematol 2005;128:690–7.
55. Samuelson S, Sandmaier BM, Heslop HE, et al. Allogeneic haematopoietic cell transplantation for myelofibrosis in 30 patients 60-78 years of age. Br J Haematol 2011;153:76–82.
56. Gupta V, Malone AK, Hari PN, et al. Reduced-intensity hematopoietic cell transplantation for patients with primary myelofibrosis: a cohort analysis from the center for international blood and marrow transplant research. Biol Blood Marrow Transplant 2014;20:89–97.
57. Merup M, Lazarevic V, Nahi H, et al. Different outcome of allogeneic transplantation in myelofibrosis using conventional or reduced-intensity conditioning regimens. Br J Haematol 2006;135:367–73.
58. Abelsson J, Merup M, Birgegard G, et al. The outcome of allo-HSCT for 92 patients with myelofibrosis in the Nordic countries. Bone Marrow Transplant 2012; 47:380–6.
59. Stewart WA, Pearce R, Kirkland KE, et al. The role of allogeneic SCT in primary myelofibrosis: a British Society for Blood and Marrow Transplantation study. Bone Marrow Transplant 2010;45:1587–93.
60. Takagi S, Ota Y, Uchida N, et al. Successful engraftment after reduced-intensity umbilical cord blood transplantation for myelofibrosis. Blood 2010;116:649–52.
61. Robin M, Ciannotti F, Deconinck E. Outcomes after unrelated cord blood transplantation for adults with primary or secondary myelofibrosis: a retrospective study on behalf of Eurocord and chronic malignancy working party-EBMT. Blood 2013;122(21):301.
62. Panagiota V, Thol F, Markus B, et al. Prognostic effect of calreticulin mutations in patients with myelofibrosis after allogeneic hematopoietic stem cell transplantation. Leukemia 2014;28(7):1552–5.
63. Verstovsek S, Kantarjian HM, Estrov Z, et al. Long-term outcomes of 107 patients with myelofibrosis receiving JAK1/JAK2 inhibitor ruxolitinib: survival advantage in comparison to matched historical controls. Blood 2012;120: 1202–9.
64. Jaekel N, Behre G, Behning A, et al. Allogeneic hematopoietic cell transplantation for myelofibrosis in patients pretreated with the JAK1 and JAK2 inhibitor ruxolitinib. Bone Marrow Transplant 2014;49:179–84.
65. Stubig T, Alchalby H, Ditschkowski M, et al. JAK inhibition with ruxolitinib as pretreatment for allogeneic stem cell transplantation in primary or post-ET/PV myelofibrosis. Leukemia 2014;28(8):1736–8.

Chronic Myeloid Leukemia–Transplantation in the Tyrosine Kinase Era

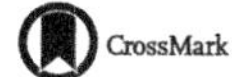

Andrew J. Innes, MBChB, MRCP, FRCPath[a],
Jane F. Apperley, MD, FRCP, FRCPath[a,b,*]

KEYWORDS

- Chronic myeloid leukemia • Allogeneic stem cell transplant
- Tyrosine kinase inhibitors

KEY POINTS

- Tyrosine kinase inhibitors have replaced hematopoietic stem cell transplantation (HSCT) in the first-line treatment of chronic myeloid leukemia (CML) in its chronic phase.
- HSCT remains a viable treatment option.
- HSCT remains the standard of care for patients with accelerated or blast-phase CML.

INTRODUCTION

Chronic myeloid leukemia (CML) is clonal stem cell disorder driven by the BCR-ABL1 fusion gene resulting from a reciprocal translocation between chromosomes 9 and 22 (the Philadelphia chromosome). It is a triphasic disease, with most patients presenting in chronic phase (CP) characterized by hepatosplenomegaly, thrombocytosis, and leukocytosis of mature granulocytes and their precursors. Until relatively recently, the natural disease history dictated that patients remained in CP for several years before progressing to the accelerated (AP) and blast (BP) phases, which were inevitably fatal. The first reports of CML date back to the mid-nineteenth century, and early treatment strategies included arsenic, splenic radiation, busulfan, and hydroxycarbamide.[1] Although these approaches were effective in symptom control, they did little to alter the natural progression of the disease to BP. During the 1980s, allogeneic hematopoietic stem cell transplantation (HSCT) became the first, and remains the only

---

Conflict-of-Interest Disclosure: J.F. Apperley has received honoraria from and serves on advisory boards for Novartis. A.J. Innes declares no competing financial interests.
[a] Centre for Haematology, Faculty of Medicine, Imperial College London, Hammersmith Hospital, Du Cane Road, London W12 0NN, UK; [b] Department of Clinical Haematology, Imperial College Healthcare NHS Trust, Hammersmith Hospital, Du Cane Road, London W12 0NN, UK
* Corresponding author. Centre for Haematology, Faculty of Medicine, Imperial College London, Hammersmith Hospital, Du Cane Road, London W12 0NN, UK.
E-mail address: j.apperley@imperial.ac.uk

Hematol Oncol Clin N Am 28 (2014) 1037–1053
http://dx.doi.org/10.1016/j.hoc.2014.08.002 **hemonc.theclinics.com**

treatment capable of consistently eradicating the malignant clonal stem cell population.[2] For several decades allogeneic HSCT remained the gold standard treatment for younger patients with suitable human leukocyte antigen (HLA)-identical donors. The identification of the BCR-ABL1 fusion gene in 1983,[3] and the understanding that this encoded a dysregulated tyrosine kinase capable of autophosphorylation and activation of downstream proteins, led to the development of the tyrosine kinase inhibitors (TKIs). Today, for most patients the ultimate goal of leukemic eradication and cure with HSCT has been superseded by a target of deep molecular remission and long-term disease control with an oral agent. Undoubtedly, the TKIs have now replaced HSCT as the first-line treatment of CP CML. Nevertheless, allogeneic HSCT remains a valuable treatment option for CML, and this review focuses on its current role.

INDICATIONS FOR TRANSPLANTATION

Chronic-Phase Chronic Myeloid Leukemia

Three of the 5 TKIs currently available are licensed for first-line treatment in CML, namely imatinib, dasatinib, and nilotinib. The goal of therapy is to induce deep and durable responses using an agent that can be tolerated in the long term, because for most patients treatment will be lifelong.

The response to TKI therapy is the most important prognostic factor, and is assessed on 3 levels; hematologic, cytogenetic, and molecular. The European Leukemia Network (ELN) have established criteria defining complete hematologic response, complete cytogenetic response (CCyR), and major molecular response (MMR), and require that these responses be achieved by certain time points.[4] Recently updated guidelines use these milestones to stratify response into categories of optimal, warning, and failure.[5] Furthermore, this recent version has incorporated the finding by several groups that an inability to achieve a 10-fold reduction in tumor load by 3 months, as indicated by a real-time, quantitative, reverse transcriptase–polymerase chain reaction (RQ-PCR) result of less than 10%, is associated with a relatively poor long-term survival.[6,7]

Imatinib is capable of inducing CCyR in the most patients and MMR in many, both of which are associated with prolonged long-term survival.[8] It is this level of efficacy that has led to its adoption as first-line therapy. However, despite its success, by 8 years more than 40% of patients will discontinue imatinib because of intolerance and/or lack or loss of response.[8] The second-generation TKIs (2GTKIs) dasatinib, nilotinib, and bosutinib have now all been used as front-line therapy. Trial data show that their higher potency in inhibiting BCR-ABL1 translates to superiority in achieving cytogenetic and molecular responses. Two large prospective, randomized clinical trials comparing one or other of these agents with imatinib demonstrated prolonged durable remissions, with nilotinib achieving MMR at 3 years in 70% to 73% of patients compared with 53% with imatinib,[9] and dasatinib achieving MMR in 69% compared with 55% with imatinib.[10] Although the data for bosutinib are less mature, similar superiority over imatinib has been demonstrated, with MMR rates of 41% at 12 months compared with 27% with imatinib.[11] In both trials of nilotinib and dasatinib, failure to achieve an RQ-PCR of less than 10% at 3 months was associated with an increased risk of treatment failure. Moreover, in both studies approximately 30% of patients had discontinued their front-line therapy at 3 years, indicating ongoing problems with longer-term efficacy and tolerability.

The 2 main reasons necessitating TKI cessation are intolerance and resistance. Toxicities such as nausea and diarrhea, muscle cramps and arthralgia, edema, and rashes can be common, particularly at the initiation of therapy. Later, patients taking imatinib complain of chronic debilitating fatigue.[12] Typically these side effects are mild and can often be managed with temporary treatment interruption or dose reduction; however, for some they are severe and intolerable, and require cessation of treatment with the particular drug. Dasatinib and nilotinib have some more serious toxicities, only rarely (or never) observed with imatinib, including pleural effusion and pulmonary arterial hypertension on dasatinib[10] and hyperglycemia, abnormal liver function tests, and vascular thrombotic events on nilotinib.[13]

Drug resistance can occur for several reasons. It may be primary, whereby from the outset there is no or little response to the drug, or it can be secondary, developing after a period of initial response. The mechanisms of resistance are beyond the remit of this review, although broadly there are 2 main categories: resistance with an associated kinase domain (KD) mutation and resistance without an identifiable KD mutation. In most cases leukemic cells containing KD mutations are thought to be present at the time of diagnosis and can be observed (or selected) only after nonmutated cells have been killed by the TKI.[14] These mutations (single-nucleotide polymorphisms) may render the protein resistant to 1 or more TKI.[15] Although knowledge of the site of a KD mutation may guide the choice of 2GTKI, many patients will be resistant to their therapy without evidence of a KD.

Patients who fail front-line treatment with imatinib may respond to a change to a 2GTKI. Second-line dasatinib is associated with a 6-year progression-free survival (PFS) of 40% to 50%, with overall survival (OS) on the order of 70%. Of note, in the largest phase II trial of 670 patients, only 28% of those treated with dasatinib remained on the study drug 6 years later.[16] Similar patterns of response are seen in patients treated with nilotinib as second-line therapy following prior imatinib. The largest phase II trial of nilotinib in imatinib-resistant or intolerant patients showed that CCyR was achieved in 45% of patients with OS and PFS at 48 months of 78% and 57%, respectively. Again at 48 months, importantly 70% of patients had discontinued treatment, the most common reason being disease progression.[17] The data from these 2 large studies show that although 2GTKI can induce a durable remission in many patients, most of those who require a 2GTKI will subsequently require an alternative therapy, one of which might be HSCT. Just as 3-month BCR-ABL1 burden is predictive of long-term survival in front-line TKI, the same is true of second-line therapy. Those patients who fail to achieve BCR-ABL1 of less than 10% after 3 months of second-line therapy have a significantly poorer long-term outlook,[18] and the predictive power of such an early assessment could be helpful in the identification of potential HSCT candidates.

Early data on the use of a third-generation TKI, ponatinib, the only drug to be active against the T315I mutation, suggest that approximately 40% of patients resistant or intolerant to multiple TKIs will achieve CCyR, with 27% achieving MMR[19]: while both CCyR and MMR are predictors of prolonged survival, mature data are awaited. In patients with the T315I mutation responses are slightly better, with CCyR and MMR rates of 66% and 56%, respectively; however, about half of these patients will still require alternative treatment.[19] In this circumstance allogeneic HSCT is the only option for long-term survival.

In summary, approximately 10% to 15% of patients presenting in CP will ultimately fail to achieve a durable remission with any TKI (**Fig. 1**). For these patients, allogeneic HSCT may offer a strategy to achieve long-term remission.

Advanced-Phase Chronic Myeloid Leukemia

The outcome for patients who present in either AP or BP, or who develop AP or BP while on treatment, is extremely poor. Frequently these patients carry multiple

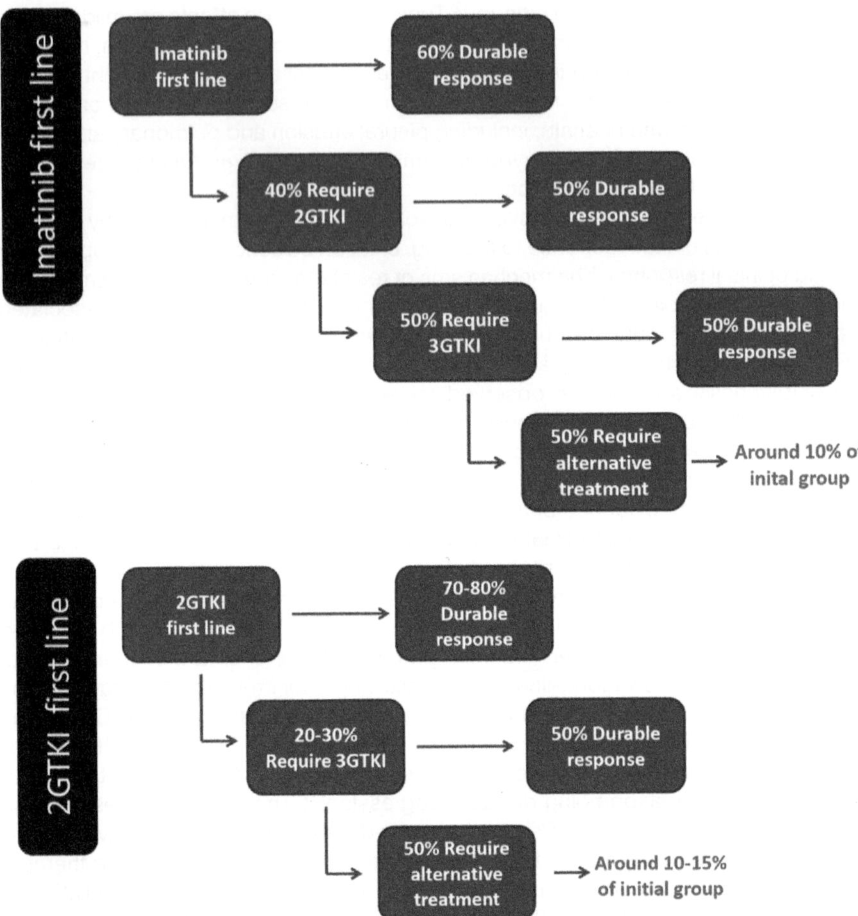

Fig. 1. Summary of predicted outcome following tyrosine kinase inhibitor (TKI) treatment in chronic phase of chronic myeloid leukemia. 2G, second-generation; 3G, third-generation.

additional nonrandom chromosomal abnormalities,[20] and those previously exposed to a TKI may also harbor KD mutations. In contrast to CP, TKIs have had less impact on the outcome of AP, and very little impact on the outcome of BP disease.

In BP, the median OS has only risen from 3 to 4 months pre-TKI to 7 to 11 months in the post-TKI era.[21] Although often these patients will initially respond to TKI therapy, almost invariably their response is partial and transient, thereby generating a window of opportunity for definitive treatment such as HSCT. HSCT in the second CP offers the best prospect of long-term survival for these patients,[22] with less than 10% achieving long-term survival if transplanted in frank BP.[23] Although TKI treatment may never achieve CCyR and MMR in patients presenting with BP, imatinib can briefly induce hematologic remission in 50% to 70%.[21] For those progressing to BP during treatment with a TKI, cytoreductive chemotherapy in combination with a 2GTKI seems to offer the best prospect of returning the patient to CP,[21,24] permitting consideration of HSCT.

For AP patients the impact of TKIs is more positive. Imatinib is capable of achieving CCyR in around 60% of patients.[25] 2GTKIs show promise in achieving better responses (MMR 76%), although with only small numbers of patients described to date.[26] At present, durable response rates remain too low to confidently withhold HSCT in eligible patients. Jiang and colleagues[27] suggested a risk-stratification algorithm capable of identifying low-risk patients in whom HSCT conferred no advantage over imatinib (6-year OS 81% vs 100%), but these patients constituted less than 1 in 3 AP patients. The outcome for high-risk patients who did not receive HSCT was dismal (5-year OS 18% vs 100%).

PREPARATION FOR TRANSPLANT

The decision to proceed to allogeneic HSCT in the TKI era must take into account several factors. As already discussed, disease-specific factors may influence the decision to transplant, such as phase of disease and probability of response to 2GTKI in imatinib-resistant patients. The second major factor to consider is fitness for transplant. Patient-specific factors such as age and comorbidities are known to predict mortality following HSCT, and the risk of transplant must be carefully balanced against the risks of disease progression.

Assessment of Transplant Risk

In the late 1990s the European Group for Blood and Marrow Transplant (EBMT) developed a risk-scoring system for patients with CML based on a data set of more than 3000 patients, at a time when CML was the commonest indication for allogeneic HSCT.[28] This system is based on 5 variables (**Table 1**) and is a powerful predictor of both survival and transplant-related mortality (TRM), with predicted 5-year OS ranging from 72% to 20% in the low- to high-risk groups, respectively. These data were accumulated from patients who had not been exposed to TKI. Of interest, a recent reanalysis of the EBMT database using patients transplanted after exposure to TKI shows that the score remains prognostic.[29] The EBMT score has been independently validated by the Center for International Blood and Marrow Transplant Research (CIBMTR),[30] and is also valuable in the assessment of patients undergoing a second allogeneic HSCT in CML.[31] In addition to the EBMT score, recent data have shown that comorbidities at the time of transplant significantly affect transplant outcome. The hematopoietic cell transplantation comorbidity index (HCT-CI)[32] has been used to predict non-relapse mortality and OS in many hematologic malignancies.[33–35] More recently, its use has been validated as an independent predictor of TRM and OS in CML patients undergoing allogeneic HSCT and, importantly, many of the patients used for its validation had been pretreated with TKIs, justifying its use in current practice.[36] This study also identified the presence of an elevated C-reactive protein at the time of admission for transplant, as an independent predictor of increased TRM and reduced OS.

Timing of Transplant

In current practice, TKIs will almost always be the first line of treatment in a newly diagnosed CML patient. However, tools now exist for identifying patients who are likely to fare poorly with first-, second-, and third-generation TKIs.[5–7] Although prediction of a poor outcome in these patients should not preclude a trial of alternative drugs, it should alert the clinician to the prospect that allogeneic HSCT may offer the best prospect of long-term remission, prompting early discussion about HSCT with the patient in addition to early identification of potential donors. For this reason, the authors would advocate HLA typing and donor identification in patients listed in **Table 2**.

In patients with AP or BC, there is no doubt that allogeneic HSCT offers the best prospect of long-term survival,[21,25] although timing of transplant is crucial. The best possible response must be sought before HSCT, and the time from achieving

Table 1
EBMT risk score

Risk Factor	Category	Score
Donor type	HLA-identical sibling	0
	Matched unrelated donor	1
Disease stage	First chronic phase	0
	Accelerated phase	1
	Blast crisis	2
Age of recipient (y)	<20	0
	20–40	1
	>40	2
Sex combination	All except:	0
	Male recipient/female donor	1
Time from diagnosis to transplant (mo)	<12	0
	>12	1

	Probability of Outcome at 5 y (%)		
Risk Score	**LFS**	**OS**	**TRM**
0	60	72	20
1	60	70	23
2	47	62	31
3	37	48	46
4	35	40	51
5	19	18	71
6	16	22	73

Abbreviations: EBMT, European Group for Blood and Marrow Transplant; HLA, human leukocyte antigen; LFS, leukemia-free survival; OS, overall survival; TRM, transplant-related mortality.

Data from Gratwohl A, Hermans J, Goldman JM, et al. Risk assessment for patients with chronic myeloid leukemia before allogeneic blood or marrow transplantation. Chronic Leukemia Working Party of the European Group for Blood and Marrow Transplantation. Lancet 1998;352:1087–92.

best response to proceeding to HSCT minimized. Ideally patients should be transplanted as soon as practical after achieving second (or higher) CP.

ALLOGENEIC TRANSPLANT OUTCOME

More than 3 decades have passed since the first reports of bone marrow transplant for CML. At the time, the eradication of the Philadelphia positive clonal cells by

Table 2
Triggers for HLA typing and donor search after discussion with patient

Triggers for Initiation of an HLA Donor Search (sibling's HLA typing, followed by unrelated donor search)	
Chronic phase	Patents failing/intolerant to imatinib (or alternative first-line TKI) and T315i mutation or Predicted poor response to 2GTKI Patients failing/intolerant to 2 or more TKI
Accelerated or blast phase	All patients deemed fit for allogeneic HSCT

Abbreviations: 2GTKI, second-generation TKI; HSCT, hematopoietic stem cell transplantation; TKI, tyrosine kinase inhibitor.

myeloablation and successful syngeneic donor transplant was revolutionary, and marked the start of a new chapter in the evolution of CML management.[2] In the following 20 years pioneering work resulted in a surge of HSCT for CML, which led to both cure from the disease for thousands of patients and the establishment of the principles on which much of the current transplant practice is based.[37] In the subsequent 15 years following the introduction of the TKIs, there has been an equally steep decline in the number of transplants. However, the legacy of data means that following careful patient selection, CML is one of the most well understood and evidence-based indications for HSCT.

Early transplant outcomes, despite offering cure for many, were hampered by high TRM. Between 1980 and 1990 more than 2600 patients underwent allogeneic HSCT in Europe for CML, and the TRM approached 40% with 20-year OS rates of 40%, 20%, and 10% for CP, AP, and BP, respectively.[38,39] More recent data show that improvements in transplant procedures and supportive care have significantly improved outcomes and have decreased TRM. Data from the CIBMTR in 2008 documented survivals of 79% and 72% at 1 and 2 years, respectively, for HSCT undertaken between 1999 and 2004,[40] and the most recently transplanted patients within the German CML study IV showed further improvements, with 3-year OS in excess of 90%.[22]

For patients in AP or BP a favorable TRM, combined with the dismal long-term outlook with alternative strategies, dictates HSCT as the best long-term strategy. For CP patients, however, one is faced with several more intricate questions regarding who and when to transplant. (1) Do transplant outcome data from the pre-imatinib era translate to patients who have tried and failed TKI therapy? (2) Does prolonging the time to transplant by trying multiple TKIs worsen transplant outcome? (3) Should HSCT remain a first-line option for any patients? Some of the questions are addressed by the recent literature on transplant outcome in CML, which is summarized in **Table 3**.[41–52]

Do Transplant Outcome Data from the Pre-Imatinib Era Translate to Patients Who Have Tried and Failed Tyrosine Kinase Inhibitor Therapy?

TKIs are not cytotoxic agents and have a mechanism of action very different to that of HSCT, so it cannot be assumed that patients who fail TKI but come to transplant still in CP have a worse outcome than patients transplanted earlier in their disease course. The impact of the use of TKIs before HSCT remains somewhat controversial. Published data have attempted to compare transplant outcomes in patients treated and not treated with TKIs, often using different time periods. However, the reason for the decision as to whether to use a TKI before transplant is often not provided, so the patient groups might not be directly comparable. Most patients coming to transplant in recent years have most probably failed 1 or more TKIs and might, therefore, be presumed to have "poor biology" disease. Perhaps the most useful information comes from a recent EBMT analysis of 5732 patients transplanted from 2000 to 2011, which showed similar 5-year OS and PFS in TKI-treated patients (n = 1247) compared with de novo transplanted patients (n = 4485) (5-year OS 59% vs 61%, 5-year PFS 42% vs 46%).[29]

Does Prolonging the Time to Transplant by Trying Multiple Tyrosine Kinase Inhibitors Worsen the Transplant Outcome?

The EBMT score from then 1990s identified time to transplant of more than 1 year as a risk factor for poorer outcome. In practice, nowadays most patients referred for HSCT have been treated with multiple TKIs, and are often more than 1 year from diagnosis at the time of transplant. The reanalysis of the EBMT data specifically probed this question. Direct comparison of patients with prior TKI therapy with those without confirmed

Table 3
Summary of published HSCT data since 2009

Authors,[Ref.] Year	Transplant Period	No. of Patients	Disease Phase (%)	Pre-HSCT TKI (%)	Donor (%)	Source: BM/PB (%)	Regimen (%)	OS	EFS/DFS	TRM	Comments
Transplantation in chronic phase											
Luo et al,[41] 2009	2005–2007	28	CP1 = 28 (100)	Imatinib = 28 (100)	Sib 13 (46) URD 15 (54)	BM = 7 (25) PB = 21 (75)	RIC = 28 (100)	81% (3 y)	67% (3 y DFS)	4%	Retrospective single-center study
Pavlů et al,[36] 2009	2000–2010	173	CP = 173 (100)	NR	NR	NR	NR	89% (If EBMT score 0 or 1) (3 y)	NR	NR	Retrospective single-center study
Liu et al,[42] 2011	1997–2009	91	CP1 = 91 (100)	Imatinib resistance = 4	Sib = 48 Related, other = 13 URD = 30	BM = 31 (34) PB = 60 (66)	MAC = 91 (100)	81.8 (5 y)	74.8 (5 y DFS)	15.9 (5 y TRM)	Retrospective single-center study
Transplantation in advanced phase											
Jiang et al,[27] 2011	2001–2008	132	AP = 132	Imatinib only = 87 (66) Imatinib + HSCT = 45 (34)	Sib = 19 (42) Other = 26 (58)	NR	MAC = 45	Low risk (6 y) Imatinib 100% HSCT 81% High risk (5 y) Imatinib 18% HSCT 100%	Low risk (6 y PFS) Imatinib 85% HSCT 95% High risk (5 y PFS) Imatinib 19% HSCT 100%	NR	Prospective single-center study (Imatinib vs HSCT)
Khoury et al,[43] 2012	1999–2004	449	CP2 = 184 (41) AP = 185 (41) BC = 80 (18)	Imatinib = 224 (50)	Sib = 121 (27) URD = 314 (70) Other = 14 (3)	BM = 234 (52) PB = 215 (48)	MAC = 350 (78) RIC = 99 (22)	CP2 = 36% AP = 43% BC = 14% (3 y)	CP2 = 27% AP = 37% BC = 10% (LFS 3 y)	CP2 = 33% AP = 34% BC = 46% (TRM 1 y)	Retrospective multicenter study (CIBMTR)
Zheng et al,[44] 2013	2002–2011	32	AP = 19 (59) BC = 15 (41)	Prior imatinib = 17 (53)	Sib = 16 (50) Cord = 16 (50)	BM = 1 (3) PB = 6 (18) BM+PB = 9 (28) Cord = 16 (50)	MAC = 30 (94) RIC = 2 (6)	Cord = 62% Sib = 49% (5 y)	Cord = 50% Sib = 40% (5 y LFS)	Cord = 37.5% Sib = 12.5% (180 d CI)	Retrospective single-center study (Cord vs Sib)

Mixed disease groups											
Shimoni et al,[45] 2009	NR	21	CP1 = 5 (24) AP = 6 (29) BC = 8 (38) ALL = 2 (10)	Dasatinib = 13 (62)[a] Nilotinib = 8 (38)[a]	Sib = 7 (33) URD = 13 (62) Haplo = 1 (5)	BM = 2 (10) PB = 19 (90)	MAC = 14 (67) RIC = 7 (33)	64% (2 y)	46% (2 y)	7%	Retrospective single-center study
Saussele et al,[22] 2010	2003–2008	84	CP1 (elective) = 19 (23) CP1 (TKI failure) = 37 (44) AP = 3 (4) BC = 25 (30)	All imatinib	Sib = 30 (36) URD = 54 (64)	BM = 20 (24) PB = 64 (76)	MAC = 57 (68) RIC = 11 (13) Other = 16 (19)	CP1 (elective) 88% CP1 (imatinib failure) 94% AP 59% (3 y)	CMR at last PCR 88%	Early TRM 8%	Prospective multicenter study (CML study IV)
Copelan et al,[46] 2009	1984–1995	335	CP = 229 (68) AP = 62 (18) BC = 44 (13)	NR	Sib = 335 (100)	BM = 335 (100)	MAC = 335 (100)	CP = 70% AP = 38% BP = 16% (3 y)	CP = 69% AP = 38% BP = 14%	Late (3 y) TRM CP = 14% AP = 41%	Retrospective multicenter study
Bacher et al,[47] 2009	1998–2004	1716	CP1 = 1084 (63) CP >1 = 203 (12) AP = 211 (12) BC = 128 (7) Unknown = 90 (5)	NR	Matched related = 683 (40) Mismatched related = 90 (5) Matched unrelated = 764 (45) Mismatched unrelated = 168 (10) Unknown = 11 (1)	BM = 604 (35) PB = 1069 (62) Unknown = 7 (1)	MAC = 1424 (83) RIC = 292 (17)	CP = 70% AP = 34% (5 y)	NR	100 d = 11% 1 y = 24% 5 y = 28%	Retrospective multicenter study (German registry report)

(continued on next page)

Table 3
(continued)

Authors,[Ref.] Year	Transplant Period	No. of Patients	Disease Phase (%)	Pre-HSCT TKI (%)	Donor (%)	Source: BM/PB (%)	Regimen (%)	OS	EFS/DFS	TRM	Comments
Sanz et al,[48] 2010	1997–2009	26	CP1 = 7 (27) CP2 = 11 (47) AP = 2 (8) BC = 6 (23)	NR	Cord = 26	Cord = 26 (100)	MAC = 26 (100)	NR	DFS 41% (8 y) (CP 59% vs non-CP 0%)	NR	Retrospective single-center study
Jabbour et al,[49] 2011	2004–2007	47	CP1 = 16 (34) CP2 = 10 (21) AP = 12 (25) BC = 9 (19)	Imatinib failure = 47 (100) + 2G TKI 29 (62)	Sib = 23 (49) Other = 24 (51)	NR	MAC = 15 (32) RIC = 32 (68)	63% (Mutation 44% vs no mutation 76%) (2 y)	49% (2 y EFS) (mutation 36% vs no mutation 58%)	13% (2 y)	Retrospective single-center study
Warlick et al,[53] 2012	2001–2007	306	CP1 = 158 (52) CP2/AP = 125 (41) BC = 25 (8)	Imatinib = 220 (72) No TKI = 79 (26) Unknown = 7 (2)	Sib = 143 (47) URD = 163 (53)	BM = 57 (19) PB = 249 (81)	RIC = 306 (100)	40–49 y = 54% 50–59 y = 52% >60 y = 41% (3 y)	40–49 y = 35% 50–59 y = 32% >60 y = 16% (2 y)	40–49 y = 13% 50–59 y = 7% >60 y = 9% (100 d)	Retrospective multicenter study (CIBMTR)
Topcuoglu et al,[50] 2012	1989–2007	84	CP1 = 66 (79) CP2 = 5 (6) AP = 13 (15)	NR	Sib = 84 (100)	BM = 8 (10) PB = 76 (90)	MAC = 56 (67) RIC = 38 (33)	56% No difference RIC vs MAC (5 y)	48% LFS No difference RIC vs MAC (5 y)	7% RIC 14% MAC	Retrospective single-center study (RIC vs MAC)

Zuckerman et al,[51] 2012	1999–2005	38	CP1 = 34 (89) AP = 4 (11)	Imatinib = 4 (11) No TKI = 34 (89)	Sib = 37 (97) URD = 1 (3)	PB = 38 (100)	MAC = 38 (100)	84% (5 y)	79% (5 y)	13% (CI at 10 y)	Single-institution long-term follow-up
Oyekunle et al,[52] 2013	2002–2009	68	CP1 = 27 (40) CP >1 = 41 (60)	Pre-HSCT TKI = 48 (71) Post-HSCT TKI = 20 (29)	Matched = 59 (87) Mismatched = 9 (13)	BM = 10 (15) PB = 58 (85)	MAC = 45 (66) RIC = 23 (33)	63% (2 y)	54% (2 y)	NR	Single-institute HSCT in TKI era
Milojkovic et al,[29] 2014	2000–2011	5732	Prior TKI: CP = 635 (51) CP >1 = 314 (25) AP = 168 (14) BC = 130 (10) Non-TKI: NR	Prior TKI = 1247 No TKI = 4485	NR	NR	NR	Non-TKI 61% Prior TKI 59% (5 y)	Non-TKI 46% Prior TKI 42%	NR	Retrospective multicenter study (EBMT)

Abbreviations: AP, accelerated phase; BC, blast crisis/phase; BM, bone marrow stem cells; CI, comorbidity index; CIBMTR, Center for International Blood and Marrow Transplant Research; CP, chronic phase; CP1, first chronic phase; CP2, second chronic phase; CP>1, second or higher chronic phase; DFS, disease-free survival; EFS, event-free survival; Haplo, haploidentical donor; HSCT, hematopoietic stem cell transplantation; MAC, myeloablative; NR, not reported; OS, overall survival; PB, peripheral blood stem cells; RIC, reduced-intensity conditioning; Sib, sibling; TKI, tyrosine kinase inhibitor; TRM, transplant-related mortality; URD, unrelated donor.

[a] Most recently used TKI.

that in the pre-TKI era, transplant more than a year from diagnosis was associated with an inferior survival. However, this was no longer true in TKI-treated patients.[29] Despite these data being difficult to fully understand, they provide some reassurance that delaying transplantation with the aim of trialing second-line or third-line TKI does not negatively affect the subsequent transplant outcome.

Should Hematopoietic Stem Cell Transplantation Remain a First-Line Option for Any Patients?

The use of HSCT as first-line therapy is now unusual in countries of high economic status where access to TKIs is relatively straightforward. In countries with less financial stability, there is still an argument to use HSCT early in the disease course, as the high cost in the short term is justified to avoid the prolonged expense of TKI therapy. Even in wealthier nations, patient choice must also be taken into account. Given the excellent long-term OS from HSCT, a young patient presenting in CP may favor HSCT over lifelong use of a TKI. Of interest, patients who elected to undergo HSCT rather than continue long-term TKI in the German CML study had a survival identical to those who underwent HSCT for imatinib failure.[22]

Conditioning regimen and stem cell source choice

Early conditioning regimens in CML often consisted of myeloablative combinations of total body irradiation and cyclophosphamide or other cytotoxic agents.[37] The subsequent introduction of T-cell depletion has permitted the use of matched and even mismatched volunteer unrelated donors with lower rates of acute and chronic graft-versus-host disease (GvHD), although this has resulted in higher rates of post-transplant relapse.[37] Recognizing that much of the curative effect of HSCT in CML relies on the graft-versus-leukemic effect led to the development of reduced-intensity protocols, often followed by preemptive donor lymphocyte infusion (DLI). Evaluating the role of myeloablative versus reduced-intensity protocols is confounded by differences in patient demographics between the 2 groups. Whereas reduced-intensity conditioning regimens are inferior to myeloablative regimens for high-risk patients because of the increased risk of relapse, for good-risk patients they improve accessibility to transplant for older patients in whom the high transplant toxicity of myeloablative regimens would otherwise preclude HSCT.[53] Data on regimen superiority are sparse, and the heterogeneity of the regimens used in the studies in **Table 3** demonstrates that in practical terms the choice of conditioning regimen, including whether they ought to include T-cell depletion, often depends on the institute or physician.

Bone marrow was traditionally the favored stem cell source, but more recently peripheral blood–derived stem cells (PBSC) are the most popular option. In 2012 a randomized controlled trial compared bone marrow and PBSC sources, and demonstrated higher rates of chronic GvHD with PBSC (53% vs 41%).[54] The rates of graft failure, however, were marginally higher with bone marrow stem cells (9% vs 3%). This study included, but was not limited to, CP CML patients. It could be argued that bone marrow should remain the first choice in CML in CP as there is no difference in OS or PFS between bone marrow and PBSC. Furthermore, if reduced-intensity regimens and/or T-cell depletion strategies are used to reduce the risk of TRM, both are associated with an increased risk of relapse, and the presence of chronic GvHD might preclude future use of DLI.

POST-TRANSPLANT MONITORING AND MANAGEMENT OF RELAPSE

Detection of BCR-ABL1 transcripts in peripheral blood by polymerase chain reaction (PCR) was developed to detect disease relapse following HSCT. Early PCR, however, was qualitative and capable only of detecting the presence of leukemic transcripts. The subsequent development of quantitative PCR allowed serial measurement of the BCR-ABL1 burden, identifying rising transcripts as an indication for intervention.[55] Serial measurement or BCR-ABL1 transcript copy numbers is therefore mandatory after transplant. In patients undergoing reduced-intensity conditioning HSCT for CML, eradication of the BCR-ABL1 clones can only be achieved once full donor chimerism exists[56]: therefore in the early post-transplant period, monitoring of the degree of donor chimerism in both whole blood and T cells is essential.

Our institution has previously established criteria for defining molecular relapse (MR), which are highly predictive of progressive disease.[57] However, immune manipulation with DLI is capable of restoring remission in most patients with MR.[58] Registry data suggest that 16% to 40% of patients undergoing HSCT will require DLI for subsequent disease management,[59] and there are established escalating dose regimens that maximize the probability of restoring remission while minimizing the risk of GvHD.[60,61] These schedules are safe and effective in sibling, HLA-matched and HLA-mismatched donors, providing a minimum of 9 months has elapsed since transplant.[58]

Some patients cannot receive DLI for post-transplant relapse because of the presence of GvHD and/or the inability to obtain additional cells from the original donor. In these situations, TKIs have been used instead and with good effect.[62] At present, however, most patients undergoing HSCT for CML are likely to have received multiple TKIs before transplant, suggesting that in the absence of acute GvHD, DLI should remain the first-line therapy for relapse.

SUMMARY

The introduction of TKIs for the management of CML has completely revolutionized clinical practice over the past 15 years. TKIs have replaced HSCT as the cornerstone of the treatment of CML. However, for the 10% to 15% of CP patients who will not remain in long-term remission on a TKI, HSCT remains an important treatment option. The data presented suggest that even in multiply pretreated patients, high rates of OS seen with HSCT in the pre-TKI era can still be expected. HSCT remains the standard of care for eligible patients in AP or BC with suitable donors.

REFERENCES

1. Goldman JM. Chronic myeloid leukemia: a historical perspective. Semin Hematol 2010;47:302–11.
2. Fefer A, Cheever MA, Thomas ED, et al. Disappearance of Ph1-positive cells in four patients with chronic granulocytic leukemia after chemotherapy, irradiation and marrow transplantation from an identical twin. N Engl J Med 1979;300: 333–7.
3. Groffen J, Stephenson JR, Heisterkarmp N, et al. Philadelphia chromosomal break points are clustered within a limited region, bcr. on chromosome 22. Cell 1984;36:93–9.
4. Baccarani M, Saglio G, Goldman J, et al, European LeukemiaNet. Evolving concepts in the management of chronic myeloid leukemia: recommendations from an expert panel on behalf of the European LeukemiaNet. Blood 2006;108: 1809–20.
5. Baccarani M, Deininger MW, Rosti G, et al. European LeukemiaNet recommendations for the management of chronic myeloid leukemia. Blood 2013; 2013(122):872–84.

6. Hanfstein B, Müller MC, Hehlmann R, et al. Early molecular and cytogenetic response is predictive for long-term progression-free and overall survival in chronic myeloid leukemia (CML). Leukemia 2012;26:2096–102.
7. Marin D, Ibrahim AR, Lucas C, et al. Assessment of BCR-ABL1 transcript levels at 3 months is the only requirement for predicting outcome for patients with chronic myeloid leukemia treated with tyrosine kinase inhibitors. J Clin Oncol 2012;30:232–8.
8. Deininger M, O'Brien SG, Guilhot F. International randomized study of interferon vs STI571 (IRIS) 8-year follow up: sustained survival and low risk for progression or events in patients with newly diagnosed chronic myeloid leukemia in chronic phase (CML-CP) treated with imatinib. 2009 114: Abstract 1126.
9. Larson RA, Hochhaus A, Hughes TP, et al. Nilotinib vs imatinib in patients with newly diagnosed Philadelphia chromosome-positive chronic myeloid leukemia in chronic phase: ENESTnd 3-year follow-up. Leukemia 2012;26:2197–203.
10. Jabbour E, Kantarjian HM, Saglio G, et al. Early response with dasatinib or imatinib in chronic myeloid leukemia: 3-year follow-up from a randomized phase 3 trial (DASISION). Blood 2014;123:494–500.
11. Cortes JE, Kim DW, Kantarjian HM, et al. Bosutinib versus imatinib in newly diagnosed chronic-phase chronic myeloid leukemia: results from the BELA trial. J Clin Oncol 2012;30:3486–92.
12. Steegmann JL, Cervantes F, le Coutre P, et al. Off-target effects of BCR-ABL1 inhibitors and their potential long-term implications in patients with chronic myeloid leukemia. Leuk Lymphoma 2012;53:2351–61.
13. Saglio G, Kim DW, Issaragrisil S, et al. Nilotinib versus imatinib for newly diagnosed chronic myeloid leukemia. N Engl J Med 2010;362:2251–9.
14. Soverini S, Hochhaus A, Nicolini FE, et al. BCR-ABL kinase domain mutation analysis in chronic myeloid leukemia patients treated with tyrosine kinase inhibitors: recommendations from an expert panel on behalf of European LeukemiaNet. Blood 2011;118:1208–15.
15. Ernst T, La Rosée P, Müller MC, et al. BCR-ABL mutations in chronic myeloid leukemia. Hematol Oncol Clin North Am 2011;25:997–1008.
16. Shah NP, Guilhot F, Cortes JE, et al. Long-term outcome with dasatinib after imatinib failure in chronic-phase chronic myeloid leukemia: follow-up of a phase 3 study. Blood 2014;123:2317–24.
17. Giles FJ, le Coutre PD, Pinilla-Ibarz J, et al. Nilotinib in imatinib-resistant or imatinib-intolerant patients with chronic myeloid leukemia in chronic phase: 48-month follow-up results of a phase II study. Leukemia 2013;27:107–12.
18. Kim DD, Lee H, Kamel-Reid S, et al. BCR-ABL1 transcript at 3 months predicts long-term outcomes following second generation tyrosine kinase inhibitor therapy in the patients with chronic myeloid leukaemia in chronic phase who failed Imatinib. Br J Haematol 2013;160:630–9.
19. Cortes JE, Kim DW, Pinilla-Ibarz J, et al. A phase 2 trial of ponatinib in Philadelphia chromosome-positive leukemias. N Engl J Med 2013;369:1783–96.
20. Griesshammer M, Heinze B, Bangerter M, et al. Karyotype abnormalities and their clinical significance in blast crisis of chronic myeloid leukemia. J Mol Med 1997;75:836–8.
21. Hehlmann R. How I treat CML blast crisis. Blood 2012;120:737–47.
22. Saussele S, Lauseker M, Gratwohl A, et al. Allogeneic hematopoietic stem cell transplantation (allo SCT) for chronic myeloid leukemia in the imatinib era: evaluation of its impact within a subgroup of the randomized German CML Study IV. Blood 2010;115:1880–5.

23. Silver RT. The blast phase of chronic myeloid leukaemia. Best Pract Res Clin Haematol 2009;22:387–94.
24. Milojkovic D, Ibrahim A, Reid A, et al. Efficacy of combining dasatinib and FLAG-IDA for patients with chronic myeloid leukemia in blastic transformation. Haematologica 2012;97:473–4.
25. Rea D, Etienne G, Nicolini F, et al. First-line imatinib mesylate in patients with newly diagnosed accelerated phase-chronic myeloid leukemia. Leukemia 2012;26:2254–9.
26. Ohanian M, Kantarjian HM, Quintas-Cardama A, et al. Tyrosine kinase inhibitors as initial therapy for patients with chronic myeloid leukemia in accelerated phase. Clin Lymphoma Myeloma Leuk 2014;14:155–62.
27. Jiang Q, Xu LP, Liu DH, et al. Imatinib mesylate versus allogeneic hematopoietic stem cell transplantation for patients with chronic myelogenous leukemia in the accelerated phase. Blood 2011;117:3032–40.
28. Gratwohl A, Hermans J, Goldman JM, et al. Risk assessment for patients with chronic myeloid leukaemia before allogeneic blood or marrow transplantation. Chronic Leukemia Working Party of the European Group for Blood and Marrow Transplantation. Lancet 1998;352:1087–92.
29. Milojkovic D, Szydlo D, Hoek J, et al. Prognostic significance of EBMT score for chronic myeloid leukaemia patients in the era of tyrosine kinase inhibitor therapy: a retrospective study from the chronic malignancy working party of the European Group For Blood and Marrow Transplantation (EBMT). Bone Marrow Transplant 2014;49:S34–5.
30. Passweg JR, Walker I, Sobocinski KA, et al. Validation and extension of the EBMT risk score for patients with chronic myeloid leukaemia (CML) receiving allogeneic haematopoietic stem cell transplants. Br J Haematol 2004;125:613–20.
31. Rezvani K, Kanfer EJ, Marin D, et al. EBMT risk score predicts outcome of allogeneic hematopoietic stem cell transplantation in patients who have failed a previous transplantation procedure. Biol Blood Marrow Transplant 2012;18:235–40.
32. Sorror ML, Maris MB, Storb R, et al. Hematopoietic cell transplantation (HCT)-specific comorbidity index: a new tool for risk assessment before allogeneic HCT. Blood 2005;106:2912–9.
33. Sorror ML, Giralt S, Sandmaier BM, et al. Hematopoietic cell transplantation specific comorbidity index as an outcome predictor for patients with acute myeloid leukemia in first remission: combined FHCRC and MDACC experiences. Blood 2007;110:4606–13.
34. Sorror M, Storer B, Sandmaier BM, et al. Hematopoietic cell transplantation-comorbidity index and Karnofsky performance status are independent predictors of morbidity and mortality after allogeneic nonmyeloablative hematopoietic cell transplantation. Cancer 2008;112:1992–2001.
35. Zipperer E, Pelz D, Nachtkamp K, et al. The hematopoietic stem cell transplantation comorbidity index is of prognostic relevance for patients with myelodysplastic syndrome. Haematologica 2009;94:729–32.
36. Pavlů J, Kew AK, Taylor-Roberts B, et al. Optimizing patient selection for myeloablative allogeneic hematopoietic cell transplantation in chronic myeloid leukemia in chronic phase. Blood 2010;115:4018–20.
37. Pavlů J, Szydlo RM, Goldman JM, et al. Three decades of transplantation for chronic myeloid leukemia: what have we learned? Blood 2011;117:755–63.
38. Gratwohl A, Brand R, Apperley J, et al. Allogeneic hematopoietic stem cell transplantation for chronic myeloid leukemia in Europe 2006: transplant activity, long-term data and current results. An analysis by the Chronic Leukemia

Working Party of the European Group for Blood and Marrow Transplantation (EBMT). Haematologica 2006;91:513–21.

39. Gratwohl A, Heim D. Current role of stem cell transplantation in chronic myeloid leukaemia. Best Pract Res Clin Haematol 2009;22:431–43.
40. Lee SJ, Kukreja M, Wang T, et al. Impact of prior imatinib mesylate on the outcome of hematopoietic cell transplantation for chronic myeloid leukemia. Blood 2008;112:3500–7.
41. Luo Y, Lai XY, Tan YM, et al. Reduced-intensity allogeneic transplantation combined with imatinib mesylate for chronic myeloid leukemia in first chronic phase. Leukemia 2009;23:1171–4.
42. Liu QF, Xu XJ, Chen YK, et al. Long-term outcomes of HLA-matched sibling compared with mismatched related and unrelated donor hematopoietic stem cell transplantation for chronic phase chronic myelogenous leukemia: a single institution experience in China. Ann Hematol 2011;90:331–41.
43. Khoury HJ, Kukreja M, Goldman JM, et al. Prognostic factors for outcomes in allogeneic transplantation for CML in the imatinib era: a CIBMTR analysis. Bone Marrow Transplant 2012;47:810–6.
44. Zheng C, Tang B, Yao W, et al. Comparison of unrelated cord blood transplantation and HLA-matched sibling hematopoietic stem cell transplantation for patients with chronic myeloid leukemia in advanced stage. Biol Blood Marrow Transplant 2013;19:1708–12.
45. Shimoni A, Leiba M, Schleuning M, et al. Prior treatment with the tyrosine kinase inhibitors dasatinib and nilotinib allows stem cell transplantation (SCT) in a less advanced disease phase and does not increase SCT Toxicity in patients with chronic myelogenous leukemia and Philadelphia positive acute lymphoblastic leukemia. Leukemia 2009;23:190–4.
46. Copelan EA, Crilley PA, Szer J, et al. Late mortality and relapse following BuCy2 and HLA-identical sibling marrow transplantation for chronic myelogenous leukemia. Biol Blood Marrow Transplant 2009;15:851–5.
47. Bacher U, Klyuchnikov E, Zabelina T, et al. The changing scene of allogeneic stem cell transplantation for chronic myeloid leukemia—a report from the German Registry covering the period from 1998 to 2004. Ann Hematol 2009; 88:1237–47.
48. Sanz J, Montesinos P, Saavedra S, et al. Single-unit umbilical cord blood transplantation from unrelated donors in adult patients with chronic myelogenous leukemia. Biol Blood Marrow Transplant 2010;16:1589–95.
49. Jabbour E, Cortes J, Santos FP, et al. Results of allogeneic hematopoietic stem cell transplantation for chronic myelogenous leukemia patients who failed tyrosine kinase inhibitors after developing BCR-ABL1 kinase domain mutations. Blood 2011;117:3641–7.
50. Topcuoglu P, Arat M, Ozcan M, et al. Case-matched comparison with standard versus reduced intensity conditioning regimen in chronic myeloid leukemia patients. Ann Hematol 2012;91:577–86.
51. Zuckerman T, Katz T, Haddad N, et al. Allogeneic stem cell transplantation for patients with chronic myeloid leukemia: risk stratified approach with a long-term follow-up. Am J Hematol 2012;87:875–9.
52. Oyekunle A, Zander AR, Binder M, et al. Outcome of allogeneic SCT in patients with chronic myeloid leukemia in the era of tyrosine kinase inhibitor therapy. Ann Hematol 2013;92:487–96.
53. Warlick E, Ahn KW, Pedersen TL, et al. Reduced intensity conditioning is superior to nonmyeloablative conditioning for older chronic myelogenous leukemia

patients undergoing hematopoietic cell transplant during the tyrosine kinase inhibitor era. Blood 2012;119:4083–90.

54. Anasetti C, Logan BR, Lee SJ, et al. Peripheral-blood stem cells versus bone marrow from unrelated donors. N Engl J Med 2012;367:1487–96.
55. Olavarria E, Kanfer E, Szydlo R, et al. Early detection of BCR-ABL transcripts by quantitative reverse transcriptase-polymerase chain reaction predicts outcome after allogeneic stem cell transplantation for chronic myeloid leukemia. Blood 2001;97:1560–5.
56. Uzunel M, Mattsson J, Brune M, et al. Kinetics of minimal residual disease and chimerism in patients with chronic myeloid leukemia after nonmyeloablative conditioning and allogeneic stem cell transplantation. Blood 2003;101:469–72.
57. Lin F, van Rhee F, Goldman JM, et al. Kinetics of increasing BCR-ABL transcript numbers in chronic myeloid leukemia patients who relapse after bone marrow transplant. Blood 1996;87:4473–8.
58. Innes AJ, Lurkins J, Szydlo R. The majority of patients receiving donor lymphocyte infusions for relapsed chronic myeloid leukemia remain PCR positive despite maintaining long-term remission. Blood 2011;118. Abstract 4103.
59. Innes AJ, Beattie R, Sergeant R, et al. Escalating-dose HLA-mismatched DLI is safe for the treatment of leukaemia relapse following alemtuzumab-based myeloablative allo-SCT. Bone Marrow Transplant 2013;48:1324–8.
60. Mackinnon S, Papadopoulos EB, Carabasi MH, et al. Adoptive immunotherapy evaluating escalating doses of donor leukocytes for relapse of chronic myeloid leukemia after bone marrow transplantation: separation of graft-versus-leukemia responses from graft-versus-host disease. Blood 1995;86:1261–8.
61. Dazzi F, Szydlo RM, Craddock C, et al. Comparison of single-dose and escalating-dose regimens of donor lymphocyte infusion for relapse after allografting for chronic myeloid leukemia. Blood 2000;95:67–71.
62. Olavarria E, Ottmann OG, Deininger M, et al. Response to imatinib in patients who relapse after allogeneic stem cell transplantation for chronic myeloid leukemia. Leukemia 2003;17:1707–12.

Transplantation in Chronic Lymphocytic Leukemia

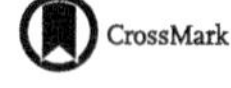

Does It Still Matter in the Era of Novel Targeted Therapies?

Fabienne McClanahan, MD[a,b],
John Gribben, MD, DSc, FRCP, FRCPath, FMedSci[a,*]

KEYWORDS

• Chronic lymphocytic leukemia • Allogeneic hematopoietic stem cell transplantation • Novel substances • High-risk patients • GvL • GvHD

KEY POINTS

- Hematopoietic stem cell transplantation (HSCT) offers the only potentially curative approach to the treatment of chronic lymphocytic leukemia (CLL) but is suitable only for a minority of patients and is associated with significant treatment-related mortality and morbidity.
- Guidelines suggest that HSCT is indicated in fit CLL patients with a suitable matched donor, del17p-/TP53 mutations, or who have relapsed shortly after chemo-immunotherapy (high-risk patients).
- HSCT must always be considered in view of other, potentially less toxic therapies.
- Several new agents demonstrate impressive and durable responses in high-risk patients who might be candidates for transplant.
- The choice of HSCT versus a novel agent is one that must be gauged on a patient-by-patient basis.

INTRODUCTION: HOW THE AVAILABILITY OF IMMUNOCHEMOTHERAPY AND NOVEL SUBSTANCES ARE CHANGING CHRONIC LYMPHOCYTIC LEUKEMIA TREATMENT

Chronic lymphocytic leukemia (CLL) is the most common leukemia in adults in the Western world and is characterized by the progressive accumulation of mature typically CD5-positive B lymphocytes within the blood, bone marrow, and secondary

[a] Centre for Haemato-Oncology, Barts Cancer Institute, Queen Mary University of London, Charterhouse Square, London EC1M6BQ, UK; [b] Division of Molecular Genetics, German Cancer Research Center (DKFZ), Im Neuenheimer Feld 580, Heidelberg 69120, Germany
* Corresponding author.
E-mail address: j.gribben@qmul.ac.uk

Hematol Oncol Clin N Am 28 (2014) 1055–1071
http://dx.doi.org/10.1016/j.hoc.2014.08.005 hemonc.theclinics.com

lymphoid organs.[1–3] Although CLL is mostly an indolent disease, there are subgroups of patients that die within a few years from diagnosis despite intensive therapy. Over the past decade, significant advances in the understanding of the pathogenesis of CLL have led to the development of a range of novel treatment options for patients requiring therapy. In young patients without significant comorbidities, immunochemotherapy with fludarabine, cyclophosphamide, and the anti-CD20 monoclonal antibody (mAb) rituximab (FCR) has been established as the first-line standard-of-care treatment.[4,5] Although this regimen leads to high overall response rates (ORR) and a long progression-free survival (PFS), it is unsuitable for certain subgroups of patients: these include patients with p53 abnormalities who respond poorly to purine-analogue-based immunochemotherapy and relapse often and early,[6–8] and elderly patients with comorbidities unable to tolerate FCR-associated toxicities.[9]

In the latter, chlorambucil is a widely accepted therapeutic option, and the combination with rituximab is generally well tolerated and improves PFS.[10,11] A recently published pivotal phase 3 trial by the German CLL Study Group showed that the type 2 anti-CD20 antibody obinutuzumab was superior to rituximab when each was combined with chlorambucil.[12] Ofatumumab is another fully humanized anti-CD20 mAb that has revealed high efficacy in untreated and relapsed/refractory patients, and even in patients pretreated with rituximab.[13–15] Several recent clinical studies indicate that novel agents interfering with B-cell receptor (BCR) signaling, such as the Bruton's tyrosine kinase (BTK) inhibitor ibrutinib, the PI3kp110δ inhibitor idelalisib, or the BCL2 inhibitor navitoclax, are well tolerated and very active, even for the treatment of relapsed and fludarabine-refractory CLL, and various combinations with immunochemotherapy are currently being tested in registration studies or are under clinical development.[16–22] Although these early results appear very encouraging, it is yet to be seen how they will translate into long-lasting remissions and disease control. In addition, a recent report indicates that patients can become resistant to ibrutinib therapy because of mutations of drug binding sites within the BCR pathway, and similar resistance mechanisms to other substances are likely.[23]

The only curative treatment option in CLL so far is allogeneic hematopoietic stem cell transplantation (HSCT).[24] HSCT takes advantage of the graft-versus-leukemia (GvL) effect mediated by differentiated transplanted effector cells, which are capable of mounting an antitumor immune response and inducing long-lasting clinical remission.[25] However, HSCT is only suitable for a selected group of patients, and the challenges that HSCT has to face in 2014 are the following:

- To identify and predict which patients and specific subgroups of patients benefit most from HSCT, and in which novel substances are unlikely to alter the biological course of their disease
- To recognize the appropriate time point when HSCT should be offered
- To determine if and how HSCT should be best combined with novel therapeutic options.

This review summarizes the current knowledge on HSCT in CLL and critically discusses its role in the era of novel treatment strategies.

THE UNMET NEED OF POOR-RISK CHRONIC LYMPHOCYTIC LEUKEMIA PATIENTS BEFORE THE AVAILABILITY OF NOVEL SUBSTANCES

Although immunochemotherapy has significantly improved the outcome for most CLL patients, there are subgroups of patients who have repeatedly been identified as having a poor response to therapy. The pivotal report by Döhner and colleagues[6] predicted that patients with del17p- typically require therapy within 1 year of diagnosis and have a median overall survival (OS) of just 32 months. This lack of chemosensitivity is biologically explained by the malfunction of the tumor suppressor protein p53, whose gene locus is located on the short arm of chromosome 17.[26] In CLL, deletion of 17p- leads to the inactivation of the TP53 gene; this is often accompanied by inactivating mutations of the second locus of TP53, leading to a complete loss of function.[27,28] Within the pivotal CLL8 trial, which demonstrated the superiority of frontline FCR over fludarabine and cyclophosphamide alone, del17p- was the strongest negative predictive factor for response to therapy and survival, and the clinical responses that were achieved were not durable. Even though there are retrospective data indicating that some patients with del17p- might experience an indolent course despite the mutation,[29] similar unfavorable outcomes have been observed in other prospective trials using combinations of rituximab with bendamustine[30] or fludarabine alone.[31]

Until recently, the only therapy that appeared to be able to overcome the negative impact of p53 abnormalities in the first-line treatment setting, in terms of both its predictive value and its effect on the response to treatment, is the anti-CD52 mAb alemtuzumab and combinations with chlorambucil, high-dose corticosteroids, rituximab, and FCR.[32–37] These approaches, however, are associated with high hematological and nonhematological toxicities and severe infectious complications and are therefore unsuitable for most elderly CLL patients. In the relapsed setting, the management of patients with TP53 abnormalities is even more challenging. Several clinical studies have demonstrated that FCR and combinations with high-dose corticosteroids, alemtuzumab, or alternative regimens consisting of rituximab, oxaliplatin, cytarabine, and fludarabine (OFAR) have only limited and short-term efficacy and are associated with high toxicity rates.[37–43] However, depending on doses and application routes, it also seems feasible that alemtuzumab-based regimens can serve as a means to “bridge” the time to HSCT.

Summary

del17p- and/or p53 abnormalities are negative predictive factors for response to therapy and survival. These abnormalities can be partly overcome by treatment with the anti-CD52 antibody alemtuzumab, alone and in combination, but it comes at the cost of high nonhematological and hematological toxicities.

INDICATION OF TRANSPLANTATION: THE 2007 EUROPEAN SOCIETY OF BLOOD AND MARROW TRANSPLANTATION CONSENSUS CRITERIA AND BEYOND

In line with the experiences from these (immuno)chemotherapy-based clinical trials, the European Society of Blood and Marrow Transplantation (EBMT) transplant consensus from 2007 states that HSCT is a reasonable treatment option in relapsed/fludarabine-refractory patients and patients with p53 abnormalities with indication for treatment.[44] This option is also reflected in the 2008 International Workshop on Chronic Lymphocytic Leukemia (iwCLL) guidelines, which recommend that patients with resistant disease, a short time to progression, and del(17p) should be offered investigative clinical protocols, including HSCT.[45] In a more recently published *Perspective*, 3 risk categories were suggested based on the predicted effectiveness of FCR-like treatment, and the “highest-risk” category included patients in which treatment with FCR is unlikely to yield acceptable response or remission rates or prolong survival.[46] Features of “highest-risk” include TP53 loss/mutation, purine analogue-refractoriness, a very short response to prior FCR, and failure to achieve complete response (CR) after FCR; these patients were considered prime candidates for investigational agents in clinical trials and HSCT. These definitions are summarized in **Table 1**.

Table 1
Patients and subgroups that should be considered for hematopoietic stem cell transplantation

EBMT criteria Dreger et al,[44] 2007	• Relapse within 24 mo after having achieved a response with intensive treatment (purine analogue combinations, autoSCT) • Detection of p53 abnormality and indication for treatment • Fludarabine resistance: nonresponse or early relapse (<12 mo after purine analogue-based therapy)
iwCLL criteria Hallek et al,[45] 2008	• Resistant disease: failure to achieve CR/PR • Relapse within 6 mo of last treatment • Detection of del(17p)-
Highest risk in risk category model Zenz et al,[46] 2012	• Fludarabine refractory CLL • Early relapse (within 24 mo) after FCR (or FCR-like) treatment • *TP53* deletion/mutation and indication for treatment

Abbreviations: CLL, chronic lymphocytic leukemia; CR, complete response; EBMT, european society of blood and marrow transplantation; FCR, fludarabine, cyclophosphamide, rituximab; iwCLL, international workshop on chronic lymphocytic leukemia; PR, partial response.

Summary

Internationally accepted guidelines suggest that HSCT is indicated in patients who are fit enough for this approach, have a suitable matched donor, have 17p deletion or TP53 mutations, or have relapsed relatively quickly after chemo-immunotherapy.

EVIDENCE FOR THE EFFICACY OF HEMATOPOIETIC STEM CELL TRANSPLANTATION IN CHRONIC LYMPHOCYTIC LEUKEMIA

The first myeloablative treatment-based transplantation strategies were developed more than 20 years ago, but were unsuitable for most patients because of their high morbidity and mortality.[47,48] After it was recognized that engraftment and GvL activity can be achieved without preceding myeloablative treatment,[49–51] nonmyeloablative reduced intensity conditioning (RIC) strategies have made HSCT accessible to a larger cohort of CLL patients, including the elderly and those with comorbidities, reflected in the number of RIC-HSCTs in the EBMT registry: according to the 2012 annual activity survey, 3% of all HSCT indications were performed in CLL (n = 475), mostly from unrelated donors, making CLL the most frequent indication for HSCT among lymphomas.[52]

Several large studies have demonstrated that in contrast to other intensive therapies, the relapse incidence after HSCT seems to decrease over time, indicating that RIC HSCT provides long-term disease control in about 40% of patients and also overcomes the negative prognostic effect of p53 abnormalities and fludarabine-refractoriness.[53–61] The results from the largest reported prospective studies are summarized in **Table 2**. The curative potential of HSCT was also confirmed in patients with SF3B1 and NOTCH1 gene mutations,[62] which have been identified as novel recurrent genetic mutations in CLL and are mostly associated with resistance or poor response to conventional treatment.[63–66] A smaller, recently published prospective trial of 40 patients using RIC with fludarabine, total body irradiation, and rituximab demonstrated a positive effect of rituximab on OS and EFS in multivariate analyses.[67]

HSCT seems particularly active in patients with complete or partial disease remission at the time of transplantation: in patients with chemosensitive disease, the 5-year OS could be increased to up to 80%.[53,57,68] To achieve a good remission state is challenging however, and as discussed before, some regimens that seem suitable happen at the cost of high toxicities. Recent studies indicate that modified OFAR

Table 2
Summary of results from the largest reported prospective studies of reduced intensity conditioning hematopoietic stem cell transplantation in chronic lymphocytic leukemia

	Fred Hutchinson Cancer Center	German CLL Study Group	MD Anderson Cancer Center	Dana Farber Cancer Institute
	Sorror et al,[54] 2008	Dreger et al,[53,62] 2010 & 2013	Khouri et al,[56] 2011	Brown et al,[57] 2013
Number of patients	82	90	86	76
Conditioning regimen	Flu/low-dose TBI	Flu/Cy ± ATG	Flu/Cy ± R	Flu/Bu
Donors, % (sibling/MUR)	63/37	41/59	50/50	37/63
Median follow-up, mo	60	72	37	61
Early mortality, % (<100 d)	<10	<3	<3	<3
NRM, %	23	23	17	16
Acute grade 3-4 GvHD, %	20	14	7	17
Severe chronic GvHD, %	53	55	56	48
Median PFS, %	39 (5 y)	38 (6 y)	36 (6 y)	43 (6 y)
Median OS, %	50 (5 y)	58 (6 y)	51 (6 y)	63 (6 y)

Abbreviations: ATG, antithymocyte globulin; Bu, busulfan; Cy, cyclophosphamide; Flu, fludarabine; MUR, matched unrelated donor; R, rituximab; TBI, total body irradiation.

and alemtuzumab-based regimens are the most favorable strategies to help prepare patients for successful HSCT by achieving good remissions.[43,69–71] In general, pretransplant characteristics as assessed by the EBMT risk score seem to be of predictive value for OS: this score uses 5 patient-specific pretransplant variables (age, disease status, time from diagnosis to transplant, donor type, and donor–recipient sex combination).[72] A retrospective EBMT analysis demonstrated that there was a significant difference in OS at 5 years between patients with score 1 to 3 and patients having a higher score and also supported the use of matched unrelated donors as equivalent alternative to HLA-matched sibling donors in CLL.[68]

Summary

RIC HSCT provides long-term disease control in about 40% of patients, including patients with adverse prognostic markers, but remission status at the time of transplantation and pretransplant characteristics are predictive of HSCT outcome.

POSTTRANSPLANTATION MONITORING BY MINIMAL RESIDUAL DISEASE KINETICS AND GRAFT-VERSUS-LEUKEMIA ACTIVITY

The curative effect of HSCT in some patients supports our current understanding of the importance of minimal residual disease (MRD) as a quantification of treatment response. MRD denotes a subclinical disease burden that remains after specific therapy. For CLL, this is defined as a contamination of 5 CLL cells or less per nanoliter of peripheral blood in the absence of clinical signs or symptoms of the disease.[73] Patients showing less than one CLL cell in 10,000 benign leukocytes in peripheral blood or bone marrow are considered MRD-negative.[45] MRD levels have been demonstrated to be an independent predictor of PFS and OS after immunochemotherapy and add significantly to the prognostic power of known pretreatment parameters.[74–76] Recent data indicate that they can potentially also be used to de-escalate treatment based on the MRD depth of response.[77] After HSCT, MRD kinetics rather than levels seem to identify patients that are at risk of clinical relapse, long before clinical signs become apparent.[53,78,79] This is most likely mediated by ongoing GvL activity of donor T lymphocytes and their continuous immunotherapeutic activity, which is highly sensitive to immunomodulation by immune suppression or donor lymphocyte infusions.[80,81]

Summary

After HSCT, MRD kinetics aid in the assessment of response and indicate the level of ongoing GvL-mediated immunotherapeutic activity.

ADVERSE EVENTS AND RISK OF GRAFT-VERSUS-HOST DISEASE IN CHRONIC LYMPHOCYTIC LEUKEMIA

GvL activity in CLL seems to be closely correlated to graft-versus-host disease (GvHD), as patients with chronic GvHD (cGvHD) have a reduced risk of relapse.[57,82] Accordingly, an increased relapse rate was observed when donor T cells were depleted.[55,60,68] However, cGvHD remains a significant problem and is largely responsible for nonrelapse mortality (NRM) rates of up to 23% and affects up to 60% of patients in the large clinical trials summarized in **Table 2**. Apart from its impact on NRM, cGVHD is the major determinant of quality of life after HSCT.[83,84] The clinical symptoms of cGVHD, however, decrease over time in many affected patients, and therapeutic immunosuppression could be terminated after 1 to 2 years in many patients in the trials summarized in **Table 2**.

Other acute side effects of RIC HSCT in the early transplant phase include nausea, mucositis, and infections. Because of substantial improvements of supportive and anti-infective treatments and the availability of dedicated transplant units, these are considerably easier to manage than in the era of myeloablative HSCT, which is reflected in very low early mortality rates of less than 10% in the first 100 days after HSCT (see **Table 2**).

Summary

HSCT is associated with significant treatment-related mortality and morbidity, largely due to chronic GvHD.

MANAGEMENT OF RELAPSE AFTER HEMATOPOIETIC STEM CELL TRANSPLANTATION

Even though HSCT can be curative in up to 40% of patients, a significant proportion still relapses after HSCT. To date, there is no standard treatment or guidelines available for patients who failed HSCT and are unresponsive to post-HSCT immunomodulation-based interventions. In a retrospective analysis of 40 patients from the MD Anderson Cancer Center (MDACC), median time to HSCT failure was 7 months, and the most common salvage treatment regimens were re-treatment with rituximab-based and alemtuzumab-based immunochemotherapy and treatment with thalidomide or lenalidomide and ibrutinib.[85] This treatment led to a median OS from time of progression of 53 months, indicating that post-HSCT relapses are sensitive to salvage therapy. Interestingly, there were no differences between FCR, alemtuzumab, or combination chemotherapy in OS, whereas most patients that received ibrutinib were still alive at the time of last follow-up.

Summary

The clinical management of relapse after HSCT is challenging but seems to be sensitive to immunochemotherapy treatment.

AUTOLOGOUS HEMATOPOIETIC STEM CELL TRANSPLANTATION

Long before the advent of fludarabine or antibody-based strategies, there was realistic hope that myeloablative therapy followed by autologous stem cell transplantation (autoSCT) might be an effective and potentially curative front-line treatment option for suitable patients with CLL. Since then, several prospective trials have demonstrated that autoSCT can prolong EFS and PFS if used as part of early front-line treatment, but fails to improve OS and lacks the potential to overcome the negative impact of biomarkers that confer resistance to chemotherapy or early relapse.[86–89] In addition, it is associated with increased risk of late adverse events such as secondary malignancies.[60,89,90] Therefore, autoSCT currently does not play a role in the treatment of CLL, and patients that have benefited from this approach in the past are also most likely to respond to conventional immunochemotherapy.

Summary

Autologous SCT no longer plays a role in the treatment of CLL.

OUTCOME OF POOR RISK CHRONIC LYMPHOCYTIC LEUKEMIA PATIENTS IN THE ERA OF NOVEL SUBSTANCES AND TREATMENTS

Because of the availability of novel substances and treatment strategies, the standard of care in CLL is changed dramatically. These new approaches include new mAbs, immune modulatory agents, substances interfering with the BCR signaling pathway, and novel cellular therapies. As extensive reviews have been published elsewhere, the impact on patients with high-risk CLL is the focus of this section.[91–93]

Although representing a “passive” immunotherapy, mAbs display enhanced antitumoral activity by engaging the immune system through increased complement-dependent cytotoxicity and antibody-dependent cellular cytotoxicity. Anti-CD20 mAbs are now integral components of CLL therapy,[5,12–15] but the new generation antibody ofatumumab seems to be more effective in refractory patients and in patients pretreated with rituximab, yielding a response rate of almost 60%.[13] Lenalidomide has been demonstrated to have pleiotropic effects on immune cells in both preclinical and clinical studies, primarily by enhancing antitumoral immunity in effector cells.[94–99] Several clinical trials have demonstrated that lenalidomide as a single agent and in combination with rituximab has activity both in untreated and relapsed/refractory CLL and in patients with del17p-, but is associated with nonnegligible toxicities such as tumor flare reaction and increased risk of opportunistic infections.[100–107] The combination of lenalidomide with ofatumumab is currently being investigated in relapsed/refractory CLL.

The most striking results have been observed in recently published prospective trials using the BCR signaling inhibitors ibrutinib and idelalisib: ibrutinib is a BTK inhibitor that primarily blocks BCR associated anti-apoptosis pathways. In addition, it affects BCR-controlled and chemokine-controlled retention and homing of CLL cells in their growth-supporting and survival-supporting lymph node and bone marrow microenvironment.[108–110] In a phase I/II study in 85 heavily pretreated patients with relapsed or refractory CLL, the ORR was 71%, with a PFS of 75% and an OS of

83% at 26 months, and response was independent of del17p-.[16] Toxicities were mild and only a few serious adverse events were observed. Idelalisib is an inhibitor of PI3K110δ, which is also a component of CLL signaling pathways involved in cell survival, clonal expansion, and malignant cells retention in lymphoid tissues.[111,112] In a phase I study conducted on 54 heavily pretreated CLL patients with relapsed/refractory disease, including patients with del17p- (24%), 81% of patients achieved nodal responses with an overall response rate of 72% and a very acceptable safety profile.[20] A phase III trial was then initiated on 220 patients with relapsed CLL receiving idelalisib in combination with rituximab versus rituximab plus placebo.[21] Because of overwhelming efficacy, the study was interrupted after the first interim analysis: the ORR was 81% for the combination therapy versus 13% for rituximab monotherapy, whereas OS at 12 months was 92% versus 80%, and PFS was 93% versus 46%. Multiple ongoing randomized and nonrandomized trials are now investigating combinations of these substances with ofatumumab, rituximab, bendamustine, and other novel agents.

BCL-2 antagonists such as navitoclax and ABT-199 mainly work by triggering apoptosis via targeting the BCL2 family. In a phase I study with 29 patients with relapsed/refractory CLL, lymphocytosis was reduced by more than 50% in 19 of 21 patients with baseline lymphocytosis, and partial response (PR) or stabilization of disease was achieved in almost half of the patients, again including patients with del17p- CLL.[22] Another promising group of agents that have shown efficacy in high-risk CLL patients are cyclin-dependent kinase inhibitors such as flavopiridol. In a recently published phase I study, the combination with cyclophosphamide and rituximab was tolerable and active in high-risk CLL patients without being associated with tumor lysis syndrome, confirming previous findings that flavopiridol can overcome the negative impact of del17p-.[113,114]

However, a recent report indicates that patients can become resistant to ibrutinib therapy because of mutations of drug-binding sites within the BCR pathway, and similar resistance mechanisms to other substances are likely are currently under investigation.[23]

A very exciting new active immunotherapy strategy is chimeric antigen receptor (CAR) T-cell therapy. CAR technology has recently emerged as a novel and promising perspective to specifically target malignant cells with precisely engineered T cells. It uses the single-chain variable fragment from an antibody molecule fused with an internal T-cell signaling domain to form a CAR, which is then transduced into T cells.[115] A major advantage of this approach is that it eliminates MHC restriction, enabling the same CAR to be used for several different patients. In a pivotal report, a heavily pretreated high-risk patient with refractory CLL received autologous T cells that had been modified with CARs directed at CD19, a B-cell surface antigen, resulting in remission induction and lasting tumor control.[116] Since then, several clinical trials have reported impressive results with anti-CD19 CARs, in both CLL and acute lymphoblastic leukemia.[116–120] However, it has also become clear that the success of CAR therapy depends on the inclusion of lymphoreducing conditioning chemotherapy and the choice of CAR design.[116,118,119,121] In addition, CAR T-cell therapy can be associated with severe complications such as cytokine release syndrome, a potentially lethal complication, and lasting normal B-cell depletion.[118,122]

Summary

There are several new agents and immunotherapy approaches that are in clinical trials or recently approved in CLL that demonstrate impressive responses and durable durations of response in high-risk patients who might be candidates for transplant.

DISCUSSION: POTENTIAL FOR THE COMBINATION OF HEMATOPOIETIC STEM CELL TRANSPLANTATION AND NOVEL THERAPIES

Recent clinical trials have taught us that novel agents are efficacious, are very tolerable, and have the ability to abrogate the negative predictive effect of fludarabine-resistance and del17p-. However, similar to targeted treatment of chronic myeloid leukemia with break point cluster region/abelson murine leukemia viral oncogene homolog 1 (BCR/ABL) antagonists, resistance mechanisms are emerging and give reasons for concern about the long-term curative effect of those substances. In addition, one has to keep in mind that most of those agents are only available in clinical trials, or once they are approved come at a very high treatment cost and only in selected countries, which makes them inaccessible for most patients in need. Patient numbers with specific mutations are also still small, and it is therefore uncertain if the observations relating to del17p- patients can be extrapolated to p53 abnormalities (ie, isolated mutations, with/without del17p-), and to other mutations known to confer an adverse prognosis or poor response to treatment. Similarly, the outcome of patients that are relapsing following novel treatments is not known, and one can only speculate how such treatment will influence the biology and chemosensitivity of the relapsed disease.

In the context of CAR therapy, although this is a very promising treatment approach and seems to be highly efficacious in patients that would have otherwise had no further therapeutic option, further studies are needed to fully investigate the clinical use of CAR T-cell therapy and treatment-related toxicities, and its optimal combination with existing treatment approaches. Similarly to novel agents, this is only available in few selected sites and within clinical trials; because of the complexity involved in cell collection, genetic manipulation, application, and clinical management, this is very likely (and desired) to stay in the hand of dedicated specialized CAR manufacturing and treatment centers.

On the other hand, long-term follow-up data from large prospective trials of HSCT reaching almost a decade in a few centers have led to the thought that despite being suitable for only selected subgroups of patients and coming at the cost of rather extensive GvHD and reduction of quality of life, HSCT has curative potential in about half of the patients undergoing this procedure. Although there is no prospective data on whether HSCT can change the natural biological course of high-risk CLL, there are some retrospective data using a donor versus no-donor comparison approach, which indicate that OS was significantly improved in patients with donor.[123] These observations indicate that HSCT does indeed have the potential to correct the natural dismal course of disease of high-risk CLL. However, HSCT should always be restricted to patients meeting the EBMT transplant/highest-risk patient criteria (see **Table 1**) and should never be part of first-line treatment in the general patient population.

As there are no direct comparisons between HSCT and novel agents, general evidence-based recommendations are very difficult to make at this point. Instead, the limitations of each approach need to be understood and the chances and risks of each procedure carefully weighed on a case-by-case basis. In general, the availability of treatments, their expected benefit and side effects, and individual treatment-histories and pretransplant characteristics as determined by the EBMT risk score need to be taken into consideration. With the data that are available up to now, it seems feasible to consider HSCT in highest-risk patients (ie, patients who are relapsed/refractory and exhibit p53 abnormalities or del11q-, are suitable for transplant in terms of age and concomitant diseases, have a well-matched donor, and are willing to undergo this procedure). As the success of HSCT is, however, highly dependent on the remission state of the time of HSCT, it seems very desirable to focus on achieving disease control first. Disease control can be facilitated by novel substances. As they are also well tolerated and show only moderate toxicities, they seem a good option to bridge the time until HSCT, and maybe even to postpone HSCT to a later point in the disease. How these substances should be best combined, if there is the option to completely eliminate the chemotherapy backbone from induction or second-line treatment, and whether they will have an affect on GvL and immunmodulation, are the major focus of ongoing preclinical and clinical studies.

Summary

The judicious choice of which patients merit this approach remains important. HSCT must always be considered in view of other, potentially less toxic therapies that could be offered. The choice of HSCT versus a novel agent is one that must be gauged on a patient-by-patient basis, and this will change as data mature on the use of novel agents in CLL.

REFERENCES

1. Chiorazzi N, Rai KR, Ferrarini M. Chronic lymphocytic leukemia. N Engl J Med 2005;352:804–15.
2. Siegel R, Ma J, Zou Z, et al. Cancer statistics, 2014. CA Cancer J Clin 2014;64: 9–29.
3. Howlader N, Noone AM, Krapcho M, et al, editors. SEER cancer statistics review, 1975-2009 (vintage 2009 populations). Bethesda (MD): National Cancer Institute; 2012. based on November 2011 SEER data submission, posted to the SEER web site. Available at: http://seer.cancer.gov/csr/1975_2009_pops09/.
4. Tam CS, O'Brien S, Wierda W, et al. Long-term results of the fludarabine, cyclophosphamide, and rituximab regimen as initial therapy of chronic lymphocytic leukemia. Blood 2008;112:975–80.
5. Hallek M, Fischer K, Fingerle-Rowson G, et al. Addition of rituximab to fludarabine and cyclophosphamide in patients with chronic lymphocytic leukaemia: a randomised, open-label, phase 3 trial. Lancet 2010;376:1164–74.
6. Döhner H, Stilgenbauer S, Benner A, et al. Genomic aberrations and survival in chronic lymphocytic leukemia. N Engl J Med 2000;343:1910–6.
7. Zenz T, Eichhorst B, Busch R, et al. TP53 mutation and survival in chronic lymphocytic leukemia. J Clin Oncol 2010;28:4473–9.
8. Fink AM, Bottcher S, Ritgen M, et al. Prediction of poor outcome in CLL patients following first-line treatment with fludarabine, cyclophosphamide and rituximab. Leukemia 2013;27:1949–52.
9. Shanafelt T. Treatment of older patients with chronic lymphocytic leukemia: key questions and current answers. Hematology Am Soc Hematol Educ Program 2013;2013:158–67.
10. Hillmen P, Gribben JG, Follows GA, et al. Rituximab plus chlorambucil as first-line treatment for chronic lymphocytic leukemia: final analysis of an open-label phase II study. J Clin Oncol 2014;32:1236–41.
11. Foà R, Del Giudice I, Cuneo A, et al. Chlorambucil plus rituximab with or without maintenance rituximab as first-line treatment for elderly chronic lymphocytic leukemia patients. Am J Hematol 2014;89:480–6.
12. Goede V, Fischer K, Busch R, et al. Obinutuzumab plus chlorambucil in patients with CLL and coexisting conditions. N Engl J Med 2014;370:1101–10.

13. Wierda WG, Kipps TJ, Mayer J, et al. Ofatumumab as single-agent CD20 immunotherapy in fludarabine-refractory chronic lymphocytic leukemia. J Clin Oncol 2010;28:1749–55.
14. Wierda WG, Kipps TJ, Durig J, et al. Chemoimmunotherapy with O-FC in previously untreated patients with chronic lymphocytic leukemia. Blood 2011;117: 6450–8.
15. Wierda WG, Padmanabhan S, Chan GW, et al. Ofatumumab is active in patients with fludarabine-refractory CLL irrespective of prior rituximab: results from the phase 2 international study. Blood 2011;118:5126–9.
16. Byrd JC, Furman RR, Coutre SE, et al. Targeting BTK with ibrutinib in relapsed chronic lymphocytic leukemia. N Engl J Med 2013;369:32–42.
17. Jaglowski SM, Jones JA, Flynn JM, et al. A phase 1b/2 study evaluating activity and tolerability of the BTK inhibitor ibrutinib in combination with ofatumumab in patients with chronic lymphocytic leukemia/small lymphocytic lymphoma (CLL/SLL) and related diseases. ASCO Meeting Abstracts 2014;32:7009.
18. Byrd JC, Brown JR, O'Brien S, et al. Ibrutinib versus ofatumumab in previously treated chronic lymphoid leukemia. N Engl J Med 2014;371:213–23.
19. Burger JA, Keating MJ, Wierda WG, et al. Safety and activity of ibrutinib plus rituximab for patients with high-risk chronic lymphocytic leukaemia: a single-arm, phase 2 study. Lancet Oncol 2014;15(10):1090–9.
20. Brown JR, Byrd JC, Coutre SE, et al. Idelalisib, an inhibitor of phosphatidylinositol 3-kinase p110delta, for relapsed/refractory chronic lymphocytic leukemia. Blood 2014;123:3390–7.
21. Furman RR, Sharman JP, Coutre SE, et al. Idelalisib and rituximab in relapsed chronic lymphocytic leukemia. N Engl J Med 2014;370:997–1007.
22. Roberts AW, Seymour JF, Brown JR, et al. Substantial susceptibility of chronic lymphocytic leukemia to BCL2 inhibition: results of a phase i study of navitoclax in patients with relapsed or refractory disease. J Clin Oncol 2012;30:488–96.
23. Woyach JA, Furman RR, Liu TM, et al. Resistance mechanisms for the Bruton's tyrosine kinase inhibitor ibrutinib. N Engl J Med 2014;370:2286–94.
24. Gribben JG, Riches JC. Immunotherapeutic strategies including transplantation: eradication of disease. Hematology Am Soc Hematol Educ Program 2013;2013:151–7.
25. Kolb HJ. Graft-versus-leukemia effects of transplantation and donor lymphocytes. Blood 2008;112:4371–83.
26. Isobe M, Emanuel BS, Givol D, et al. Localization of gene for human p53 tumour antigen to band 17p13. Nature 1986;320:84–5.
27. Zenz T, Kröber A, Scherer K, et al. Monoallelic TP53 inactivation is associated with poor prognosis in chronic lymphocytic leukemia: results from a detailed genetic characterization with long-term follow-up. Blood 2008;112:3322–9.
28. Dicker F, Herholz H, Schnittger S, et al. The detection of TP53 mutations in chronic lymphocytic leukemia independently predicts rapid disease progression and is highly correlated with a complex aberrant karyotype. Leukemia 2008;23:117–24.
29. Tam CS, Shanafelt TD, Wierda WG, et al. De novo deletion 17p13.1 chronic lymphocytic leukemia shows significant clinical heterogeneity: the M. D. Anderson and Mayo Clinic experience. Blood 2009;114:957–64.
30. Fischer K, Cramer P, Busch R, et al. Bendamustine in combination with rituximab for previously untreated patients with chronic lymphocytic leukemia: a multicenter phase II Trial of the German Chronic Lymphocytic Leukemia Study Group. J Clin Oncol 2012;30:3209–16.

31. Woyach JA, Ruppert AS, Heerema NA, et al. Chemoimmunotherapy with fludarabine and rituximab produces extended overall survival and progression-free survival in chronic lymphocytic leukemia: long-term follow-up of CALGB study 9712. J Clin Oncol 2011;29:1349–55.
32. Hillmen P, Skotnicki AB, Robak T, et al. Alemtuzumab compared with chlorambucil as first-line therapy for chronic lymphocytic leukemia. J Clin Oncol 2007; 25:5616–23.
33. Zent CS, Call TG, Shanafelt TD, et al. Early treatment of high-risk chronic lymphocytic leukemia with alemtuzumab and rituximab. Cancer 2008;113:2110–8.
34. Pettitt AR, Jackson R, Carruthers S, et al. Alemtuzumab in combination with methylprednisolone is a highly effective induction regimen for patients with chronic lymphocytic leukemia and deletion of TP53: final results of the national cancer research institute CLL206 trial. J Clin Oncol 2012;30:1647–55.
35. Parikh SA, Keating MJ, O'Brien S, et al. Frontline chemoimmunotherapy with fludarabine, cyclophosphamide, alemtuzumab, and rituximab for high-risk chronic lymphocytic leukemia. Blood 2011;118:2062–8.
36. Stilgenbauer S, Zenz T, Winkler D, et al. Subcutaneous alemtuzumab in fludarabine-refractory chronic lymphocytic leukemia: clinical results and prognostic marker analyses from the CLL2H study of the German Chronic Lymphocytic Leukemia Study Group. J Clin Oncol 2009;27:3994–4001.
37. Zent CS, Taylor RP, Lindorfer MA, et al. Chemoimmunotherapy for relapsed/refractory and progressive 17p13-deleted chronic lymphocytic leukemia (CLL) combining pentostatin, alemtuzumab, and low-dose rituximab is effective and tolerable and limits loss of CD20 expression by circulating CLL cells. Am J Hematol 2014;89:757–65.
38. Bowen DA, Call TG, Jenkins GD, et al. Methylprednisolone-rituximab is an effective salvage therapy for patients with relapsed chronic lymphocytic leukemia including those with unfavorable cytogenetic features. Leuk Lymphoma 2007; 48:2412–7.
39. Badoux XC, Keating MJ, Wang X, et al. Cyclophosphamide, fludarabine, alemtuzumab, and rituximab as salvage therapy for heavily pretreated patients with chronic lymphocytic leukemia. Blood 2011;118:2085–93.
40. Badoux XC, Keating MJ, Wang X, et al. Fludarabine, cyclophosphamide, and rituximab chemoimmunotherapy is highly effective treatment for relapsed patients with CLL. Blood 2011;117:3016–24.
41. Keating MJ, Flinn I, Jain V, et al. Therapeutic role of alemtuzumab (Campath-1H) in patients who have failed fludarabine: results of a large international study. Blood 2002;99:3554–61.
42. Tsimberidou AM, Wierda WG, Plunkett W, et al. Phase I-II study of oxaliplatin, fludarabine, cytarabine, and rituximab combination therapy in patients with richter's syndrome or fludarabine-refractory chronic lymphocytic leukemia. J Clin Oncol 2008;26:196–203.
43. Brown JR, Messmer B, Werner L, et al. A phase I study of escalated dose subcutaneous alemtuzumab given weekly with rituximab in relapsed chronic lymphocytic leukemia/small lymphocytic lymphoma. Haematologica 2013;98: 964–70.
44. Dreger P, Corradini P, Kimby E, et al. Indications for allogeneic stem cell transplantation in chronic lymphocytic leukemia: the EBMT transplant consensus. Leukemia 2007;21:12–7.
45. Hallek M, Cheson BD, Catovsky D, et al. Guidelines for the diagnosis and treatment of chronic lymphocytic leukemia: a report from the International Workshop

on Chronic Lymphocytic Leukemia updating the National Cancer Institute Working Group 1996 guidelines. Blood 2008;111:5446–56.
46. Zenz T, Gribben JG, Hallek M, et al. Risk categories and refractory CLL in the era of chemoimmunotherapy. Blood 2012;119:4101–7.
47. Rabinowe S, Soiffer R, Gribben J, et al. Autologous and allogeneic bone marrow transplantation for poor prognosis patients with B-cell chronic lymphocytic leukemia. Blood 1993;82:1366–76.
48. Khouri IF, Keating MJ, Vriesendorp HM, et al. Autologous and allogeneic bone marrow transplantation for chronic lymphocytic leukemia: preliminary results. J Clin Oncol 1994;12:748–58.
49. Khouri IF, Keating M, Körbling M, et al. Transplant-lite: induction of graft-versus-malignancy using fludarabine-based nonablative chemotherapy and allogeneic blood progenitor-cell transplantation as treatment for lymphoid malignancies. J Clin Oncol 1998;16:2817–24.
50. Slavin S, Nagler A, Naparstek E, et al. Nonmyeloablative stem cell transplantation and cell therapy as an alternative to conventional bone marrow transplantation with lethal cytoreduction for the treatment of malignant and nonmalignant hematologic diseases. Blood 1998;91:756–63.
51. McSweeney PA, Niederwieser D, Shizuru JA, et al. Hematopoietic cell transplantation in older patients with hematologic malignancies: replacing high-dose cytotoxic therapy with graft-versus-tumor effects. Blood 2001;97:3390–400.
52. Passweg JR, Baldomero H, Peters C, et al. Hematopoietic SCT in Europe: data and trends in 2012 with special consideration of pediatric transplantation. Bone Marrow Transplant 2014;49:744–50.
53. Dreger P, Doehner H, Ritgen M, et al. Allogeneic stem cell transplantation provides durable disease control in poor-risk chronic lymphocytic leukemia: long-term clinical and MRD results of the German CLL Study Group CLL3X trial. Blood 2010;116:2438–47.
54. Sorror ML, Storer BE, Sandmaier BM, et al. Five-year follow-up of patients with advanced chronic lymphocytic leukemia treated with allogeneic hematopoietic cell transplantation after nonmyeloablative conditioning. J Clin Oncol 2008;26:4912–20.
55. Schetelig J, van Biezen A, Brand R, et al. Allogeneic hematopoietic cell transplantation for chronic lymphocytic leukemia with 17p- deletion: a retrospective EBMT analysis. J Clin Oncol 2008;26:5094–100.
56. Khouri IF, Bassett R, Poindexter N, et al. Nonmyeloablative allogeneic stem cell transplantation in relapsed/refractory chronic lymphocytic leukemia: long-term follow-up, prognostic factors, and effect of human leukocyte histocompatibility antigen subtype on outcome. Cancer 2011;117:4679–88.
57. Brown JR, Kim HT, Armand P, et al. Long-term follow-up of reduced-intensity allogeneic stem cell transplantation for chronic lymphocytic leukemia: prognostic model to predict outcome. Leukemia 2013;27:362–9.
58. Moreno C, Villamor N, Colomer D, et al. Allogeneic stem-cell transplantation may overcome the adverse prognosis of unmutated VH gene in patients with chronic lymphocytic leukemia. J Clin Oncol 2005;23:3433–8.
59. Dreger P, Brand R, Hansz J, et al. Treatment-related mortality and graft-versus-leukemia activity after allogeneic stem cell transplantation for chronic lymphocytic leukemia using intensity-reduced conditioning. Leukemia 2003;17:841–8.
60. Gribben JG, Zahrieh D, Stephans K, et al. Autologous and allogeneic stem cell transplantations for poor-risk chronic lymphocytic leukemia. Blood 2005;106:4389–96.

61. Schetelig J, Thiede C, Bornhauser M, et al. Evidence of a graft-versus-leukemia effect in chronic lymphocytic leukemia after reduced-intensity conditioning and allogeneic stem-cell transplantation: the Cooperative German Transplant Study Group. J Clin Oncol 2003;21:2747–53.
62. Dreger P, Schnaiter A, Zenz T, et al. TP53, SF3B1, and NOTCH1 mutations and outcome of allotransplantation for chronic lymphocytic leukemia: six-year follow-up of the GCLLSG CLL3X trial. Blood 2013;121:3284–8.
63. Wang L, Lawrence MS, Wan Y, et al. SF3B1 and other novel cancer genes in chronic lymphocytic leukemia. N Engl J Med 2011;365:2497–506.
64. Quesada V, Conde L, Villamor N, et al. Exome sequencing identifies recurrent mutations of the splicing factor SF3B1 gene in chronic lymphocytic leukemia. Nat Genet 2012;44:47–52.
65. Stilgenbauer S, Schnaiter A, Paschka P, et al. Gene mutations and treatment outcome in chronic lymphocytic leukemia: results from the CLL8 trial. Blood 2014;123:3247–54.
66. Baliakas P, Hadzidimitriou A, Sutton LA, et al. Recurrent mutations refine prognosis in chronic lymphocytic leukemia. Leukemia 2014. [Epub ahead of print].
67. Michallet M, Socié G, Mohty M, et al. Rituximab, fludarabine, and total body irradiation as conditioning regimen before allogeneic hematopoietic stem cell transplantation for advanced chronic lymphocytic leukemia: long-term prospective multicenter study. Exp Hematol 2013;41:127–33.
68. Michallet M, Sobh M, Milligan D, et al. The impact of HLA matching on long-term transplant outcome after allogeneic hematopoietic stem cell transplantation for CLL: a retrospective study from the EBMT registry. Leukemia 2010;24:1725–31.
69. Tsimberidou AM, Wierda WG, Wen S, et al. Phase I-II clinical trial of oxaliplatin, fludarabine, cytarabine, and rituximab therapy in aggressive relapsed/refractory chronic lymphocytic leukemia or Richter syndrome. Clin Lymphoma Myeloma Leuk 2013;13:568–74.
70. Stilgenbauer S, Cymbalista F, Leblond V, et al. Subcutaneous alemtuzumab combined with oral dexamethasone, followed by alemtuzumab maintenance or allo-SCT In CLL with 17p- or refractory to fludarabine - interim analysis of the CLL2O trial of the GCLLSG and FCGCLL/MW. ASH Annual Meeting Abstracts 2010;116:920.
71. Krejci M, Doubek M, Brychtova Y, et al. Fludarabine with cytarabine followed by reduced-intensity conditioning and allogeneic hematopoietic stem cell transplantation in patients with poor-risk chronic lymphocytic leukemia. Ann Hematol 2013;92:249–54.
72. Gratwohl A, Stern M, Brand R, et al. Risk score for outcome after allogeneic hematopoietic stem cell transplantation. Cancer 2009;115:4715–26.
73. Boettcher S, Ritgen M, Dreger P. Allogeneic stem cell transplantation for chronic lymphocytic leukemia: lessons to be learned from minimal residual disease studies. Blood Rev 2011;25:91–6.
74. Moreton P, Kennedy B, Lucas G, et al. Eradication of minimal residual disease in B-cell chronic lymphocytic leukemia after alemtuzumab therapy is associated with prolonged survival. J Clin Oncol 2005;23:2971–9.
75. Boettcher S, Ritgen M, Fischer K, et al. Minimal residual disease quantification is an independent predictor of progression-free and overall survival in chronic lymphocytic leukemia: a multivariate analysis from the randomized GCLLSG CLL8 trial. J Clin Oncol 2012;30:980–8.

76. Santacruz R, Villamor N, Aymerich M, et al. The prognostic impact of minimal residual disease in patients with chronic lymphocytic leukemia requiring first-line therapy. Haematologica 2014;99:873–80.
77. Strati P, Keating MJ, O'Brien SM, et al. Eradication of bone marrow minimal residual disease may prompt early treatment discontinuation in CLL. Blood 2014; 123:3727–32.
78. Farina L, Carniti C, Dodero A, et al. Qualitative and quantitative polymerase chain reaction monitoring of minimal residual disease in relapsed chronic lymphocytic leukemia: early assessment can predict long-term outcome after reduced intensity allogeneic transplantation. Haematologica 2009;94:654–62.
79. Logan AC, Zhang B, Narasimhan B, et al. Minimal residual disease quantification using consensus primers and high-throughput IGH sequencing predicts post-transplant relapse in chronic lymphocytic leukemia. Leukemia 2013;27:1659–65.
80. Richardson SE, Khan I, Rawstron A, et al. Risk-stratified adoptive cellular therapy following allogeneic hematopoietic stem cell transplantation for advanced chronic lymphocytic leukaemia. Br J Haematol 2013;160:640–8.
81. Machaczka M, Johansson JE, Remberger M, et al. Allogeneic hematopoietic stem cell transplant with reduced-intensity conditioning for chronic lymphocytic leukemia in Sweden: does donor T-cell engraftment 3 months after transplant predict survival? Leuk Lymphoma 2012;53:1699–705.
82. Toze CL, Galal A, Barnett MJ, et al. Myeloablative allografting for chronic lymphocytic leukemia: evidence for a potent graft-versus-leukemia effect associated with graft-versus-host disease. Bone Marrow Transplant 2005;36:825–30.
83. Dreger P. The evolving role of stem cell transplantation in chronic lymphocytic leukemia. Hematol Oncol Clin North Am 2013;27:355–69.
84. Pidala J, Kurland B, Chai X, et al. Patient-reported quality of life is associated with severity of chronic graft-versus-host disease as measured by NIH criteria: report on baseline data from the Chronic GVHD Consortium. Blood 2009;117: 4651–7.
85. Benjamini O, Rozovski U, Jain P, et al. Outcome of chronic lymphocytic leukemia (CLL) patients that failed allogeneic stem cell transplantation. Blood ASH Annual Meeting Abstracts 2013;122:2880.
86. Michallet M, Dreger P, Sutton L, et al. Autologous hematopoietic stem cell transplantation in chronic lymphocytic leukemia: results of European intergroup randomized trial comparing autografting versus observation. Blood 2010;117: 1516–21.
87. Sutton L, Chevret S, Tournilhac O, et al. Autologous stem cell transplantation as a first-line treatment strategy for chronic lymphocytic leukemia: a multicenter, randomized, controlled trial from the SFGM-TC and GFLLC. Blood 2011;117: 6109–19.
88. Brion A, Mahe B, Kolb B, et al. Autologous transplantation in CLL patients with B and C Binet stages: final results of the prospective randomized GOELAMS LLC 98 trial. Bone Marrow Transplant 2012;47:542–8.
89. Dreger P, Doehner H, McClanahan F, et al. Early autologous stem cell transplantation for chronic lymphocytic leukemia: long-term follow-up of the German CLL Study Group CLL3 trial. Blood 2012;119:4851–9.
90. Milligan DW, Kochethu G, Dearden C, et al. High incidence of myelodysplasia and secondary leukaemia in the UK Medical Research Council Pilot of autografting in chronic lymphocytic leukaemia. Br J Haematol 2006;133:173–5.
91. Hallek M. Signaling the end of chronic lymphocytic leukemia: new frontline treatment strategies. Blood 2013;122:3723–34.

92. Jones JA, Byrd JC. How will B-cell-receptor-targeted therapies change future CLL therapy? Blood 2014;123:1455–60.
93. Davila M, Bouhassira DG, Park J, et al. Chimeric antigen receptors for the adoptive T cell therapy of hematologic malignancies. Int J Hematol 2014;99:361–71.
94. Ramsay AG, Johnson AJ, Lee AM, et al. Chronic lymphocytic leukemia T cells show impaired immunological synapse formation that can be reversed with an immunomodulating drug. J Clin Invest 2008;118:2427–37.
95. Shanafelt TD, Ramsay AG, Zent CS, et al. Long-term repair of T-cell synapse activity in a phase II trial of chemoimmunotherapy followed by lenalidomide consolidation in previously untreated chronic lymphocytic leukemia (CLL). Blood 2013;121:4137–41.
96. Ramsay AG, Clear AJ, Fatah R, et al. Multiple inhibitory ligands induce impaired T-cell immunologic synapse function in chronic lymphocytic leukemia that can be blocked with lenalidomide: establishing a reversible immune evasion mechanism in human cancer. Blood 2012;120:1412–21.
97. Ramsay AG, Evans R, Kiaii S, et al. Chronic lymphocytic leukemia cells induce defective LFA-1-directed T-cell motility by altering Rho GTPase signaling that is reversible with lenalidomide. Blood 2013;121:2704–14.
98. Aue G, Njuguna N, Tian X, et al. Lenalidomide-induced upregulation of CD80 on tumor cells correlates with T-cell activation, the rapid onset of a cytokine release syndrome and leukemic cell clearance in chronic lymphocytic leukemia. Haematologica 2009;94:1266–73.
99. Lapalombella R, Andritsos L, Liu Q, et al. Lenalidomide treatment promotes CD154 expression on CLL cells and enhances production of antibodies by normal B cells through a PI3-kinase-dependent pathway. Blood 2010;115:2619–29.
100. Chanan-Khan A, Miller KC, Musial L, et al. Clinical efficacy of lenalidomide in patients with relapsed or refractory chronic lymphocytic leukemia: results of a phase II study. J Clin Oncol 2006;24:5343–9.
101. Witzig TE, Wiernik PH, Moore T, et al. Lenalidomide oral monotherapy produces durable responses in relapsed or refractory indolent non-Hodgkin's Lymphoma. J Clin Oncol 2009;27:5404–9.
102. Badoux XC, Keating MJ, Wen S, et al. Phase II study of lenalidomide and rituximab as salvage therapy for patients with relapsed or refractory chronic lymphocytic leukemia. J Clin Oncol 2013;31:584–91.
103. Andritsos LA, Johnson AJ, Lozanski G, et al. Higher doses of lenalidomide are associated with unacceptable toxicity including life-threatening tumor flare in patients with chronic lymphocytic leukemia. J Clin Oncol 2008;26:2519–25.
104. Ferrajoli A, Lee BN, Schlette EJ, et al. Lenalidomide induces complete and partial remissions in patients with relapsed and refractory chronic lymphocytic leukemia. Blood 2008;111:5291–7.
105. Chen CI, Bergsagel PL, Paul H, et al. Single-agent lenalidomide in the treatment of previously untreated chronic lymphocytic leukemia. J Clin Oncol 2011;29:1175–81.
106. Badoux XC, Keating MJ, Wen S, et al. Lenalidomide as initial therapy of elderly patients with chronic lymphocytic leukemia. Blood 2011;118:3489–98.
107. Strati P, Keating MJ, Wierda WG, et al. Lenalidomide induces long-lasting responses in elderly patients with chronic lymphocytic leukemia. Blood 2013;122:734–7.
108. Ponader S, Chen SS, Buggy JJ, et al. The Bruton tyrosine kinase inhibitor PCI-32765 thwarts chronic lymphocytic leukemia cell survival and tissue homing in vitro and in vivo. Blood 2012;119:1182–9.

109. Herman SE, Gordon AL, Hertlein E, et al. Bruton tyrosine kinase represents a promising therapeutic target for treatment of chronic lymphocytic leukemia and is effectively targeted by PCI-32765. Blood 2011;117:6287–96.
110. de Rooij MF, Kuil A, Geest CR, et al. The clinically active BTK inhibitor PCI-32765 targets B-cell receptor- and chemokine-controlled adhesion and migration in chronic lymphocytic leukemia. Blood 2012;119:2590–4.
111. Hoellenriegel J, Meadows SA, Sivina M, et al. The phosphoinositide 3'-kinase delta inhibitor, CAL-101, inhibits B-cell receptor signaling and chemokine networks in chronic lymphocytic leukemia. Blood 2011;118:3603–12.
112. Herman SE, Lapalombella R, Gordon AL, et al. The role of phosphatidylinositol 3-kinase-delta in the immunomodulatory effects of lenalidomide in chronic lymphocytic leukemia. Blood 2011;117:4323–7.
113. Stephens DM, Ruppert AS, Maddocks K, et al. Cyclophosphamide, alvocidib (flavopiridol), and rituximab, a novel feasible chemoimmunotherapy regimen for patients with high-risk chronic lymphocytic leukemia. Leuk Res 2013;37: 1195–9.
114. Woyach JA, Lozanski G, Ruppert AS, et al. Outcome of patients with relapsed or refractory chronic lymphocytic leukemia treated with flavopiridol: impact of genetic features. Leukemia 2012;26:1442–4.
115. June CH, Blazar BR, Riley JL. Engineering lymphocyte subsets: tools, trials and tribulations. Nat Rev Immunol 2009;9:704–16.
116. Porter DL, Levine BL, Kalos M, et al. Chimeric antigen receptor-modified T cells in chronic lymphoid leukemia. N Engl J Med 2011;365:725–33.
117. Kochenderfer JN, Dudley ME, Feldman SA, et al. B-cell depletion and remissions of malignancy along with cytokine-associated toxicity in a clinical trial of anti-CD19 chimeric-antigen-receptor-transduced T cells. Blood 2012;119: 2709–20.
118. Brentjens RJ, Riviere I, Park JH, et al. Safety and persistence of adoptively transferred autologous CD19-targeted T cells in patients with relapsed or chemotherapy refractory B-cell leukemias. Blood 2011;118:4817–28.
119. Kalos M, Levine BL, Porter DL, et al. T cells with chimeric antigen receptors have potent antitumor effects and can establish memory in patients with advanced leukemia. Sci Transl Med 2011;3:95ra73.
120. Grupp SA, Kalos M, Barrett D, et al. Chimeric antigen receptor-modified T cells for acute lymphoid leukemia. N Engl J Med 2013;368:1509–18.
121. Kochenderfer JN, Dudley ME, Carpenter RO, et al. Donor-derived CD19-targeted T cells cause regression of malignancy persisting after allogeneic hematopoietic stem cell transplantation. Blood 2013;122:4129–39.
122. Xu XJ, Tang YM. Cytokine release syndrome in cancer immunotherapy with chimeric antigen receptor engineered T cells. Cancer Lett 2014;343:172–8.
123. Herth I, Dietrich S, Benner A, et al. The impact of allogeneic stem cell transplantation on the natural course of poor-risk chronic lymphocytic leukemia as defined by the EBMT consensus criteria: a retrospective donor versus no donor comparison. Ann Oncol 2014;25:200–6.

Hematopoietic Stem Cell Transplantation for Non-Hodgkin Lymphoma

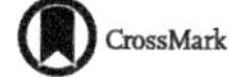

Vijaya Raj Bhatt, MBBS, Julie M. Vose, MD, MBA*

KEYWORDS

- Non-Hodgkin lymphoma • Diffuse large B-cell lymphoma • Follicular lymphoma
- Mantle cell lymphoma • Peripheral T-cell lymphoma
- Autologous hematopoietic stem cell transplantation
- Allogeneic hematopoietic stem cell transplantation

KEY POINTS

- Autologous stem cell transplantation can improve survival in primary refractory or relapsed aggressive B-cell lymphoma and mantle cell lymphoma as well as in relapsed follicular or peripheral T-cell lymphoma.
- Autologous stem cell transplantation in first remission in selected patients with high-risk aggressive B-cell lymphoma, mantle cell lymphoma, and peripheral T-cell lymphoma is associated with improved progression-free survival.
- Allogeneic stem cell transplantation offers a lower relapse rate but a higher nonrelapse mortality resulting in overall survival similar to autologous stem cell transplantation.
- Allogeneic stem cell transplantation can be considered in select patients who fail induction therapy, autologous stem cell transplantation, or are ineligible for autologous transplant.

INTRODUCTION

With the lifetime probability of developing non-Hodgkin lymphoma (NHL) of approximately 2%, NHL is a leading cause of cancer with an estimated 70,800 new diagnoses in the United States in 2014. Although the 5-year survival of NHL has improved from 47% (1975–1977) to 71% (2003–2009) in the last 3 decades, NHL is estimated to account for 18,990 deaths in the United States in 2014.[1] This finding highlights a need for an improvement in up-front and salvage therapy for NHL. Hematopoietic stem cell transplantation (SCT) is a therapeutic option, which may offer a survival benefit to select patients, as described later.

Conflict of interest: The authors have nothing to disclose.
Division of Hematology-Oncology, Department of Internal Medicine, University of Nebraska Medical Center, 987680 Nebraska Medical Center, Omaha, NE 68198-7680, USA
* Corresponding author.
E-mail address: jmvose@unmc.edu

Hematol Oncol Clin N Am 28 (2014) 1073–1095
http://dx.doi.org/10.1016/j.hoc.2014.08.015 hemonc.theclinics.com
0889-8588/14/$ – see front matter

PATIENT EVALUATION OVERVIEW

A multidisciplinary approach to patient selection may reduce transplant-related mortality (TRM) and morbidity (**Table 1**). Hematopoietic cell transplantation comorbidity index (HCT CI) predicts nonrelapse mortality (NRM) and survival in allogeneic SCT (alloSCT) for hematologic malignancy[2] as well as autologous SCT (autoSCT) for lymphoma.[3] HCT CI is more sensitive and has a better survival prediction than the Charlson Comorbidity Index. Additionally, elevated lactate dehydrogenase (LDH) and the absence of chemosensitivity also predict higher NRM.[2,3] Patients who are older than 60 years are frequently not considered good candidates for myeloablative alloSCT but may be eligible for nonmyeloablative alloSCT. The presence of human immunodeficiency virus (HIV) or hepatitis B or C does not preclude autoSCT but may require further evaluation and close monitoring. The role of alloSCT in patients with HIV is currently not established.

INDICATIONS OF TRANSPLANTATION

High-risk aggressive B-cell lymphoma, mantle cell lymphoma (MCL), relapsed or refractory B-cell lymphoma, and peripheral T-cell lymphoma (TCL) have poor overall survival (OS) with conventional chemotherapy and are candidates for high-dose chemotherapy (HDT) followed by autoSCT or alloSCT (**Fig. 1**, **Table 2**).

TRANSPLANTATION IN AGGRESSIVE NON-HODGKIN LYMPHOMA

Diffuse large B-cell lymphoma (DLBCL) consisting of approximately one-third of all NHL is the most common aggressive NHL.[4] It can arise de novo or as a transformation of indolent lymphoma, such as follicular lymphoma (FL).[5] Although rituximab-based immunochemotherapy has improved OS in DLBCL, high-intermediate–risk or high-risk disease is associated with a 4-year OS of 49% to 59%.[6] SCT has been extensively investigated in both up-front and salvage settings.

Up-front Autologous Stem Cell Transplantation for Aggressive Non-Hodgkin Lymphoma

Several trials have failed to show an OS benefit with up-front HDT/autoSCT in DLBCL or other aggressive NHL. A meta-analysis of 15 randomized controlled trials (n = 3079) highlighted a similar TRM ($P = .14$) and higher complete remission rate ($P = .004$) but no improvement in event-free survival (EFS) ($P = .31$) or OS ($P = .58$) with HDT/autoSCT,

Table 1
Patient evaluation for hematopoietic SCT for NHL

Rational	Evaluation
Restaging of NHL	CT or PET scan, bone marrow and lymph node biopsies
Risk assessment for TRM	Performance status, nutritional and psychosocial status, viral serologies (particularly for alloSCT), cardiopulmonary, renal and liver function tests
Key eligibility criteria	Karnofsky performance score ≥70%, ejection fraction ≥40%, DLCO ≥50%, and serum creatinine clearance of ≥50 mL/min for autoSCT; also serum total bilirubin <2 times the upper limit of normal for alloSCT

Abbreviations: alloSCT, allogeneic stem cell transplantation; autoSCT, autologous stem cell transplantation; CT, computed tomography; DLCO, diffusion capacity for carbon monoxide corrected for hemoglobin; PET, positron emission tomography.

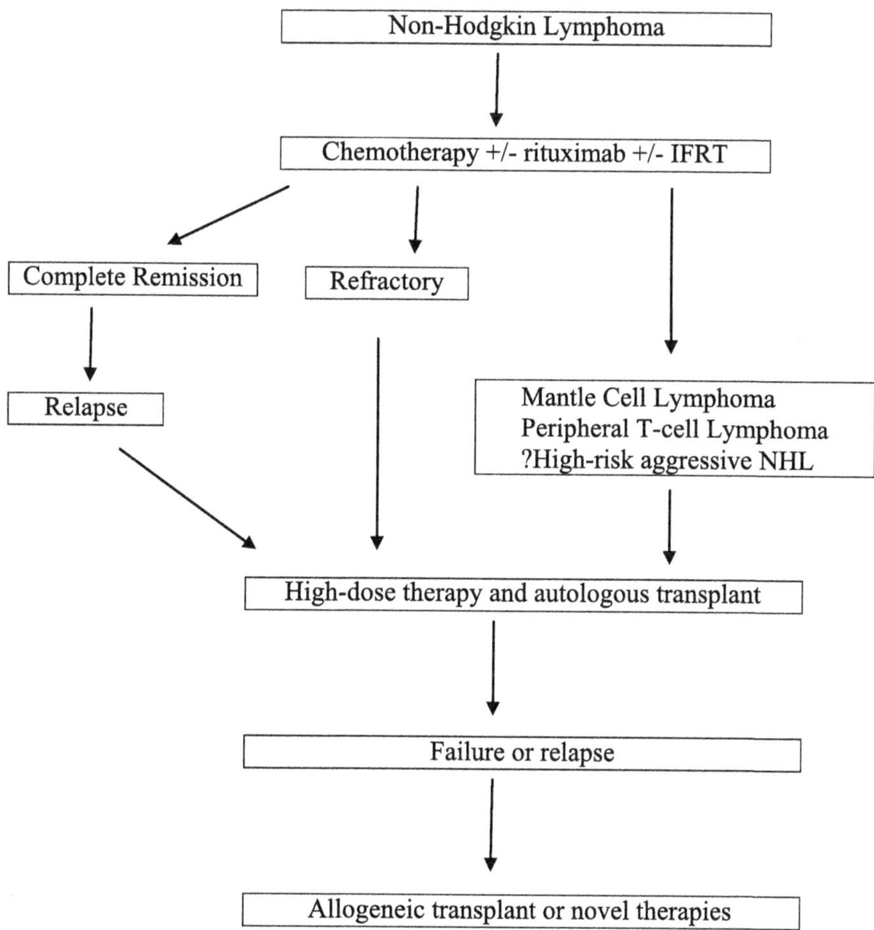

Fig. 1. Algorithm for management of NHL outside of a trial. IFRT, involved field radiation.

compared with conventional chemotherapy, in aggressive NHL.[7] Therefore, up-front autoSCT is not indicated in an unselected population of aggressive NHL. High-intermediate–risk or high-risk DLBCL is associated with an EFS of approximately 50% at 3 to 4 years.[6,8] Hence, several studies have explored the possibility of a survival increment with up-front HDT/autoSCT in this subgroup of patients. In one of the first trials, LNH-87, up-front autoSCT in aggressive lymphomas offered no OS benefit; however, a retrospective subgroup analysis showed improved progression-free survival (PFS) and OS in high-intermediate–risk and high-risk patients.[9] A recently reported multicenter Southwest Oncology Group trial 9704 randomized high-intermediate–risk or high-risk aggressive NHL to one additional cycle of chemotherapy, followed by autoSCT (n = 125) or 3 additional cycles of chemotherapy (n = 128). Eligible patients had received and responded to 5 cycles of cyclophosphamide, doxorubicin, vincristine and prednisone (CHOP) or CHOP-rituximab (CHOP-R). Grade 3 to 4 toxicities were significantly higher with autoSCT. At 2 years, there was an improvement in PFS (69% vs 55%, *P* = .005) but no difference in OS (74% vs 71%, *P* = .30) with autoSCT compared with chemotherapy. A higher success rate of salvage therapy in patients, who relapsed after initial chemotherapy, explains the lack of OS advantage. A subset analysis showed

Table 2
Indication for hematopoietic SCT for NHL outside of a clinical trial

Lymphoma Type	Indication for AutoSCT	Indication for AlloSCT
Diffuse large B-cell lymphoma	• Primary induction failure • Relapsed disease • High-risk CR1/PR1	• Failure of autoSCT • Primary induction failure • Relapsed with persistent bone marrow disease
Follicular/indolent lymphoma	• Relapsed diseased	• Primary induction failure • Second or higher CR/PR
MCL	• Primary induction failure • Relapsed diseased • CR1/PR1	• Relapsed diseased • CR1/PR1
Peripheral TCL	• Relapsed diseased • CR1/PR1	• Primary induction failure • CR1/PR1
Burkitt	• Relapsed diseased • CR1/PR1	• Primary induction failure • Relapsed diseased • CR1/PR1

For nonmyeloablative alloSCT, there should be no evidence of bulky disease or greater than 30% bone marrow involvement.

Abbreviations: CR, complete remission; PR, partial remission.

improved OS with autoSCT for the high-international prognostic index (IPI) group (82% vs 64%, $P = .01$).[10] Several prior trials, with important differences in their designs, have not shown an OS advantage with HDT/autoSCT in high-risk disease.[11–13] Improved risk stratification based on the cell of origin, the presence of double-hit rearrangement or gray-zone lymphomas, and interim positron emission tomography (PET) positivity may enhance patient selection in addition to IPI for future trials.[14] Conversely, improvement in up-front therapy may reduce the benefit of consolidation HDT/autoSCT.

Autologous Stem Cell Transplantation for Refractory or Relapsed Aggressive Non-Hodgkin Lymphoma

Approximately 10% to 15% of patients are refractory to primary rituximab-based therapy or progress soon afterward. An additional one-third of patients relapse within 2 to 3 years after the initial therapy.[15,16] Outcomes are generally poor in these patients with chemotherapy alone. Patients who respond to salvage therapy have chemosensitive disease and are taken to HDT/autoSCT if they are transplant candidates (**Table 3**).[17–19,24]

AutoSCT in patients with primary refractory NHL have worse outcomes than relapsed patients who had previously achieved complete remission.[24] However, select patients with primary refractory disease still benefit from autoSCT.[18,19] An Autologous Blood and Marrow Transplant Registry study among primary refractory diffuse aggressive NHL (n = 184) treated with HDT/autoSCT demonstrated a complete remission rate of 44% as well as 5-year PFS and OS of 31% and 37%, respectively. Adverse prognostic factors included chemotherapy resistance, a Karnofsky performance status score less than 80 at autoSCT, 55 years of age or older at autoSCT, history of 3 or more prior chemotherapy regimens, and no delivery of involved-field radiation therapy (IFRT) before or after autoSCT.[18] In another study among primary refractory aggressive NHL (n = 85), autoSCT resulted in 3-year EFS and OS of 44% and 52%, respectively. An extranodal site of disease greater than 1 and a second-line age-adjusted IPI of 3 to 4 predicted poor outcomes.[19] Thus, autoSCT should be considered in select transplant-eligible primary refractory patients who have chemosensitive disease to salvage therapy.

Table 3
AutoSCT in relapsed or refractory diffuse large B-cell lymphoma

Author,[Ref.] Year	N	Characteristics	Salvage Therapy	OS
Philip et al,[17] 1995	215	Relapsed	Chemotherapy vs HDT/autoSCT	53% vs 32% at 5 y
Vose et al,[18] 2001	184	Induction failure	Various before HDT/autoSCT	37% at 5 y
Kewalramani et al,[19] 2000	85	Induction failure	ICE before HDT/autoSCT	52% at 3 y among patients who underwent transplant
Kewalramani et al,[20] 2004	36	Refractory or relapsed	RICE before HDT/autoSCT	67% at 2 y among patients who underwent transplant
Khouri et al,[21] 2005	67	Relapsed	High-dose R plus chemotherapy before HDT/autoSCT	80% at 2 y
Vose et al,[22] 2004	429	First relapse vs second complete remission	Various or none before HDT/autoSCT	38% vs 55% at 3 y
Gisselbrecht et al,[23] 2010	396	Refractory or relapsed	RICE vs RDHAP before HDT/autoSCT	47% vs 51% (P = .4) at 3 y

Abbreviations: ICE, ifosfamide, etoposide, and carboplatin; R, rituximab; RDHAP, rituximab, dexamethasone, high-dose cytarabine, and cisplatin; RICE, rituximab, ifosfamide, etoposide, and carboplatin.

Several studies have established the benefit of autoSCT in relapsed aggressive NHL, which is the current standard in transplant-eligible patients.[17,23] The PARMA trial of relapsed NHL (n = 215) randomized chemosensitive patients treated with 2 cycles of conventional chemotherapy to radiation and HDT/autoSCT (n = 55) versus 4 cycles of chemotherapy and radiation (n = 54). The response rates (84% vs 44%), 5-year EFS (46% vs 12%), and 5-year OS (53% vs 32%) were significantly higher in the autoSCT group.[17] The Collaborative Trial in Relapsed Aggressive Lymphoma (CORAL) trial compared 2 salvage regimens before autoSCT for CD20+ DLBCL in first relapse or primary refractory disease (n = 396). There was no significant difference in response rates after 3 cycles of chemotherapy (63% vs 62%), 3-year PFS (31% vs 42%, P = .4), and OS (47% vs 51%, P = .4) for the rituximab, ifosfamide, etoposide, and carboplatin (RICE) and the rituximab, dexamethasone, high-dose cytarabine, and cisplatin (RDHAP) arms, respectively. Prognostic factors included refractory disease or early relapse within 12 months after diagnosis, high IPI, and prior rituximab use. Patients with an early relapse after rituximab-based therapy had a poor prognosis, whereas prior rituximab use did not affect EFS in patients who relapsed greater than 12 months after the diagnosis.[23] A subsequent analysis of the CORAL trial assessed the impact of the cell of origin (by Hans algorithm) on the outcomes of salvage therapy and autoSCT. Among the patients treated with RDHAP, the 3-year PFS (52% vs 32%, P = .01) and OS (61% vs 45%) were higher for the germinal center B-cell (GCB) type compared with non-GCB DLBCL. However, the 3-year PFS (31% vs 27%, P = .81) and OS (50% vs 49%) did not differ for GCB and non-GCB DLBCL treated with RICE therapy. The prognostic relevance of the cell of origin was maintained in a multivariate analysis. This study suggests that RDHAP may be a better salvage regimen for patients with relapsed/refractory GCB DLBCL who are fit to tolerate this therapy.[25] In 2 studies using salvage chemotherapy followed by HDT/ASCT, the cell of origin of relapsed or refractory DLBCL, as determined by immunohistochemistry, did not predict outcomes.[26,27] The prognostic role of the cell of origin is debated in the setting of HDT/autoSCT; however, the authors' current approach is to offer RDHAP as a preferred salvage therapy to young and fit patients with GCB DLBCL.

Improving the Outcomes of Autologous Stem Cell Transplantation

Several strategies including radioimmunotherapy, radiotherapy, and rituximab have been investigated to improve the outcomes of autoSCT. Multiple phase I and II trials have evaluated the role of radioimmunotherapy (^{131}I-tositumomab or ^{90}Y-ibritumomab tiuxetan) with HDT before autoSCT and shown promising results.[28–33] A subsequent phase III Blood and Marrow Transplant Clinical Trials Network (BMT CTN) 0401 trial compared rituximab–carmustine, etoposide, cytarabine, and melphalan (BEAM) and ^{131}I-tositumomab–BEAM in chemosensitive persistent or relapsed DLBCL (n = 224). The results showed no difference in the 2-year PFS (48% vs 47%, *P* = .94) and OS (65% vs 61%, *P* = .38) between the two groups.[34] The use of radioimmunotherapy, therefore, cannot be recommended outside of a clinical trial.

The role of IFRT before autoSCT was addressed by a retrospective study among 164 patients with relapsed or refractory DLBCL. IFRT (30 Gy as 1.5-Gy fractions twice daily) was delivered to involved sites greater than 5 cm or areas with residual disease greater than 2 cm. The addition of IFRT was associated with low local relapse and minimal TRM and morbidity.[35] The delivery of IFRT before or after autoSCT has been shown to be prognostic among primary refractory patients treated with autoSCT.[19] IFRT should be used before or after autoSCT in patients with bulky or residual disease.

Among patients without prior rituximab exposure, rituximab use during salvage therapy before HDT/autoSCT may improve PFS and OS.[36] Additionally, rituximab use with HDT before autoSCT has been demonstrated to improve outcomes in high-risk treatment-naïve aggressive NHL as well as in relapsed/refractory settings; however, in these studies, first-line chemotherapy did not include rituximab, thus, limiting the applicability of these studies in the rituximab era.[37–39] Rituximab maintenance after autoSCT has shown conflicting results[21,40] and remains investigational.

Predicting the Outcomes of Autologous Stem Cell Transplantation

Various clinical factors, such as age-adjusted IPI,[19,23,40,41] an extranodal site of disease greater than 1,[19] increased LDH at diagnosis,[22] older age,[18,22] and poor performance status[18] predict poor outcomes. Primary refractory disease,[23,24] refractory relapse,[18,22] and disease relapse within 12 months of the diagnosis[22,23,40] are important predictors of poor outcomes. A history of 3 or more prior chemotherapy regimens has also been shown to correlate with poor outcomes.[18] Hence, transplant-eligible patients should undergo HDT/autoSCT in the first relapse. In addition to the clinical factors, retrospective studies have shown better outcomes in patients with a negative PET scan before autoSCT.[42–44] In one study, however, there was no difference in EFS among patients with a negative pre-autoSCT and post-autoSCT PET scan compared with patients with a positive pre-autoSCT but negative post-autoSCT PET scan. The author concluded that HDT/autoSCT can improve the poor prognosis conferred by positive pre-autoSCT PET in select patients who attain a negative PET status after autoSCT.[44] Although a positive pre-autoSCT PET scan may be prognostic, whether a positive PET should change the management remains unanswered.

Allogeneic Stem Cell Transplantation for Diffuse Large B-Cell lymphoma

Patients with DLBCL who fail multiple chemotherapies or autoSCT have poor outcomes, with a median OS of approximately 10 months in the rituximab era.[45] These patients may be candidates for alloSCT. A Center for International Blood and Marrow Transplant Research (CIBMTR) study compared the outcomes of first autoSCT (n = 837) or matched sibling myeloablative alloSCT (n = 79) performed between 1995 and 2003 in patients with DLBCL who were older than 18 years. AlloSCT recipients, compared with autoSCT recipients, were more likely to have a higher stage (stage III/IV disease 80% vs 66%), marrow involvement at diagnosis (42% vs 17%), more prior chemotherapy regimens (≥3 prior regimens 51% vs 41%), and resistant disease (42% vs 15%). The risk of grades 2 to 4 acute graft-versus-host disease (GVHD) at 100 days of alloSCT was 42%, whereas the risk of chronic GVHD at 5 years was 26%. At 5 years, the risk of TRM (45% vs 18%) was higher and progression or relapse (33% vs 40%) was lower with alloSCT compared with autoSCT. The 5-year PFS and OS with alloSCT, compared with autoSCT, were 22% versus 43% and 22% versus 49%, respectively. In this retrospective analysis, the high TRM offset the lower disease progression or relapse with alloSCT. Nonetheless, alloSCT can result in meaningful 5-year OS in high-risk patients, including heavily pretreated and chemoresistant patients.[46]

A European Bone Marrow Transplantation Registry (EBMTR) study assessed the outcomes of matched-related donor or matched-unrelated donor (MUD) alloSCT with a myeloablative conditioning regimen (n = 37) or reduced intensity conditioning (RIC) (n = 64) for DLBCL relapsed after autoSCT. The 3-year NRM, relapse rate, PFS, and OS were 28%, 30%, 41%, and 53%, respectively. NRM was significantly higher for patients older than 45 years and for those with an early relapse (<12 months) after autoSCT. The relapse rate was higher in refractory patients; PFS was lower among early relapsers (<12 months) after autoSCT. Thus, alloSCT is a therapeutic option after failure of autoSCT particularly among younger patients with a long remission after autoSCT.[47]

Another CIBMTR study among refractory or relapsed DLBCL treated with myeloablative (n = 165), RIC (n = 143) and nonmyeloablative (n = 88) conditioning before alloSCT demonstrated a higher 5-year NRM (56% vs 47% vs 36%, $P = .007$), lower 5-year relapse/progression (26% vs 38% vs 40%, $P = .031$), and similar 5-year PFS (15%–25%) and OS (18%–26%) with myeloablative compared with RIC and nonmyeloablative conditioning. NRM was lower with nonmyeloablative conditioning and more recent transplant year and higher with lower Karnofsky performance status (<90), prior relapse-resistant disease, and use of MUD. Nonmyeloablative conditioning, no prior use of rituximab, and prior relapse-resistant disease were associated with a higher rate of relapse/progression.[48] Taken together, these studies indicate that alloSCT is associated with higher TRM but lower relapse rates than autoSCT. AlloSCT is a viable option in young patients with relapsed DLBCL, including those who have failed autoSCT. The outcomes are better among patients with good performance status, young age, chemosensitive disease, and who relapse greater than 12 months after autoSCT. RIC or nonmyeloablative conditioning may reduce NRM, possibly expanding its utilization to older patients.

TRANSPLANTATION IN INDOLENT AND FOLLICULAR LYMPHOMAS

FL, composing approximately 22% of all NHL,[49] is the most frequent indolent lymphoma.[4] Despite achieving complete remission with initial therapy, patients with FL have frequent relapses and are frequently incurable with conventional therapy. In one study, approximately 10% of the patients with FL were primary refractory to first-line rituximab-based therapy and an additional one-third relapsed within 3 years.[50] SCT has been attempted in both up-front and relapse settings to improve survival.

Up-front Autologous Stem Cell Transplantation for Follicular Lymphomas

Several studies have shown an improved PFS with consolidating autoSCT in first remission. In the German Low Grade Lymphoma Study Group (GLSG) trial, patients with advanced FL (n = 240) received CHOP-like induction therapy and then were randomized to autoSCT or interferon-α maintenance until disease progression. The 5-year PFS was significantly higher (64% vs 33%, $P<.0001$) in the autoSCT group; the relatively short follow-up precluded the determination of OS.[51] In the French Groupe Ouest-Est d'Etude des Leucémies et Autres Maladies du Sang (GOELAMS) study, patients with advanced FL (n = 172) were randomized to immunochemotherapy or HDT/autoSCT with an ex vivo purged graft. AutoSCT resulted in a higher response rate (81% vs 69%, $P = .045$) and 5-year EFS (60% vs 48%, $P = .05$) but similar 5-year OS (84% vs 78%, $P = .49$). The lack of OS advantage was related to an 18% risk of secondary malignancies within 5 years after autoSCT.[52] A longer follow-up of the study showed a plateau in PFS 7 years after HDT/autoSCT, suggesting the possibility of cure in a subgroup of patients; however, the 9-year OS remained similar in the two groups.[53] In the Groupe d'Etude des Lymphomes de l'Adulte (GELA) trial, patients with advanced FL (n = 401) were randomized to CHOP-like chemotherapy with or without autoSCT. AutoSCT, compared with chemotherapy alone, did not improve 7-year EFS (38% vs 28%, $P = .11$) or OS (76% vs 71%, $P = .53$).[54] These studies from the prerituximab era indicate a possible improvement in PFS with autoSCT; however, the results are less relevant in the rituximab era.

In the Gruppo Italiano Trapianto di Midollo Osseo (GITMO) trial, high-risk patients with FL (n = 134) were randomized to R-CHOP versus rituximab-supplemented HDT/autoSCT. AutoSCT, compared with chemotherapy, resulted in a higher complete remission rate (85% vs 62%, $P<.001$) and 4-year EFS (61% vs 28%, $P<.001$) but similar OS (81% vs 80%, $P = .96$). Molecular remission, more commonly seen with autoSCT, was the strongest predictor of outcomes. Seventy-one percent of patients who relapsed after R-CHOP received HDT/ASCT, which resulted in a complete remission rate of 85% and a 3-year EFS of 68%.[55] Given these results and the possibility of secondary malignancies,[52] in the rituximab era, HDT/autoSCT may be best used in the relapsed setting in FL.

Autologous Stem Cell Transplantation for Refractory or Relapsed Follicular Lymphomas

AutoSCT has been associated with excellent OS in patients with relapsed FL (**Table 4**).[56–58] In the randomized European CUP trial among patients with relapsed FL (n = 140), the 2-year PFS and 4-year OS were significantly higher with unpurged (58% and 71%) or purged (55% and 77%) autoSCT compared with CHOP chemotherapy alone (26% and 46%); however, there was no benefit with purging.[56] In another study, the survival advantage with autoSCT was observed regardless of the frontline rituximab exposure.[57] In a study done at the University of Nebraska Medical Center, a histologic grade of FL 3, a high-risk FLIPI score at the time of autoSCT, and prior exposure to 3 or more chemotherapy regimens predicted worse OS and PFS. The use of a conditioning regimen incorporating monoclonal antibody decreased the risk of progressive FL. Thus, SCT earlier in the disease course and the use of a monoclonal antibody-based conditioning regimen may improve outcomes.[58] An EBMTR study demonstrated that an age of 45 years and older,

Table 4
AutoSCT in relapsed or refractory FL

Author,[Ref.] Year	N	Characteristics	Salvage Therapy	OS
Schouten et al,[56] 2003	140	Relapsed	Conventional chemotherapy vs HDT/autoSCT	46% vs 70+%[a] at 4 y
Le Gouill et al,[57] 2011	175	Relapsed or refractory after rituximab-based induction	Conventional chemotherapy vs HDT/autoSCT	92% vs 63% at 3 y
Vose et al,[58] 2008	248	Relapsed or refractory	HDT/autoSCT	63% at 5 y
Montoto et al,[59] 2007	693	First remission, relapsed or refractory	HDT/autoSCT	52% at 10 y
Evens et al,[60] 2013	135	Relapsed or refractory after rituximab-based induction	HDT/autoSCT	87% at 3 y

[a] 70+%=71% and 77% for unpurged and purged HDT/autoSCT respectively.

chemoresistant disease, and total body irradiation (TBI)-containing regimens are predictive of shorter OS. The 5-year NRM was 9%, which was higher among patients aged 45 years and older, refractory disease, and TBI-containing regimens. At a median of 7 years, 9% developed a second malignancy, including secondary myeloid neoplasms (5.7%), mainly in patients who had received TBI. A plateau in the PFS curve was seen with a long follow-up, suggesting a possibility of cure in a subset of patients.[59] Thus, HDT/autoSCT improves outcomes in patients with relapsed FL; young patients with chemosensitive disease should undergo HDT/autoSCT in second remission following the use of a non-TBI monoclonal antibody-based conditioning regimen.

Improving the Outcomes of Autologous Stem Cell Transplantation

Two commonly used techniques to improve the outcomes of autoSCT in FL include graft purging[61,62] and the use of rituximab therapy.[63–66] The achievement of molecular remission and long-term complete remission with graft purging are encouraging; however, a high incidence of secondary malignancy[61] and the lack of benefit with purging in the European CUP trial[56] mandates further exploration of its utility.

Rituximab has been successfully used before and after autoSCT to improve outcomes.[63–65] In a prospective single-arm study of patients with relapsed FL (n = 23), in vivo rituximab graft purging and post-autoSCT rituximab maintenance resulted in a time to progression, which was greater than the last prior therapy. Molecular remission after autoSCT correlated with a prolonged PFS.[65] Rituximab has also been successfully used for control of clinically or molecularly detectable residual disease after autoSCT in patients with FL with minimal residual disease.[66] Thus, rituximab may be useful for the prolongation of response after autoSCT.

Predicting the Outcomes of Autologous Stem Cell Transplantation

Several factors, such as a histologic grade of FL 3, a high-risk FLIPI score at autoSCT,[58] age of 45 years or older,[59] poor performance status ($\geq$2 vs <2), multiple nodal involvement (>4 vs $\leq$4),[67] prior exposure to 3 or more chemotherapy regimens,[58] chemoresistant disease, and the use of TBI-containing regimens,[59] have been shown to predict poor OS. Molecular remission after HDT/autoSCT may also predict prolonged disease-free survival (DFS).[68]

Allogeneic Stem Cell Transplantation for Follicular Lymphomas

AlloSCT is associated with high TRM; therefore, it is reserved for multiply relapsed patients, primary refractory disease, or after failure of autoSCT. In an International Bone Marrow Transplant Registry/Autologous Blood and Marrow Transplant Registry study of patients with FL undergoing SCT (n = 904), the 5-year OS was 51%, 62%, and 55%, after alloSCT, purged ASCT, and unpurged autoSCT. AlloSCT, compared with autoSCT, resulted in higher 5-year TRM (30% vs 8%–14%) and a lower 5-year relapse risk (21% vs 43%–58%). Purged autoSCT resulted in 26% lower 5-year relapse risk (43% vs 58%) compared with unpurged autoSCT. Graft purging was associated with improved OS. Age greater than 40 years, prolonged time interval from diagnosis to SCT (>1 year), chemoresistant disease, elevated LDH, poor performance status, SCT late in the disease course (after first or second remission or first relapse), and year of SCT (1990–1993 vs more recent) predicted poor OS. Additionally, bone marrow involvement at SCT predicted a higher risk of relapse, whereas a TBI-containing regimen predicted higher TRM and lower recurrence. There was no correlation between GVHD and recurrence.[69] High TRM associated with myeloablative alloSCT has led to the exploration of RIC alloSCT.

A BMT CTN multicenter trial (n = 30) comparing the outcomes of autoSCT versus RIC alloSCT within relapsed chemosensitive FL was closed early because of slow accrual but demonstrated a 3-year PFS and OS of 63% and 73% in autoSCT and 86% and 100% in RIC alloSCT.[70] In a CIBMTR study of FL (n = 208), RIC alloSCT, compared with myeloablative alloSCT, resulted in similar 3-year PFS (55% vs 67%, *P* = .07) and OS (62% vs 71%, *P* = .15). Lower performance status and chemoresistant disease, but not conditioning regimen, was associated with higher TRM and lower OS and PFS. Multivariate analysis revealed a nearly 3-fold increased risk of disease progression after RIC alloSCT.[71] Whether RIC alloSCT, compared with myeloablative alloSCT, improves outcomes in FL is not established; but the outcomes are comparable, making RIC an acceptable therapeutic option in elderly patients. Similarly, T-cell depleted RIC alloSCT with the use of donor lymphocyte infusion (DLI) for any relapses has shown promising results to reduce TRM and improve outcomes in multiply relapsed FL patients.[72,73]

TRANSPLANTATION IN MANTLE CELL LYMPHOMA

MCL composes approximately 6% of NHL,[49] is incurable with conventional chemotherapy, and has a median remission duration of 1.5 to 3.0 years and a median OS of 3 to 6 years with conventional chemotherapy.[74] HDT/autoSCT was initially studied in a relapse setting and subsequently in a frontline setting with a goal to improve outcomes.

Up-front Autologous Stem Cell Transplantation for Mantle Cell Lymphoma

Several studies, predominantly nonrandomized trials and retrospective studies, have evaluated the role of up-front autoSCT in young patients with symptomatic MCL following various induction regimens. The European MCL network randomized patients with MCL aged 65 years or younger in first complete remission (n = 122) following a CHOP-like regimen to myeloablative radiochemotherapy and autoSCT or α-interferon maintenance. The autoSCT arm, compared with the interferon arm, had a significantly prolonged median PFS (39 vs 17 months, *P* = .01) but similar 3-year OS (83% vs 77%, *P* = .18).[75] This study suggests that consolidation therapy with HDT/autoSCT may improve PFS in young patients with MCL.

The second Nordic MCL trial (n = 160) demonstrated a 6-year OS and EFS of 70% and 56%, respectively, among patients with untreated MCL aged younger than

66 years in a phase II protocol with dose-intensified induction immunochemotherapy with maxi-R-CHOP, alternating with rituximab and high-dose cytarabine, followed by HDT and rituximab–in vivo purged autoSCT among the responders. A significantly higher proportion of patients achieved polymerase chain reaction negativity for molecular marker (translocation [11;14]) or clonal immunoglobulin H rearrangement 2 months after the therapy compared with the historical control in the first Nordic MCL trial (92% vs 38%, *P*<.001).[67] An updated result highlighted both Ki-67 and MCL IPI (MIPI) to be the independent predictors of EFS and OS.[76] Cancer and Leukemia Group B (CALGB) 59909 used an intensive immunochemotherapy regimen in patients with newly diagnosed MCL at up to 69 years of age (n = 78). The therapy included 2 to 3 cycles of rituximab combined with methotrexate and augmented CHOP followed by high doses of cytarabine and etoposide combined with rituximab. Following stem cell mobilization, patients then received HDT/autoSCT and 2 doses of rituximab. The 5-year PFS and OS were 56% and 64%, respectively.[77] A phase II French trial (n = 60) among patients with newly diagnosed stage III/IV MCL aged younger than 66 years used 3 cycles of R-CHOP at the third cycle and 3 cycles of RDHAP, followed by HDT/ASCT. The 5-year EFS and OS were 64% and 75%, respectively.[78] The results of these studies with HDT/autoSCT are better than the historical outcomes seen in MCL; however, selection bias and differences in induction therapy may also play a role.

The intensity of initial therapy before autoSCT may play an important role in MCL. In a National Comprehensive Cancer Network's NHL database study, patients with MCL younger than 65 years treated with R-CHOP alone (18%) had a worse 3-year PFS compared with more aggressive regimens, which included rituximab and hyperfractionated cyclophosphamide, vincristine, doxorubicin, and dexamethasone (R-HyperCVAD) (58%, *P*<.001), R-CHOP and autoSCT (56%, *P*<.001), and R-HyperCVAD and autoSCT (55%, *P* = .004). PFS did not differ between the 3 aggressive regimens. There was no difference in 3-year OS between R-CHOP alone (69%), R-HyperCVAD (85%, *P*<.07), and R-CHOP and autoSCT (87%, *P*<.20). In multivariable models, R-CHOP alone had a poorer OS compared with R-HyperCVAD (hazard ratio [HR] 2.5, 95% confidence interval [CI] 1.0–6.2) but not with R-CHOP and autoSCT (HR 1.9, 95% CI 0.6–5.7).[79] However, another study determined that MIPI, but not the type of induction therapy or timing of therapy (initial observation >3 months), predicted OS in patients with MCL treated with HDT/ASCT (n = 118). An intensive induction regimen containing high-dose cytarabine (HyperCVAD), compared with other regimens, improved the PFS for all patients with MCL (*P* = .01) but not for patients who received HDT/ASCT as the initial therapy (*P* = .26).[80] These studies indicated that young patients with MCL may have improved PFS when treated with R-HyperCVAD with or without autoSCT or R-CHOP and autoSCT compared with R-CHOP alone as the initial therapy.

Autologous Stem Cell Transplantation for Refractory or Relapsed Mantle Cell Lymphoma

Young patients with symptomatic MCL are currently offered an up-front HDT/ASCT; however, historically, the role of HDT/autoSCT was initially studied as a consolidation therapy after salvage therapy. At the University of Nebraska Medical Center, 40 patients with MCL, who were predominantly primary refractory/relapsed (88%), underwent HDT/autoSCT. At 2 years, the median EFS and OS were 36% and 65%, respectively. Patients who received 3 or more prior therapies, compared with those who received less than 3 prior therapies, had a worse 2-year EFS (0% vs 45%, *P* = .004).[81] A subsequent comparison (n = 33) indicated that the use of a more intense induction regimen, such as R-HyperCVAD, before autoSCT may result in lower relapse rates (*P* = .07) but similar PFS and OS.[82] In another study (n = 16), patients with relapsed or refractory MCL received ^{131}I-tositumomab (1.7 mg/kg) followed 10 days later by HDT/autoSCT. The complete response rate was 91%, whereas the 3-year PFS and OS were 61% and 93%, respectively, thus demonstrating the radiosensitive nature of MCL.[83] Patients with relapsed/refractory MCL who have not received autoSCT as an up-front therapy may be considered for HDT/autoSCT after salvage therapy, if they are transplant eligible.

Improving the Outcomes of Autologous Stem Cell Transplantation

Rituximab has been successfully used before and after autoSCT to improve the outcomes.[63,64,84,85] In a German study, incorporation of rituximab to the conditioning regimen in patients with newly diagnosed MCL (n = 34) resulted in significantly higher 4-year EFS (83% vs 47%, *P* = .04) but similar OS (87% vs 77%), compared with historical control.[84] Rituximab has been used as a preemptive therapy to prevent clinical relapse. In a study, preemptive rituximab therapy (375 mg/m^2 weekly for 4 weeks) for molecular relapse after autoSCT resulted in a reinduction of molecular remission in 92% and a median molecular and clinical relapse-free survival of 1.5 and 3.7 years, respectively.[86] A few studies have also indicated a role of rituximab maintenance in improving PFS (but not OS) in select patients with MCL after R-HyperCVAD or autoSCT.[79,87,88] Although rituximab use can increase the risk of prolonged neutropenia or hypogammaglobulinemia, it may not increase the risk of major infections.[64]

Predicting the Outcomes of Autologous Stem Cell Transplantation

As discussed earlier, MIPI has been shown to be one of the most important prognostic factors for OS and PFS.[76,80,89,90] Disease status at SCT[91] and molecular remission[92,93] also influences outcomes. Among patients with relapsed or refractory MCL, a simplified MIPI score before autoSCT, B symptoms at diagnosis, and remission quotient predict PFS and OS. Remission quotient is defined as the time in months from diagnosis to autoSCT divided by the number of prior therapies.[90] Additionally, high Ki-67[76,94] and expression of PIM1 (moderate or strong expression), a serine/threonine kinase and proto-oncogene, by immunohistochemistry has been shown to predict poor PFS.[94]

Allogeneic Stem Cell Transplantation for Mantle Cell Lymphoma

AlloSCT in MCL has been empirically used in young patients with multiply relapsed MCL in the absence of any large-scale randomized trial. In a retrospective study comparing autoSCT and alloSCT (n = 97), patients who underwent alloSCT were younger but more heavily pretreated. Conversely, patients with autoSCT, compared with patients with alloSCT, were more likely to be in first complete remission (34% vs 18%). Overall, alloSCT resulted in higher 100-day mortality (19% vs 0%, *P*<.01), statistically insignificant lower relapse rate (21% vs 56%, *P* = .11), and similar EFS (44% vs 39%, *P* = .85) and OS (49% vs 47%, *P* = .51) at 5 years.[82] High TRM has led to the utilization of RIC alloSCT. A study of the British Society for Blood and Marrow Transplantation explored the utility of RIC alloSCT among patients with relapsed and refractory MCL (n = 70), of which 34% patients had a history of prior autoSCT. Approximately 80% of patients received an alemtuzumab-containing regimen. At 5 years, NRM, PFS, and OS were 21%, 14%, and 37%, respectively. The cumulative risk of relapse was 65% at 5 years, which was significantly influenced by disease status at SCT and chemosensitivity. Fifteen of the 18 relapsed patients underwent DLI or a second RIC alloSCT, with 73% in complete remission at the last follow-up. A prior history of less than 2 lines of therapy influenced PFS and OS, whereas age at SCT and use of an alemtuzumab-containing regimen influenced OS.[95] In another study (n = 33), alloSCT in patients with relapsed and refractory MCL using nonmyeloablative conditioning with fludarabine and 2-Gy TBI resulted in an 85% overall response rate and a 2-year NRM, DFS, and OS of 24%, 60%, and 65%, respectively.[96] The high response rate and OS in relapsed and refractory MCL with RIC and nonmyeloablative alloSCT make such treatment strategies attractive.

A recent report compared the outcomes of RIC alloSCT and autoSCT. In this CIBMTR study of patients with chemosensitive MCL (n = 519), patients received autoSCT or RIC alloSCT in the first partial or complete remission with no more than 2 lines of chemotherapy (early SCT), or later in the disease course after the patients relapsed, or in second or subsequent complete remission (late SCT). RIC alloSCT, compared with autoSCT, resulted in lower relapse/progression but higher NRM. Consequently, the 5-year OS was similar between alloSCT and autoSCT in both the early SCT (62% vs 61%, P = .95) and later SCT (31% vs 44%, P = .20) group. Early SCT resulted in a survival benefit, with the highest OS and PFS in patients who received autoSCT in the first complete remission.[97] Better results with autoSCT may be related to the utilization of alloSCT in patients, who were thought not to be good candidates for autoSCT eg, heavily pre-treated or chemoresistant patients. Nonetheless, this study validates the current practice of autoSCT in patients with MCL in first complete remission. The role of alloSCT is limited mainly by high NRM, but alloSCT can be used in eligible patients with multiple relapses or those who fail autoSCT. DLI may be considered in patients who relapse following alloSCT.

TRANSPLANTATION IN T-CELL LYMPHOMA

TCL, which composes approximately 10% to 15% of NHL, has wide geographic variation in incidence, the highest being in Asia.[98] Peripheral TCL (PTCL), which includes several subtypes, portends an overall poor prognosis with a 5-year OS of approximately 30% or less.[98] SCT has been used in both an up-front and relapsed setting in PTCL. The lack of randomized trials prevents accurate assessment of the benefit of HDT/autoSCT in patients with PTCL; however, the current studies indicate a possible benefit with autoSCT. In a large prospective phase II Nordic Lymphoma Group trial (NLG-T-01), patients with PTCL (n = 160) received a dose-dense induction regimen of 6 cycles of biweekly CHOP and etoposide (CHOEP) (etoposide was omitted in patients aged >60 years) followed by HDT/autoSCT in patients who achieved complete or partial remission. Initial chemotherapy resulted in an overall response rate of 82%. Twenty-six percent of patients could not be taken to autoSCT mainly because of primary refractory or progressive disease. At 3 months after autoSCT, 86% were in partial or complete remission. TRM was 4%, whereas the 5-year PFS and OS were 44% and 51%, respectively. Anaplastic lymphoma kinase-negative anaplastic large cell lymphoma (ALK-negative ALCL) histology (P = .031) and female sex (P = .069) predicted better OS, whereas age as a continuous variable (P = .041) and a World Health Organization performance status of 2 or more (P = .041) predicted worse OS. Bone marrow involvement predicted worse PFS (P = .027) but not OS.[99] In another large prospective multicenter study, patients with PTCL (n = 83) underwent 4 to 6 cycles of CHOP followed by HDT/autoSCT in patients who achieve partial or complete remission. Only 66% of patients underwent autoSCT; the main reason for not receiving autoSCT was progressive disease. TRM was 3.6%, whereas the 3-year OS and PFS were 48% and 36%, respectively. The prognostic index for PTCL correlated with OS in a univariate analysis.[100] Several other studies have shown a fairly high early progressive disease and similar outcomes with HDT/autoSCT.[101–103] The benefit of autoSCT, compared with historical controls treated with conventional chemotherapy, was observed in an Asian study of natural killer/TCL also.[104] Overall, the outcomes of these studies, compared with existing literature, suggest the usefulness of such strategy. However, nearly one-third of patients with PTCL can progress rapidly before SCT.

The timing of the HDT/autoSCT has been explored in a study from the City of Hope medical center. In the study, patients with PTCL (n = 67) underwent HDT/autoSCT in the first partial or complete remission (n = 12) or relapsed/primary refractory setting (n = 55). The 5-year PFS and OS of the entire cohort was 40% and 54%. The 5-year PFS (75% vs 32%, *P* = .01) of patients transplanted in the first remission was significantly higher than those transplanted in a relapsed/primary refractory setting. Patients with high-risk disease, identified by the prognostic index for PTCL, had a 5-year PFS of 8%. This study indicates that up-front HDT/autoSCT may improve outcomes in PTCL, compared with autoSCT in the relapse setting.[105] However, HDT/autoSCT has an important role in the management of patients with relapsed PTCL. The Memorial Sloan-Kettering Cancer Center compared autoSCT for relapsed or refractory PTCL responding to salvage therapy (n = 24) with chemosensitive relapsed or refractory DLBCL (n = 86). The 5-year PFS (24% vs 34%, *P* = .14) and OS (33% vs 39%, *P* = .64) were similar between PTCL and DLBCL. In a multivariate analysis, only second-line age-adjusted IPI predicted PFS (*P* = .01) and OS (*P*<.01).[106] Similar 5-year OS of 34% to 48% has been seen in other studies of autoSCT in relapsed PTCL.[107–109] Although the outcome of relapsed PTCL is poor, chemosensitive patients may benefit from HDT/autoSCT.

AlloSCT may be useful in multiply relapsed PTCL or after failure of autoSCT. In a CIBMTR study, outcomes of patients with PTCL (n = 241) who underwent autoSCT were compared with those who underwent alloSCT. Patients with autoSCT, compared with patients with alloSCT, were more likely to be in first complete remission, have chemosensitive disease, 2 or fewer prior therapies, and anaplastic large-cell histology. AutoSCT, compared with myeloablative and nonmyeloablative/RIC alloSCT, had lower NRM (11% vs 27%–32%, *P*<.001), similar PFS (47% vs 33%–36%, *P* = .18) and lower OS (59% vs 39%–52%, *P* = .03) at 3 years. The results were similar for patients transplanted beyond the first complete remission. NRM (32% vs 27%) and PFS (36% vs 33%) at 3 years were similar for myeloablative and nonmyeloablative/RIC alloSCT. In multivariate analysis, chemosensitivity and 2 or fewer lines of pre-SCT therapy were prognostic of OS.[110] Although alloSCT is associated with higher NRM, the long-term survival results of alloSCT are comparable with autoSCT. Proper patient selection and RIC alloSCT may reduce NRM. In an Italian study, RIC alloSCT in relapsed or refractory PTCL (n = 52) resulted in NRM of 12%, PFS of 50%, and OS of 40% at 5 years. Sixty-six percent of patients with disease progression (n = 12) responded to DLI. In a multivariate analysis, refractory disease and an age greater than 45 years predicted poor prognosis.[111] In another study, 17 patients with PTCL or natural killer/T-cell lymphoma (NK/TCL) underwent nonmyeloablative alloSCT. The patients were heavily treated, with a median of 3 prior therapies and a history of autoSCT in 35%. The 3-year NRM, PFS, and OS were 19%, 53%, and 59%, respectively.[112] These studies suggest that RIC alloSCT with graft-versus-lymphoma activity can result in long-term disease control in PTCL.

POSTTRANSPLANTATION MONITORING

Patients with a history of autoSCT or alloSCT are at risk of disease relapse as well as long-term complications of SCT. Monitoring for disease relapse includes clinical evaluation, complete hemogram, blood chemistry, and serum LDH. An imaging may be repeated at the end of therapy for a new baseline, beyond which there is no role for routine surveillance scans. In patients who are several years out of SCT, NRM may be more common than relapse mortality.[113] Patients who have undergone a transplant, therefore, should be closely monitored and treated for long-term complications, which include therapy-related myeloid neoplasms (particularly in autoSCT);[114] solid malignancies; infections; and cardiac, pulmonary, endocrine, and renal complications, particularly in patients with alloSCT.[115,116]

REFERENCES

1. Siegel R, Ma J, Zou Z, et al. Cancer statistics, 2014. CA Cancer J Clin 2014; 64(1):9–29.
2. Sorror ML, Maris MB, Storb R, et al. Hematopoietic cell transplantation (HCT)-specific comorbidity index: a new tool for risk assessment before allogeneic HCT. Blood 2005;106(8):2912–9.
3. Sorror M, Storer B, Gopal A, et al. Comorbidity, lactate dehydrogenase (LDH), and chemosensitivity are independent predictors of mortality after autologous hematopoietic cell transplantation (HCT) for patients (pts) with lymphoma. ASH Annual Meeting Abstracts 2007;110(11):616.
4. Morton LM, Wang SS, Devesa SS, et al. Lymphoma incidence patterns by WHO subtype in the United States, 1992-2001. Blood 2006;107(1):265–76.
5. Armitage JO. How I treat patients with diffuse large B-cell lymphoma. Blood 2007;110(1):29–36.
6. Sehn LH, Berry B, Chhanabhai M, et al. The Revised International Prognostic Index (R-IPI) is a better predictor of outcome than the standard IPI for patients with diffuse large B-cell lymphoma treated with R-CHOP. Blood 2007;109(5): 1857–61.
7. Greb A, Bohlius J, Schiefer D, et al. High-dose chemotherapy with autologous stem cell transplantation in the first line treatment of aggressive non-Hodgkin lymphoma (NHL) in adults. Cochrane Database Syst Rev 2008;(1):CD004024.
8. Ziepert M, Hasenclever D, Kuhnt E, et al. Standard international prognostic index remains a valid predictor of outcome for patients with aggressive CD20+ B-cell lymphoma in the rituximab era. J Clin Oncol 2010;28(14):2373–80.
9. Haioun C, Lepage E, Gisselbrecht C, et al. Survival benefit of high-dose therapy in poor-risk aggressive non-Hodgkin's lymphoma: final analysis of the prospective LNH87-2 protocol–a groupe d'Etude des lymphomes de l'Adulte study. J Clin Oncol 2000;18(16):3025–30.
10. Stiff PJ, Unger JM, Cook JR, et al. Autologous transplantation as consolidation for aggressive non-Hodgkin's lymphoma. N Engl J Med 2013;369(18): 1681–90.
11. Vitolo U, Chiappella A, Brusamolino E, et al. A randomized multicentre phase III study for first line treatment of young patients with high risk (aaIPI 2-3) diffuse large B-cell lymphoma (DLBCL): rituximab plus dose-dense chemotherapy CHOP-14/MEGACHOP 14 with or without intensified high-dose chemotherapy (HDC) and autologous stem cell transplantation (ASCT): results of DLCL04 trial of Italian lymphoma foundation (FIL). Ann Oncol 2011;22(suppl 4):106.
12. Milpied NJ, Legouill S, Lamy T, et al. No benefit of first-line rituximab (R) - high-dose therapy (R-HDT) over R-CHOP14 for young adults with diffuse large B-cell lymphoma. Preliminary results of the GOELAMS 075 prospective multicentre randomized trial. ASH Annual Meeting Abstracts 2010;116(21):685.

13. Schmitz N, Nickelsen M, Ziepert M, et al. Conventional chemotherapy (CHOEP-14) with rituximab or high-dose chemotherapy (MegaCHOEP) with rituximab for young, high-risk patients with aggressive B-cell lymphoma: an open-label, randomised, phase 3 trial (DSHNHL 2002-1). Lancet Oncol 2012;13(12):1250–9.
14. Milpied N. Myeloablation for lymphoma–question answered? N Engl J Med 2013;369(18):1750–1.
15. Coiffier B, Lepage E, Brière J, et al. CHOP chemotherapy plus rituximab compared with CHOP alone in elderly patients with diffuse large-B-cell lymphoma. N Engl J Med 2002;346(4):235–42.
16. Pfreundschuh M, Schubert J, Ziepert M, et al. Six versus eight cycles of biweekly CHOP-14 with or without rituximab in elderly patients with aggressive CD20+ B-cell lymphomas: a randomised controlled trial (RICOVER-60). Lancet Oncol 2008;9(2):105–16.
17. Philip T, Guglielmi C, Hagenbeek A, et al. Autologous bone marrow transplantation as compared with salvage chemotherapy in relapses of chemotherapy-sensitive non-Hodgkin's lymphoma. N Engl J Med 1995;333(23):1540–5.
18. Vose JM, Zhang MJ, Rowlings PA, et al. Autologous transplantation for diffuse aggressive non-Hodgkin's lymphoma in patients never achieving remission: a report from the Autologous Blood and Marrow Transplant Registry. J Clin Oncol 2001;19(2):406–13.
19. Kewalramani T, Zelenetz AD, Hedrick EE, et al. High-dose chemoradiotherapy and autologous stem cell transplantation for patients with primary refractory aggressive non-Hodgkin lymphoma: an intention-to-treat analysis. Blood 2000; 96(7):2399–404.
20. Kewalramani T, Zelenetz AD, Nimer SD, et al. Rituximab and ICE as second-line therapy before autologous stem cell transplantation for relapsed or primary refractory diffuse large B-cell lymphoma. Blood 2004;103(10):3684–8.
21. Khouri IF, Saliba RM, Hosing C, et al. Concurrent administration of high-dose rituximab before and after autologous stem-cell transplantation for relapsed aggressive B-cell non-Hodgkin's lymphomas. J Clin Oncol 2005;23(10):2240–7.
22. Vose JM, Rizzo DJ, Tao-Wu J, et al. Autologous transplantation for diffuse aggressive non-Hodgkin lymphoma in first relapse or second remission. Biol Blood Marrow Transplant 2004;10(2):116–27.
23. Gisselbrecht C, Glass B, Mounier N, et al. Salvage regimens with autologous transplantation for relapsed large B-cell lymphoma in the rituximab era. J Clin Oncol 2010;28(27):4184–90.
24. Philip T, Armitage JO, Spitzer G, et al. High-dose therapy and autologous bone marrow transplantation after failure of conventional chemotherapy in adults with intermediate-grade or high-grade non-Hodgkin's lymphoma. N Engl J Med 1987;316(24):1493–8.
25. Thieblemont C, Briere J, Mounier N, et al. The germinal center/activated B-cell subclassification has a prognostic impact for response to salvage therapy in relapsed/refractory diffuse large B-cell lymphoma: a bio-CORAL study. J Clin Oncol 2011;29(31):4079–87.
26. Moskowitz CH, Zelenetz AD, Kewalramani T, et al. Cell of origin, germinal center versus nongerminal center, determined by immunohistochemistry on tissue microarray, does not correlate with outcome in patients with relapsed and refractory DLBCL. Blood 2005;106(10):3383–5.
27. Gu K, Weisenburger DD, Fu K, et al. Cell of origin fails to predict survival in patients with diffuse large B-cell lymphoma treated with autologous hematopoietic stem cell transplantation. Hematol Oncol 2012;30(3):143–9.

28. Winter JN, Inwards DJ, Spies S, et al. Yttrium-90 ibritumomab tiuxetan doses calculated to deliver up to 15 Gy to critical organs may be safely combined with high-dose BEAM and autologous transplantation in relapsed or refractory B-cell non-Hodgkin's lymphoma. J Clin Oncol 2009;27(10):1653–9.
29. Nademanee A, Forman S, Molina A, et al. A phase 1/2 trial of high-dose yttrium-90-ibritumomab tiuxetan in combination with high-dose etoposide and cyclophosphamide followed by autologous stem cell transplantation in patients with poor-risk or relapsed non-Hodgkin lymphoma. Blood 2005;106(8):2896–902.
30. Press OW, Eary JF, Gooley T, et al. A phase I/II trial of iodine-131-tositumomab (anti-CD20), etoposide, cyclophosphamide, and autologous stem cell transplantation for relapsed B-cell lymphomas. Blood 2000;96(9):2934–42.
31. Decaudin D, Mounier N, Tilly H, et al. (90)Y ibritumomab tiuxetan (Zevalin) combined with BEAM (Z -BEAM) conditioning regimen plus autologous stem cell transplantation in relapsed or refractory low-grade CD20-positive B-cell lymphoma. A GELA phase II prospective study. Clin Lymphoma Myeloma Leuk 2011;11(2):212–8.
32. Vose JM, Bierman PJ, Loberiza FR, et al. Phase II trial of 131-Iodine tositumomab with high-dose chemotherapy and autologous stem cell transplantation for relapsed diffuse large B cell lymphoma. Biol Blood Marrow Transplant 2013;19(1):123–8.
33. Briones J, Novelli S, Garcia-Marco JA, et al. Autologous stem cell transplantation after conditioning with yttrium-90 ibritumomab tiuxetan plus beam in refractory non-Hodgkin diffuse large B-cell lymphoma: results of a prospective, multicenter, phase II clinical trial. Haematologica 2014;99(3):505–10.
34. Vose JM, Carter S, Burns LJ, et al. Phase III randomized study of rituximab/carmustine, etoposide, cytarabine, and melphalan (BEAM) compared with iodine-131 tositumomab/BEAM with autologous hematopoietic cell transplantation for relapsed diffuse large B-cell lymphoma: results from the BMT CTN 0401 trial. J Clin Oncol 2013;31(13):1662–8.
35. Hoppe BS, Moskowitz CH, Filippa DA, et al. Involved-field radiotherapy before high-dose therapy and autologous stem-cell rescue in diffuse large-cell lymphoma: long-term disease control and toxicity. J Clin Oncol 2008;26(11):1858–64.
36. Vellenga E, van Putten WL, van 't Veer MB, et al. Rituximab improves the treatment results of DHAP-VIM-DHAP and ASCT in relapsed/progressive aggressive CD20+ NHL: a prospective randomized HOVON trial. Blood 2008;111(2): 537–43.
37. Glass B, Ziepert M, Reiser M, et al. High-dose therapy followed by autologous stem-cell transplantation with and without rituximab for primary treatment of high-risk diffuse large B-cell lymphoma. Ann Oncol 2010;21(11):2255–61.
38. Coso D, Sebban C, Boulat O, et al. A phase II trial of rituximab as adjuvant to intensive sequential chemotherapy in patients under 60 years with untreated poor-prognosis diffuse large B-cell lymphoma. Bone Marrow Transplant 2006; 38(3):217–22.
39. Sieniawski M, Staak O, Glossmann JP, et al. Rituximab added to an intensified salvage chemotherapy program followed by autologous stem cell transplantation improved the outcome in relapsed and refractory aggressive non-Hodgkin lymphoma. Ann Hematol 2007;86(2):107–15.
40. Gisselbrecht C, Schmitz N, Mounier N, et al. Rituximab maintenance therapy after autologous stem-cell transplantation in patients with relapsed CD20(+) diffuse large B-cell lymphoma: final analysis of the collaborative trial in relapsed aggressive lymphoma. J Clin Oncol 2012;30(36):4462–9.

41. Hamlin PA, Zelenetz AD, Kewalramani T, et al. Age-adjusted International Prognostic Index predicts autologous stem cell transplantation outcome for patients with relapsed or primary refractory diffuse large B-cell lymphoma. Blood 2003; 102(6):1989–96.
42. Filmont JE, Gisselbrecht C, Cuenca X, et al. The impact of pre- and post-transplantation positron emission tomography using 18-fluorodeoxyglucose on poor-prognosis lymphoma patients undergoing autologous stem cell transplantation. Cancer 2007;110(6):1361–9.
43. Dickinson M, Hoyt R, Roberts AW, et al. Improved survival for relapsed diffuse large B cell lymphoma is predicted by a negative pre-transplant FDG-PET scan following salvage chemotherapy. Br J Haematol 2010;150(1):39–45.
44. Roland V, Bodet-Milin C, Moreau A, et al. Impact of high-dose chemotherapy followed by auto-SCT for positive interim [18F] FDG-PET diffuse large B-cell lymphoma patients. Bone Marrow Transplant 2011;46(3):393–9.
45. Nagle SJ, Woo K, Schuster SJ, et al. Outcomes of patients with relapsed/refractory diffuse large B-cell lymphoma with progression of lymphoma after autologous stem cell transplantation in the rituximab era. Am J Hematol 2013; 88(10):890–4.
46. Lazarus HM, Zhang MJ, Carreras J, et al. A comparison of HLA-identical sibling allogeneic versus autologous transplantation for diffuse large B cell lymphoma: a report from the CIBMTR. Biol Blood Marrow Transplant 2010;16(1): 35–45.
47. van Kampen RJ, Canals C, Schouten HC, et al. Allogeneic stem-cell transplantation as salvage therapy for patients with diffuse large B-cell non-Hodgkin's lymphoma relapsing after an autologous stem-cell transplantation: an analysis of the European Group for Blood and Marrow Transplantation Registry. J Clin Oncol 2011;29(10):1342–8.
48. Bacher U, Klyuchnikov E, Le-Rademacher J, et al. Conditioning regimens for allotransplants for diffuse large B-cell lymphoma: myeloablative or reduced intensity? Blood 2012;120(20):4256–62.
49. A clinical evaluation of the International Lymphoma Study Group classification of non-Hodgkin's lymphoma. The Non-Hodgkin's Lymphoma Classification Project. Blood 1997;89(11):3909–18.
50. Federico M, Luminari S, Dondi A, et al. R-CVP versus R-CHOP versus R-FM for the initial treatment of patients with advanced-stage follicular lymphoma: results of the FOLL05 trial conducted by the Fondazione Italiana Linfomi. J Clin Oncol 2013;31(12):1506–13.
51. Lenz G, Dreyling M, Schiegnitz E, et al. Myeloablative radiochemotherapy followed by autologous stem cell transplantation in first remission prolongs progression-free survival in follicular lymphoma: results of a prospective, randomized trial of the German Low-Grade Lymphoma Study Group. Blood 2004;104(9):2667–74.
52. Deconinck E, Foussard C, Milpied N, et al. High-dose therapy followed by autologous purged stem-cell transplantation and doxorubicin-based chemotherapy in patients with advanced follicular lymphoma: a randomized multicenter study by GOELAMS. Blood 2005;105(10):3817–23.
53. Gyan E, Foussard C, Bertrand P, et al. High-dose therapy followed by autologous purged stem cell transplantation and doxorubicin-based chemotherapy in patients with advanced follicular lymphoma: a randomized multicenter study by the GOELAMS with final results after a median follow-up of 9 years. Blood 2009;113(5):995–1001.

54. Sebban C, Mounier N, Brousse N, et al. Standard chemotherapy with interferon compared with CHOP followed by high-dose therapy with autologous stem cell transplantation in untreated patients with advanced follicular lymphoma: the GELF-94 randomized study from the Groupe d'Etude des Lymphomes de l'Adulte (GELA). Blood 2006;108(8):2540–4.
55. Ladetto M, De Marco F, Benedetti F, et al. Prospective, multicenter randomized GITMO/IIL trial comparing intensive (R-HDS) versus conventional (R-CHOP) chemoimmunotherapy in high-risk follicular lymphoma at diagnosis: the superior disease control of R-HDS does not translate into an overall survival advantage. Blood 2008;111(8):4004–13.
56. Schouten HC, Qian W, Kvaloy S, et al. High-dose therapy improves progression-free survival and survival in relapsed follicular non-Hodgkin's lymphoma: results from the randomized European CUP trial. J Clin Oncol 2003;21(21):3918–27.
57. Le Gouill S, De Guibert S, Planche L, et al. Impact of the use of autologous stem cell transplantation at first relapse both in naive and previously rituximab exposed follicular lymphoma patients treated in the GELA/GOELAMS FL2000 study. Haematologica 2011;96(8):1128–35.
58. Vose JM, Bierman PJ, Loberiza FR, et al. Long-term outcomes of autologous stem cell transplantation for follicular non-Hodgkin lymphoma: effect of histological grade and Follicular International Prognostic Index. Biol Blood Marrow Transplant 2008;14(1):36–42.
59. Montoto S, Canals C, Rohatiner AZ, et al. Long-term follow-up of high-dose treatment with autologous haematopoietic progenitor cell support in 693 patients with follicular lymphoma: an EBMT registry study. Leukemia 2007; 21(11):2324–31.
60. Evens AM, Vanderplas A, LaCasce AS, et al. Stem cell transplantation for follicular lymphoma relapsed/refractory after prior rituximab: a comprehensive analysis from the NCCN lymphoma outcomes project. Cancer 2013;119(20):3662–71.
61. Brown JR, Feng Y, Gribben JG, et al. Long-term survival after autologous bone marrow transplantation for follicular lymphoma in first remission. Biol Blood Marrow Transplant 2007;13(9):1057–65.
62. Arcaini L, Montanari F, Alessandrino EP, et al. Immunochemotherapy with in vivo purging and autotransplant induces long clinical and molecular remission in advanced relapsed and refractory follicular lymphoma. Ann Oncol 2008;19(7): 1331–5.
63. Brugger W, Hirsch J, Grunebach F, et al. Rituximab consolidation after high-dose chemotherapy and autologous blood stem cell transplantation in follicular and mantle cell lymphoma: a prospective, multicenter phase II study. Ann Oncol 2004;15(11):1691–8.
64. Kasamon YL, Jones RJ, Brodsky RA, et al. Immunologic recovery following autologous stem-cell transplantation with pre- and posttransplantation rituximab for low-grade or mantle cell lymphoma. Ann Oncol 2010;21(6):1203–10.
65. Hicks LK, Woods A, Buckstein R, et al. Rituximab purging and maintenance combined with auto-SCT: long-term molecular remissions and prolonged hypogammaglobulinemia in relapsed follicular lymphoma. Bone Marrow Transplant 2009;43(9):701–8.
66. Morschhauser F, Recher C, Milpied N, et al. A 4-weekly course of rituximab is safe and improves tumor control for patients with minimal residual disease persisting 3 months after autologous hematopoietic stem-cell transplantation: results of a prospective multicenter phase II study in patients with follicular lymphoma. Ann Oncol 2012;23(10):2687–95.

67. Geisler CH, Kolstad A, Laurell A, et al. Long-term progression-free survival of mantle cell lymphoma after intensive front-line immunochemotherapy with in vivo-purged stem cell rescue: a nonrandomized phase 2 multicenter study by the Nordic Lymphoma Group. Blood 2008;112(7):2687–93.
68. Corradini P, Ladetto M, Zallio F, et al. Long-term follow-up of indolent lymphoma patients treated with high-dose sequential chemotherapy and autografting: evidence that durable molecular and clinical remission frequently can be attained only in follicular subtypes. J Clin Oncol 2004;22(8):1460–8.
69. van Besien K, Loberiza FR Jr, Bajorunaite R, et al. Comparison of autologous and allogeneic hematopoietic stem cell transplantation for follicular lymphoma. Blood 2003;102(10):3521–9.
70. Tomblyn MR, Ewell M, Bredeson C, et al. Autologous versus reduced-intensity allogeneic hematopoietic cell transplantation for patients with chemosensitive follicular non-Hodgkin lymphoma beyond first complete response or first partial response. Biol Blood Marrow Transplant 2011;17(7):1051–7.
71. Hari P, Carreras J, Zhang MJ, et al. Allogeneic transplants in follicular lymphoma: higher risk of disease progression after reduced-intensity compared to myeloablative conditioning. Biol Blood Marrow Transplant 2008;14(2): 236–45.
72. Ingram W, Devereux S, Das-Gupta EP, et al. Outcome of BEAM-autologous and BEAM-alemtuzumab allogeneic transplantation in relapsed advanced stage follicular lymphoma. Br J Haematol 2008;141(2):235–43.
73. Thomson KJ, Morris EC, Milligan D, et al. T-cell-depleted reduced-intensity transplantation followed by donor leukocyte infusions to promote graft-versus-lymphoma activity results in excellent long-term survival in patients with multiply relapsed follicular lymphoma. J Clin Oncol 2010;28(23):3695–700.
74. Vose JM. Mantle cell lymphoma: 2013 Update on diagnosis, risk-stratification, and clinical management. Am J Hematol 2013;88(12):1082–8.
75. Dreyling M, Lenz G, Hoster E, et al. Early consolidation by myeloablative radiochemotherapy followed by autologous stem cell transplantation in first remission significantly prolongs progression-free survival in mantle-cell lymphoma: results of a prospective randomized trial of the European MCL Network. Blood 2005; 105(7):2677–84.
76. Geisler CH, Kolstad A, Laurell A, et al. Nordic MCL2 trial update: six-year follow-up after intensive immunochemotherapy for untreated mantle cell lymphoma followed by BEAM or BEAC + autologous stem-cell support: still very long survival but late relapses do occur. Br J Haematol 2012;158(3):355–62.
77. Damon LE, Johnson JL, Niedzwiecki D, et al. Immunochemotherapy and autologous stem-cell transplantation for untreated patients with mantle-cell lymphoma: CALGB 59909. J Clin Oncol 2009;27(36):6101–8.
78. Delarue R, Haioun C, Ribrag V, et al. CHOP and DHAP plus rituximab followed by autologous stem cell transplantation in mantle cell lymphoma: a phase 2 study from the Groupe d'Etude des Lymphomes de l'Adulte. Blood 2013; 121(1):48–53.
79. LaCasce AS, Vandergrift JL, Rodriguez MA, et al. Comparative outcome of initial therapy for younger patients with mantle cell lymphoma: an analysis from the NCCN NHL Database. Blood 2012;119(9):2093–9.
80. Budde LE, Guthrie KA, Till BG, et al. Mantle cell lymphoma international prognostic index but not pretransplantation induction regimen predicts survival for patients with mantle-cell lymphoma receiving high-dose therapy and autologous stem-cell transplantation. J Clin Oncol 2011;29(22):3023–9.

81. Vose JM, Bierman PJ, Weisenburger DD, et al. Autologous hematopoietic stem cell transplantation for mantle cell lymphoma. Biol Blood Marrow Transplant 2000;6(6):640–5.
82. Ganti AK, Bierman PJ, Lynch JC, et al. Hematopoietic stem cell transplantation in mantle cell lymphoma. Ann Oncol 2005;16(4):618–24.
83. Gopal AK, Rajendran JG, Petersdorf SH, et al. High-dose chemo-radioimmunotherapy with autologous stem cell support for relapsed mantle cell lymphoma. Blood 2002;99(9):3158–62.
84. Dreger P, Rieger M, Seyfarth B, et al. Rituximab-augmented myeloablation for first-line autologous stem cell transplantation for mantle cell lymphoma: effects on molecular response and clinical outcome. Haematologica 2007; 92(1):42–9.
85. Mangel J, Buckstein R, Imrie K, et al. Immunotherapy with rituximab following high-dose therapy and autologous stem-cell transplantation for mantle cell lymphoma. Semin Oncol 2002;29(1 Suppl 2):56–69.
86. Andersen NS, Pedersen LB, Laurell A, et al. Pre-emptive treatment with rituximab of molecular relapse after autologous stem cell transplantation in mantle cell lymphoma. J Clin Oncol 2009;27(26):4365–70.
87. Ahmadi T, McQuade J, Porter D, et al. Potential prolongation of PFS in mantle cell lymphoma after R-HyperCVAD: auto-SCT consolidation or rituximab maintenance. Bone Marrow Transplant 2012;47(8):1082–6.
88. Dietrich S, Weidle J, Rieger M, et al. Rituximab maintenance therapy after autologous stem cell transplantation prolongs progression-free survival in patients with mantle cell lymphoma. Leukemia 2014;28(3):708–9.
89. Hoster E, Klapper W, Hermine O, et al. Confirmation of the Mantle-Cell Lymphoma International Prognostic Index in Randomized Trials of the European Mantle-Cell Lymphoma Network. J Clin Oncol 2014;32(13):1338–46.
90. Cassaday RD, Guthrie KA, Budde EL, et al. Specific features identify patients with relapsed or refractory mantle cell lymphoma benefitting from autologous hematopoietic cell transplantation. Biol Blood Marrow Transplant 2013;19(9): 1403–6.
91. Vandenberghe E, Ruiz de Elvira C, Loberiza FR, et al. Outcome of autologous transplantation for mantle cell lymphoma: a study by the European Blood and Bone Marrow Transplant and Autologous Blood and Marrow Transplant Registries. Br J Haematol 2003;120(5):793–800.
92. Pott C, Hoster E, Delfau-Larue MH, et al. Molecular remission is an independent predictor of clinical outcome in patients with mantle cell lymphoma after combined immunochemotherapy: a European MCL intergroup study. Blood 2010; 115(16):3215–23.
93. Liu H, Johnson JL, Koval G, et al. Detection of minimal residual disease following induction immunochemotherapy predicts progression free survival in mantle cell lymphoma: final results of CALGB 59909. Haematologica 2012; 97(4):579–85.
94. Hsi ED, Jung SH, Lai R, et al. Ki67 and PIM1 expression predict outcome in mantle cell lymphoma treated with high dose therapy, stem cell transplantation and rituximab: a Cancer and Leukemia Group B 59909 correlative science study. Leuk Lymphoma 2008;49(11):2081–90.
95. Cook G, Smith GM, Kirkland K, et al. Outcome following Reduced-Intensity Allogeneic Stem Cell Transplantation (RIC AlloSCT) for relapsed and refractory mantle cell lymphoma (MCL): a study of the British Society for Blood and Marrow Transplantation. Biol Blood Marrow Transplant 2010;16(10):1419–27.

96. Maris MB, Sandmaier BM, Storer BE, et al. Allogeneic hematopoietic cell transplantation after fludarabine and 2 Gy total body irradiation for relapsed and refractory mantle cell lymphoma. Blood 2004;104(12):3535–42.
97. Fenske TS, Zhang MJ, Carreras J, et al. Autologous or reduced-intensity conditioning allogeneic hematopoietic cell transplantation for chemotherapy-sensitive mantle-cell lymphoma: analysis of transplantation timing and modality. J Clin Oncol 2014;32(4):273–81.
98. Armitage JO. The aggressive peripheral T-cell lymphomas: 2013. Am J Hematol 2013;88(10):910–8.
99. d'Amore F, Relander T, Lauritzsen GF, et al. Up-front autologous stem-cell transplantation in peripheral T-cell lymphoma: NLG-T-01. J Clin Oncol 2012;30(25):3093–9.
100. Reimer P, Rudiger T, Geissinger E, et al. Autologous stem-cell transplantation as first-line therapy in peripheral T-cell lymphomas: results of a prospective multicenter study. J Clin Oncol 2009;27(1):106–13.
101. Mercadal S, Briones J, Xicoy B, et al. Intensive chemotherapy (high-dose CHOP/ESHAP regimen) followed by autologous stem-cell transplantation in previously untreated patients with peripheral T-cell lymphoma. Ann Oncol 2008;19(5):958–63.
102. Nickelsen M, Ziepert M, Zeynalova S, et al. High-dose CHOP plus etoposide (MegaCHOEP) in T-cell lymphoma: a comparative analysis of patients treated within trials of the German High-Grade Non-Hodgkin Lymphoma Study Group (DSHNHL). Ann Oncol 2009;20(12):1977–84.
103. Ahn JS, Yang DH, Jung SH, et al. Autologous stem cell transplantation with busulfan, cyclophosphamide, and etoposide as an intensifying frontline treatment in patients with peripheral T cell lymphomas: a multicenter retrospective trial. Ann Hematol 2013;92(6):789–97.
104. Lee J, Au WY, Park MJ, et al. Autologous hematopoietic stem cell transplantation in extranodal natural killer/T cell lymphoma: a multinational, multicenter, matched controlled study. Biol Blood Marrow Transplant 2008;14(12):1356–64.
105. Nademanee A, Palmer JM, Popplewell L, et al. High-dose therapy and autologous hematopoietic cell transplantation in peripheral T cell lymphoma (PTCL): analysis of prognostic factors. Biol Blood Marrow Transplant 2011;17(10):1481–9.
106. Kewalramani T, Zelenetz AD, Teruya-Feldstein J, et al. Autologous transplantation for relapsed or primary refractory peripheral T-cell lymphoma. Br J Haematol 2006;134(2):202–7.
107. Rodriguez J, Conde E, Gutierrez A, et al. The adjusted International Prognostic Index and beta-2-microglobulin predict the outcome after autologous stem cell transplantation in relapsing/refractory peripheral T-cell lymphoma. Haematologica 2007;92(8):1067–74.
108. Chen AI, McMillan A, Negrin RS, et al. Long-term results of autologous hematopoietic cell transplantation for peripheral T cell lymphoma: the Stanford experience. Biol Blood Marrow Transplant 2008;14(7):741–7.
109. Smith SD, Bolwell BJ, Rybicki LA, et al. Autologous hematopoietic stem cell transplantation in peripheral T-cell lymphoma using a uniform high-dose regimen. Bone Marrow Transplant 2007;40(3):239–43.
110. Smith SM, Burns LJ, van Besien K, et al. Hematopoietic cell transplantation for systemic mature T-cell non-Hodgkin lymphoma. J Clin Oncol 2013;31(25):3100–9.

111. Dodero A, Spina F, Narni F, et al. Allogeneic transplantation following a reduced-intensity conditioning regimen in relapsed/refractory peripheral T-cell lymphomas: long-term remissions and response to donor lymphocyte infusions support the role of a graft-versus-lymphoma effect. Leukemia 2012;26(3):520–6.
112. Shustov AR, Gooley TA, Sandmaier BM, et al. Allogeneic haematopoietic cell transplantation after nonmyeloablative conditioning in patients with T-cell and natural killer-cell lymphomas. Br J Haematol 2010;150(2):170–8.
113. Hill BT, Rybicki L, Bolwell BJ, et al. The non-relapse mortality rate for patients with diffuse large B-cell lymphoma is greater than relapse mortality 8 years after autologous stem cell transplantation and is significantly higher than mortality rates of population controls. Br J Haematol 2011;152(5):561–9.
114. Akhtari M, Bhatt VR, Tandra PK, et al. Therapy-related myeloid neoplasms after autologous hematopoietic stem cell transplantation in lymphoma patients. Cancer Biol Ther 2013;14(12):1077–88.
115. Savani BN, Griffith ML, Jagasia S, et al. How I treat late effects in adults after allogeneic stem cell transplantation. Blood 2011;117(11):3002–9.
116. Burns LJ. Late effects after autologous hematopoietic cell transplantation. Biol Blood Marrow Transplant 2009;15(1 Suppl):21–4.

Stem Cell Transplantation in Hodgkin Lymphoma

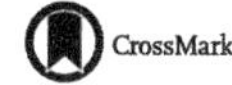

Nishitha M. Reddy, MD, MSCI[a], Miguel-Angel Perales, MD[b,*]

KEYWORDS

- Hodgkin lymphoma • Stem cell transplantation • Brentuximab-vedotin
- Donor-lymphocyte infusion

KEY POINTS

- Autologous stem cell transplantation (ASCT) should be offered to patients who fail to respond to initial treatment and/or as salvage therapy.
- Patients who relapse early (<12 months) after initial therapy are a biologically poor prognostic group.
- A negative functional imaging (PET) before transplantation is associated with improved outcome.
- Reduced-intensity conditioning allogeneic SCT should be offered for patients who relapse after ASCT.

INTRODUCTION

Hodgkin lymphoma (HL) is a rare malignancy that has a bimodal distribution of incidence, with most patients diagnosed at between 15 and 30 years of age and another peak in those older than 55 years. It is estimated that in 2014, approximately 9190 people will be diagnosed with HL in the United States.[1] Despite high success rates with initial chemotherapy, relapse occurs in 10% to 20% of patients with HL and a small minority is nonresponsive to initial chemotherapy. The standard management of these patients includes high-dose chemotherapy (HDT) followed by autologous stem cell transplantation (ASCT). For patients who relapse after ASCT, eligible candidates may be offered allogeneic SCT (allo-SCT). In this article, we discuss the indications of SCT (autologous and allogeneic) in HL and also discuss the management of patients who relapse after transplantation. In addition, we review newer agents that are being incorporated into the routine management of HL and may impact indications for SCT as they are used earlier in the treatment course.

[a] Division of Hematology/Oncology, Vanderbilt University Medical Center, 3927 The Vanderbilt Clinic, Vanderbilt-Ingram Cancer Center, Nashville, TN 37232, USA; [b] Memorial Sloan Kettering Cancer Center, 1275 York Avenue, Box 298, New York, NY 10065, USA
* Corresponding author.
E-mail address: peralesm@MSKCC.ORG

Hematol Oncol Clin N Am 28 (2014) 1097–1112
http://dx.doi.org/10.1016/j.hoc.2014.08.011 **hemonc.theclinics.com**
0889-8588/14/$ – see front matter

INDICATIONS FOR TRANSPLANTATION

ASCT is the standard of care for eligible patients with relapsed HL. Approximately half of these patients are rescued by this regimen intensity.

Current indications of ASCT in HL include the following:

1. HDT/ASCT should be offered to patients as salvage therapy.
2. HDT/ASCT may be offered as first-line therapy for patients who fail to achieve a complete response.

Current indications of allo-SCT in HL include the following:

1. Allo-SCT should be offered to eligible patients who relapse following ASCT

SALVAGE REGIMENS

Several studies have shown the importance of cytoreduction before proceeding with SCT (**Table 1**). There is moderate evidence to support a single best salvage regimen as a recommended treatment option for patients with disease relapse before ASCT. Achieving a complete remission, as defined by the absence of any detectable disease using PET with fludeoxyglucose (FDG-PET) functional imaging before ASCT, has been shown to improve event-free survival (EFS).[10] An ideal salvage regimen should therefore produce a high rate of response, with acceptable toxicity and should not hinder stem cell mobilization. Multiple combination therapies have been evaluated in phase II studies for pretransplantation salvage in patients with relapsed HL. Historically, Europeans have favored aggressive pretransplantation regimens, such as mini-BEAM or Dexa-BEAM (carmustine, etoposide, cytarabine, and melphalan).[3] These regimens are, however, associated with significant treatment-related hematologic toxicities, including 5% treatment-related mortality. In the United States, platinum-based regimens with non–cross-resistant drugs, such as ICE (ifosfamide, carboplatin, and etoposide), ESHAP (etoposide, solumederol, cytarabine, and prednisone), or

Table 1
Commonly used salvage regimens

		Response Rates (%)		
Regimen	**n**	**ORR**	**CR**	**Author**
ICE	65	88	26	Moskowitz et al,[2] 2001
mini-BEAM	55	84	51	Martin et al,[3] 2001
DHAP	102	88	21	Josting et al,[4] 2002
GDP	23	69	17	Baetz et al,[5] 2003
IGEV	91	81	54	Santoro et al,[6] 2007
GND	90	70	19	Bartlett et al,[7] 2007
IVOX	34	76	32	Sibon et al,[8] 2011
GV	31	72	36	Suyani et al,[9] 2011
ICE/aICE GVD	97		60 (ICE) 52 (GVD)	Moskowitz et al,[10] 2012

Abbreviations: aICE, augmented ICE; CR, complete response; DHAP, dexamethasone, cisplatin, cytarabine; GDP, gemcitabine, dexamethasone, cisplatin; GV, gemcitabine, vinorelbine; GV(N)D, gemcitabine, vinorelbine, and pegylated liposomal doxorubicin; ICE, ifosfamide, carboplatin, etoposide; IGEV, ifosfamide, gemcitabine, vinorelbine; IVOX, ifosfamide, etoposide, oxaliplatin; mini-BEAM, carmustine, etoposide, cytarabine, melphalan; ORR, overall response rate.

DHAP (dexamethasone, cytarabine, cisplatin) are preferred. The current salvage regimens induce a complete response (CR) rate of 19%–41% depending on the regimen used.[2,7,11] There are no published randomized trials comparing the effectiveness of combination regimens.

Based on available data and current practice in US centers, we recommend ICE salvage as an effective choice in the absence of randomized studies or in the absence of a clinical trial. Other alternative regimens include gemcitabine-based regimens. It is also important to note that a diagnostic biopsy is mandatory to confirm relapse or progressive disease before salvage treatment.

CONDITIONING REGIMENS

Preparative regimens before ASCT contain a combination of drugs with antilymphoma activity (**Table 2**). Several regimens that include cyclophosphamide, busulfan, etoposide, melphalan, and lymphoid radiation have been widely used as conditioning regimens.[10,12–18] The reported 100-day mortality is approximately 3% to 5%. The later treatment complications specifically in HL are of importance, as patients with HL are relatively younger at diagnosis and are susceptible to cumulative risks of developing secondary malignancies.

ROLE OF FUNCTIONAL IMAGING BEFORE STEM CELL TRANSPLANTATION

FDG-PET is highly sensitive in predicting outcome in HL. PET/computed tomography (CT) performed at the end of initial treatment in advanced HL has a sensitivity of 43% to 100% in discriminating residual lymphoma from fibrotic masses.[19] Therefore, PET/CT is a promising tool for predicting tumor response and progression-free

Table 2
Conditioning regimens for ASCT

			Outcomes (%)				
Regimen	n	TRM (%)	OS	PFS	EFS	2nd Malignancy (%)	Author
TBI/Cy/Et	28	0	61	43		0	Stiff et al,[12] 2003
BCNU/Cy/Et	46	6.5	50	39		2.2	
Total	74	4.1	54	41		1.3	
Bu/Cy/Et	127	5.5	51	48		3.1	Wadhera et al,[13] 2006
TLI/CCE	32		61		63		Evens et al,[14] 2007
CCE	16		27		6		
Total	48	4.2	48		44	4.2	
LACE	67	3	68		64	3.8	Perz et al,[15] 2007
CBV	43	7	57	63	53	2.3	Benekli et al,[16] 2008
Bu/Cy	19	5	41	31		11	Lane et al,[17] 2011
Bu/Mel	49		85		57		Kebriaei et al,[18] 2011
TLI/Cy/Et	56	0	88			1.2	Moskowitz et al,[10] 2012
CBV	29				79	0	
Total	85		88			3.4	

Abbreviations: BCNU, bis-chloroethylnitrosourea; Bu, busulfan; CBV, cyclophosphamide, carmustine, etoposide; CCE, carboplatin, cyclophosphamide, etoposide; Cy, cyclophosphamide; EFS, event-free survival; Et, etoposide; LACE, lomustine, cytarabine, cyclophosphamide and etoposide; Mel, melphalan; OS, overall survival; PFS, progression-free survival; TBI, total body irradiation; TLI, total lymphoid irradiation; TRM, treatment-related mortality.

survival (PFS).[20–22] A few studies have addressed the role of FDG/PET in patients treated with salvage chemotherapy before stem cell transplantation, and have shown improved outcomes in patients who achieve a CR before HDT/ASCT. In a study by Moskowitz and colleagues,[10] patients with pre-ASCT negative PET after 1 or 2 salvage regimens had an EFS greater than 80% as compared with 26% in patients with a positive PET pre-ASCT, highlighting the importance of pre-ASCT negative PET scan. Similarly, Sirohi and colleagues[23] reported that the 5-year PFS and overall survival (OS) were 69% versus 44% and 79% versus 59%, respectively, for patients who were in CR or partial response (PR) at the time of HDT/SCT. Based on the currently available data, we recommend the use of standardized methods (Deauville scoring system) while reporting PET/CT.[24] We favor proceeding with ASCT in patients who achieve a PR and preferably a CR.

AUTOLOGOUS STEM CELL TRANSPLANTATION

Autologous Stem Cell Transplantation at Disease Relapse

The role of HDT/ASCT has been evaluated in both randomized and nonrandomized trials.[25–27] To date, ASCT as salvage for HL has been shown to improve EFS, freedom from treatment failure (FFTF), and PFS, but not OS.[28] Two randomized trials comparing ASCT with conventional chemotherapy have been performed and show similar outcomes. In the study by Schmitz and colleagues,[26] 161 patients with relapsed HL were randomly assigned to 4 cycles of Dexa-BEAM or 2 cycles of Dexa-BEAM followed by ASCT. Only patients with chemosensitive disease following 2 cycles of Dexa-BEAM proceeded to SCT. At a median follow-up of 39 months, the study met the primary end point of FFTF for patients with chemosensitive disease (55% for ASCT cohort vs 34% in chemotherapy cohort, $P = .019$). The British National Lymphoma Investigation performed a prospective study in 40 patients who were randomized to HDT-BEAM followed by ASCT or lower doses of the same regimen (mini-BEAM). This study demonstrated a statistically significant improvement in EFS and PFS (P = .025 and .005, respectively) favoring ASCT.[25] These findings were further supported by the recently published Cochrane meta-analysis.[28]

Autologous Stem Cell Transplantation in Patients After Induction Therapy for Advanced Hodgkin Lymphoma

The inclusion of HDT/SCT in the initial treatment plan in patients with unfavorable HL who achieved CR with conventional chemotherapy was an attractive idea and an area of initial debate.[29] However, results from randomized studies support that ASCT should not be performed as consolidation in patients with high-risk or advanced HL who have attained a CR to induction treatment. The long-term follow-up of a randomized study of 163 patients with unfavorable HL showed a similar 10-year OS of 85% compared with 84% for patients treated with conventional chemotherapy.[30–32] Therefore, based on the current data, ASCT cannot be routinely recommended as consolidation after initial therapy in poor-risk patients with chemoresponsive disease.[33]

Autologous Stem Cell Transplantation in Patients with Induction Failure

Several of the retrospective studies of ASCT for HL have included patients with relapsed disease and patients with primary induction failure. There is an apparent benefit in patients with primary induction failure, with reported PFS of 40% to 45% and OS of 30% to 70%.[12,27,34–38] It should be noted that this indication remains controversial, as it is supported only by retrospective data. Furthermore, as noted previously, these data also precede the introduction of newer agents, such as brentuximab vedotin.

ALLOGENEIC HEMATOPOIETIC STEM CELL TRANSPLANTATION

Allogeneic hematopoietic SCT is a potentially curative treatment for patients with relapsed or refractory HL.[39,40] Initial studies of allo-SCT in patients with HL reported high treatment-related mortality (TRM) and low OS, likely as a result of the use of myeloablative conditioning in a heavily pretreated group of patients.[41–47] In an analysis of 100 patients performed by the Center for International Blood and Marrow Transplant Research (CIBMTR), 3-year OS and disease-free survival (DFS) were 21% and 15%, respectively.[43] Similar outcomes were reported by the European Society for Blood and Marrow Transplantation (EBMT) in a retrospective comparison of myeloablative and reduced-intensity conditioning (RIC).[47] The 5-year OS was 20% in the ablative group and 28% in the RIC group. Patients in the RIC cohort had significantly decreased nonrelapse mortality (NRM) (hazard ratio [HR] 2.85; 95% confidence interval [CI] 1.62–5.02; $P<.001$) and improved OS (HR 2.05; 95% CI 1.27–3.29; $P = .04$). There was also a trend for better PFS in the RIC group (HR 1.53; 95% CI 0.97–2.40; $P = .07$). The data in this retrospective analysis are consistent with improved outcomes and decreased TRM in other prospective and retrospective studies in which patients with HL were transplanted with RIC or nonablative cytoreduction.[47–53] Although registry data from the CIBMTR reported PFS and OS of 30% and 56% at 1 year, and 20% and 37% at 2 years, respectively, in patients with HL receiving reduced-intensity allo-SCT from unrelated donors,[54] single-institution studies typically report better outcomes. Regarding graft source, a recent systematic review concluded that all stem cell sources, including related and unrelated donors, haploidentical donors, and cord blood, were a reasonable consideration for allo-SCT in patients with HL.[55]

Overall, these studies support the role of graft versus lymphoma (GVL) effect after nonmyeloablative allo-SCT in patients with HL. In particular, a number of studies have documented responses to donor lymphocyte infusions (DLIs).[50,52,56] In a study by Peggs and colleagues,[50] the overall response rate (ORR) to DLI for persistent disease or progression in 16 patients was 56% (CR = 8, PR = 1). These results were further supported by a study of the UK Cooperative Group in which the ORR was 79% in 24 patients receiving DLI for relapse (CR = 14, PR = 5).[56] It should be noted that both of these studies used alemtuzumab as part of the conditioning regimen, which results in in vivo T-cell depletion and increased mixed chimerism, for which patients were also given DLI.

Although NRM has decreased with the use of RIC allo-SCT in patients with HL, it does appear to be associated with a higher rate of relapse, although this has not been validated in a prospective randomized study. Nevertheless, relapse remains a significant cause of failure after allo-SCT, and strategies to decrease the risk of relapse, either through preemptive DLI or with the use of post transplant maintenance therapy, as after ASCT, warrant further investigation (**Table 3**).

IMPACT OF PROGNOSTIC FACTORS

Unlike predictive prognostic scores for advanced-stage HL, none of the presumed prognostic factors have been studied in a prospective manner in the setting of SCT. Several prognostic markers, such as age, site of relapse, bulky disease, and performance status, have been reported to influence outcome in patients with relapsed disease.[4,58–60] However, the data are limited to small studies and may therefore be confounded by several factors. The most important predictor of outcome for relapsed disease is the duration of initial remission. In addition, the response to salvage therapy given before ASCT is a major determinant of eventual outcome.

Greaves and colleagues[58] compared early relapse (less than 12 months) with late relapse in 103 patients with relapsed refractory classical Hodgkin lymphoma and found

Table 3
Outcomes of allo-SCT in HL

Reference	n	TRM	Relapse	PFS	OS
Myeloablative					
Anderson et al,[41] 1993	53	58% (4 y)	48% (4 y)	22% (5 y)	21% (5 y)
Gajewski et al,[43] 1996	100	13% (30 d) 61% (3 y)	65% (3 y)	15% (3 y)	21% (3 y)
Milpied et al,[42] 1996	45	31% (100 d) 48% (4 y)	61% (4 y)	15% (4 y)	25% (4 y)
Akpek et al,[44] 2001	53	32% (100 d) 43% (total)	53% (10 y)	26% (10 y)	30% (10 y)
Peniket et al,[45] 2003	167	52% (4 y)	65% (5 y)	16% (4 y)	25% (4 y)
Sureda et al,[47] 2008	79	28 (3 mo) 46 (1 y)	30.4% (5 y)	20% (5 y)	22% (5 y)
Reduced intensity					
Sureda et al,[47] 2008	89	15% (3 mo) 23% (1 y)	57.3% (5 y)	28% (5 y)	18% (5 y)
Robinson et al,[48] 2009	311	17% (100 d) 24% (1 y) 27% (2 y)	48% (1 y) 64% (2 y)	26% (2 y)	46% (2 y)
Devetten et al,[54] 2009	143	33% (2 y)	47% (2 y)	20% (2 y)	37% (2 y)
Peggs et al,[50] 2005	49	4% (100 d) 16% (2 y)	43%	32% (4 y)	55% (4 y)
Burroughs et al,[49] 2008	90 RD 38 UD 24 Haplo 28	200 d 16% 0 0	2 y 56% 63% 40%	2 y 23% 29% 51%	2 y 53% 58% 58%
Alvarez et al,[53] 2006	40	12% (100 d) 25% (1 y)	NA	32% (2 y)	48% (2 y)
Anderlini et al,[52] 2005	40	5% (100 d) 22% (18 mo)	55% (18 mo)	32% (18 mo)	61% (18 mo)
Sureda et al,[57] 2012	78	8% (100 d) 15% (1 y)	59% (4 y)	24% (4 y)	43% (4 y)

Abbreviations: allo-SCT, allogeneic stem cell transplantation; Haplo, haplo-identical donor; HL, Hodgkin lymphoma; OS, overall survival; PFS, progression-free survival; RD, related donor; TRM, treatment-related mortality; UD, unrelated donor.

that the 5-year OS was 50% for patients with early relapse compared with 73% for patients with late relapse ($P = .012$). However, in patients who responded to salvage treatment and received HDT/ACT, there was no difference in OS, suggesting that patients with early relapse or failure to first-line treatment remain a population with poor prognosis, thus highlighting the need for more effective salvage for regimens for patients with early relapse.[58,59] In a study of 187 patients with relapsed HL, Brice and colleagues[60] identified 2 prognostic factors associated with outcome in a multivariate analysis: duration of first remission (<12 months) and stage at relapse. Finally, in the large German Hodgkin Lymphoma Study Group (GHSG) study, which included 422 patients with early (n = 170) or late (n = 252) relapsed HL, the duration of first remission, stage at relapse, and anemia (variable by gender) were assigned a scoring system and associated with outcome. Patients with all 3 risk factors had an OS of 27% compared with 83% in patients without any risk factors.[4]

Chemosensitivity before undergoing stem cell transplantation has also been shown to predict outcome.[61–63] Patients who achieve a CR have a better outcome with ASCT compared with those who achieve a PR.[61] In a multivariate analysis reported by Sureda and colleagues,[62] the presence of active disease at transplantation or having received 2 or more lines of therapy before ASCT were adverse prognostic factors for outcome. Similar results were reported in another retrospective study in which patients who received 3 or more lines of therapy and had less than a PR were associated with risk of disease relapse after ASCT.[63]

There is a paucity of data regarding prognostic factors after ASCT. A retrospective analysis of 511 adult patients with relapsed HL after ASCT from EBMT-Gruppo Italiano Trapianto di Midollo Osseo (GITMO) databases reported an OS of 32% at 5 years after a median follow-up of 49 months.[64] Most patients (64%) were treated with chemotherapy and/or radiotherapy, whereas 29% had an allo-SCT and 8% a second ASCT. The authors identified the following risk factors for OS: relapse less than 6 months after ASCT, stage IV, bulky disease, poor performance status, and age ≥50 years at relapse. Patients with no risk factors had OS at 5 years of 62%, whereas those with 1 and ≥2 factors had 5-year OS of 37% and 12%, respectively.

In summary, prognostic factors play an important role in identifying the poor-risk group and we therefore recommend incorporating such factors when designing clinical trials. When evaluating prognostic factors in HL, it is, however, important to note that most of the patients included in these studies received the intended procedure; in this case, ASCT. This can therefore lead to a bias of positive selection, which would be corrected by evaluating patients at the time of relapse on an intent-to-treat basis. In particular, patients with primary refractory HL who received salvage chemotherapy had a poor outcome, suggesting that primary refractory patients undergo considerable selection bias and a significant proportion of patients did not receive ASCT because of progressive disease.[65]

POST TRANSPLANTATION DISEASE MONITORING

There are no recommended guidelines for monitoring patients after SCT for HL. For monitoring of disease relapse, we do not recommend routine surveillance PET scan after documentation of complete remission. After completion of the treatment plan with high-dose therapy, routine surveillance studies with CT scan alone may be sufficient for disease monitoring for the first 2 years after therapy. Such imaging should not be performed any more frequently than every 6 to 12 months in an asymptomatic patient. In a recent retrospective study, 241 patients either had routine imaging studies performed at follow-up intervals or were monitored clinically after achieving a first CR. At 5-year follow-up, there was no difference in OS in these 2 groups, suggesting that patients following completion of therapy for HL can be monitored by clinical signs and symptoms alone.[66]

MANAGEMENT OF RELAPSES AFTER TRANSPLANTATION

Salvage options following an ASCT include consideration of radiation alone, allo-SCT, monoclonal antibodies, and other novel agents.[67] We do not recommend consideration of a second ASCT in patients who relapse after HDT/ASCT. Patients who relapse after ASCT may still be cured by an allo-SCT. Although myeloablative allo-SCT may have higher cure rates, it has been associated with increased toxicities and risk of TRM. As a result, as noted previously, RIC allo-SCT is a preferred approach because of its lower TRM. In patients who relapse after ASCT and who are not candidates for allo-SCT, achieving a cure is highly unlikely. The treatment plan offered in this situation is often not curative. Several novel agents show encouraging results, but unfortunately such responses are often short lived.

NOVEL THERAPIES AND THEIR INTEGRATION IN TRANSPLANTATION

For patients relapsing after HDT/ASCT who are not candidates for an allo-SCT or for those who relapse after allo-SCT, alternative treatment options include consideration of conventional chemotherapy/or novel agents.

Targeted Antibodies

Several monoclonal antibodies have been studied in patients with relapsed/refractory HL. To date, only one monoclonal antibody, brentuximab-vedotin, has been approved for use in patients with relapsed refractory HL.

Brentuximab vedotin

Brentuximab vedotin (BV) is an antibody drug conjugate that consists of a chimeric anti-CD30 antibody. In a large single-arm phase II study, 102 heavily pretreated patients with relapsed disease after ASCT were treated at a dose of 1.8 mg/kg administered every 3 weeks.[68] The ORR was 75%, with 34% of patients experiencing a complete remission. The median PFS and OS were 5.6 months and 22.4 months, respectively. BV enabled a few patients to proceed to allo-SCT.[69] BV was also found to be effective in patients who relapse after ASCT with a 50% ORR and a median PFS of 7.8 months.[70] A maintenance study evaluating the efficacy and safety of BV compared with placebo in patients at high risk of residual disease after ASCT has completed accrual and the results are pending (NCT01100502). BV is also being investigated in earlier lines of treatment in patients with HL, and in particular in 2 ongoing studies that incorporate BV in the salvage setting before ASCT (NCT01508312, NCT01393717).

Bendamustine

Bendamustine is a bifunctional alkylating agent with partial cross-resistance to other alkylating agents. In a phase 2 study by Moskowitz and colleagues,[71] patients with relapsed and refractory HL who were in eligible for ASCT received bendamustine at a dose of 120 mg/m^2 on days 1 and 2 every 28 days. Of the 36 patients enrolled, 12 patients experienced a CR. The ORR was 53%. Responses were also noted in patients who had disease relapse following ASCT. Thus, bendamustine appears to be a promising agent for patients with disease relapse after SCT.

Novel Agents

This term applies to drugs that specifically target a cell pathway. Most of these agents have shown only modest activity as single agents. However, combinations of these agents may hold promise by targeting different pathways that are dysregulated.

Histone deacetylase inhibitors

Histone deacetylase inhibitors play a crucial in interfering with cell proliferation and cell cycles that function as driving forces in several malignancies, including HL. Panobinostat, a potent Histone deacetylases (HDAC) inhibitor that was evaluated in a phase 2 study in patients with relapsed refractory HL, demonstrated encouraging clinical activity with an ORR of 27% and a median PFS of 6.1 months.[72] Panobinostat was also evaluated in a phase 3 trial as a maintenance therapy after HDT but was closed due to accrual.

Farnesyl transferase inhibitors

Farnesyl transferase inhibitors are a class of drugs that induce apoptosis and diminish cell proliferation. Nineteen patients with relapsed HL were included in a phase 2 study of tipifarnib. The ORR was 21% and 2 patients achieved a CR. The median OS was

14.8 months. Although the single-agent activity is modest, patients would likely benefit from a combination of these novel agents.[73]

Immunomodulators

Lenalidomide is an *immunomodulatory agent* with activity in myeloma and Non-Hodgkin lymphoma (NHL). This drug was evaluated in a phase 2 study in 38 patients with relapsed refractory HL who had undergone prior SCT. Only modest responses were reported in the study, with 1 patient achieving a CR and 6 patients achieving a PR.[74]

Check-point blockade drugs

PD-L1 expression has been identified on Hodgkin Reed-Sternberg cells,[75,76] making Hodgkin a potential target for antibodies targeting PD-1. Nivolumab (BMS-936558) is a monoclonal anti-PD-1 antibody currently being studied in hematologic malignancies, including patients with relapsed HL (NCT02181738), and recently received Food and Drug Administration Breakthrough Therapy Designation for this indication.

LONG-TERM FOLLOW-UP

As there are few data available on the follow-up and monitoring of late effects in patients with HL, the follow-up schedule is highly individualized and the treating physician should be vigilant about the treatment delivered to the patient and be aware of the risk of late complications, including secondary cancers and cardiovascular disease, particularly in patients with HL who have had previous radiation therapy. Patients also should be educated on the risk of long-term effects and receive appropriate counseling.[77] The general guidelines on monitoring secondary effects of treatment are described in the paragraph that follow.

Secondary Malignancies and Myelodysplastic Syndrome

The risk of secondary solid tumor malignancies has been reported in patients receiving extended fields of radiation. Combined modality treatments are associated with gastrointestinal malignancies and lung and breast cancer, with lung and breast cancer being the most common secondary cancers in patients with HL.[78] Annual breast screening, beginning no later than 8 to 10 years after completion of therapy or at age 40, is recommended for women who receive chest/axillary radiation. Smoking cessation should be reinforced to reduce the risk of lung cancer and chest imaging may be considered in a select group of patients.[79,80] Patients receiving intensive induction chemotherapy regimens, pelvic radiation, and/or ASCT are at an increased risk of developing secondary hematological malignancies, such as myelodysplastic syndrome and/or secondary acute leukemia.[81] Routine follow-up also should include monitoring complete blood counts.

Endocrine Disorders

Patients who received radiation therapy to the neck should be screened annually with thyroid function tests to assess for hypothyroidism. Gonadal function and fertility in survivors of HL allows for risk-adapted fertility preservation during therapy and in follow-up.[82,83]

Cardiopulmonary Toxicity

Radiation-induced cardiotoxicity is observed following the median of 5 to 10 years posttreatment. Aggressive management of cardiovascular risk reduction factors is highly recommended. In patients who have received radiation therapy to the neck, a carotid ultrasound should be considered. The history of use of bleomycin treatment and radiation to the mediastinum is associated with increased pulmonary toxicity. After SCT with the above risk factors patients should be counseled extensively on smoking cessation.[84–86]

SUMMARY

To summarize, we recommend the following:

1. ASCT should be offered to patients who fail to respond to initial treatment and/or as salvage therapy
2. Patients who relapse early (<12 months) after initial therapy are biologically a poor prognostic group
3. A negative functional imaging (PET) before transplantation is associated with improved outcome
4. RIC allo-SCT should be offered for patients who relapse after ASCT

Patients with chemosensitive disease (ie, responding to second-line chemotherapy), appear to have a much better outcome than patients with refractory disease. Functional imaging (PET/CT) plays an important role as a prognostic tool. Patients who are PET positive at the end of induction therapy appear to be the worst predictors of outcome. With the relatively high rates of cure that can be achieved in HL, the focus of initial therapy has recently shifted toward decreasing toxicity while improving remission rates by incorporating novel agents. As newer agents that target pathways such as PI3-kinase, histone deacetylase, programmed death ligand, or immunomodulators and monoclonal antibodies show efficacy in HL, the role and timing of SCT becomes even more complex. Incorporating these agents as a maintenance strategy after ASCT is certainly attractive. We believe that future clinical trials should aim to consider these novel agents in the peritransplant and post transplant periods.

REFERENCES

1. Siegel R, Ma J, Zou Z, et al. Cancer statistics, 2014. CA Cancer J Clin 2014; 64(1):9–29.
2. Moskowitz CH, Nimer SD, Zelenetz AD, et al. A 2-step comprehensive high-dose chemoradiotherapy second-line program for relapsed and refractory Hodgkin disease: analysis by intent to treat and development of a prognostic model. Blood 2001;97(3):616–23.
3. Martin A, Fernandez-Jimenez MC, Caballero MD, et al. Long-term follow-up in patients treated with Mini-BEAM as salvage therapy for relapsed or refractory Hodgkin's disease. Br J Haematol 2001;113(1):161–71.
4. Josting A, Franklin J, May M, et al. New prognostic score based on treatment outcome of patients with relapsed Hodgkin's lymphoma registered in the database of the German Hodgkin's lymphoma study group. J Clin Oncol 2002;20(1): 221–30.
5. Baetz T, Belch A, Couban S, et al. Gemcitabine, dexamethasone and cisplatin is an active and non-toxic chemotherapy regimen in relapsed or refractory Hodgkin's disease: a phase II study by the National Cancer Institute of Canada Clinical Trials Group. Ann Oncol 2003;14(12):1762–7.
6. Santoro A, Magagnoli M, Spina M, et al. Ifosfamide, gemcitabine, and vinorelbine: a new induction regimen for refractory and relapsed Hodgkin's lymphoma. Haematologica 2007;92(1):35–41.

7. Bartlett NL, Niedzwiecki D, Johnson JL, et al. Gemcitabine, vinorelbine, and pegylated liposomal doxorubicin (GVD), a salvage regimen in relapsed Hodgkin's lymphoma: CALGB 59804. Ann Oncol 2007;18(6):1071–9.
8. Sibon D, Ertault M, Al Nawakil C, et al. Combined ifosfamide, etoposide and oxaliplatin chemotherapy, a low-toxicity regimen for first-relapsed or refractory Hodgkin lymphoma after ABVD/EBVP: a prospective monocentre study on 34 patients. Br J Haematol 2011;153(2):191–8.
9. Suyani E, Sucak GT, Aki SZ, et al. Gemcitabine and vinorelbine combination is effective in both as a salvage and mobilization regimen in relapsed or refractory Hodgkin lymphoma prior to ASCT. Ann Hematol 2011;90(6):685–91.
10. Moskowitz CH, Matasar MJ, Zelenetz AD, et al. Normalization of pre-ASCT, FDG-PET imaging with second-line, non-cross-resistant, chemotherapy programs improves event-free survival in patients with Hodgkin lymphoma. Blood 2012;119(7):1665–70.
11. Aparicio J, Segura A, Garcera S, et al. ESHAP is an active regimen for relapsing Hodgkin's disease. Ann Oncol 1999;10(5):593–5.
12. Stiff PJ, Unger JM, Forman SJ, et al. The value of augmented preparative regimens combined with an autologous bone marrow transplant for the management of relapsed or refractory Hodgkin disease: a Southwest Oncology Group phase II trial. Biol Blood Marrow Transplant 2003;9(8):529–39.
13. Wadehra N, Farag S, Bolwell B, et al. Long-term outcome of Hodgkin disease patients following high-dose busulfan, etoposide, cyclophosphamide, and autologous stem cell transplantation. Biol Blood Marrow Transplant 2006; 12(12):1343–9.
14. Evens AM, Altman JK, Mittal BB, et al. Phase I/II trial of total lymphoid irradiation and high-dose chemotherapy with autologous stem-cell transplantation for relapsed and refractory Hodgkin's lymphoma. Ann Oncol 2007;18(4): 679–88.
15. Perz JB, Giles C, Szydlo R, et al. LACE-conditioned autologous stem cell transplantation for relapsed or refractory Hodgkin's lymphoma: treatment outcome and risk factor analysis in 67 patients from a single centre. Bone Marrow Transplant 2007;39(1):41–7.
16. Benekli M, Smiley SL, Younis T, et al. Intensive conditioning regimen of etoposide (VP-16), cyclophosphamide and carmustine (VCB) followed by autologous hematopoietic stem cell transplantation for relapsed and refractory Hodgkin's lymphoma. Bone Marrow Transplant 2008;41(7):613–9.
17. Lane AA, McAfee SL, Kennedy J, et al. High-dose chemotherapy with busulfan and cyclophosphamide and autologous stem cell rescue in patients with Hodgkin lymphoma. Leuk Lymphoma 2011;52(7):1363–6.
18. Kebriaei P, Madden T, Kazerooni R, et al. Intravenous busulfan plus melphalan is a highly effective, well-tolerated preparative regimen for autologous stem cell transplantation in patients with advanced lymphoid malignancies. Biol Blood Marrow Transplant 2011;17(3):412–20.
19. Terasawa T, Nihashi T, Hotta T, et al. 18F-FDG PET for posttherapy assessment of Hodgkin's disease and aggressive Non-Hodgkin's lymphoma: a systematic review. J Nucl Med 2008;49(1):13–21.
20. Hutchings M, Loft A, Hansen M, et al. FDG-PET after two cycles of chemotherapy predicts treatment failure and progression-free survival in Hodgkin lymphoma. Blood 2006;107(1):52–9.
21. Gallamini A, Rigacci L, Merli F, et al. The predictive value of positron emission tomography scanning performed after two courses of standard therapy on

treatment outcome in advanced stage Hodgkin's disease. Haematologica 2006; 91(4):475–81.
22. Zinzani PL, Rigacci L, Stefoni V, et al. Early interim 18F-FDG PET in Hodgkin's lymphoma: evaluation on 304 patients. Eur J Nucl Med Mol Imaging 2012; 39(1):4–12.
23. Sirohi B, Cunningham D, Powles R, et al. Long-term outcome of autologous stem-cell transplantation in relapsed or refractory Hodgkin's lymphoma. Ann Oncol 2008;19(7):1312–9.
24. Biggi A, Gallamini A, Chauvie S, et al. International validation study for interim PET in ABVD-treated, advanced-stage Hodgkin lymphoma: interpretation criteria and concordance rate among reviewers. J Nucl Med 2013;54(5):683–90.
25. Linch DC, Winfield D, Goldstone AH, et al. Dose intensification with autologous bone-marrow transplantation in relapsed and resistant Hodgkin's disease: results of a BNLI randomised trial. Lancet 1993;341(8852):1051–4.
26. Schmitz N, Pfistner B, Sextro M, et al. Aggressive conventional chemotherapy compared with high-dose chemotherapy with autologous haemopoietic stem-cell transplantation for relapsed chemosensitive Hodgkin's disease: a randomised trial. Lancet 2002;359(9323):2065–71.
27. Ferme C, Mounier N, Divine M, et al. Intensive salvage therapy with high-dose chemotherapy for patients with advanced Hodgkin's disease in relapse or failure after initial chemotherapy: results of the Groupe d'Etudes des Lymphomes de l'Adulte H89 Trial. J Clin Oncol 2002;20(2):467–75.
28. Rancea M, von Tresckow B, Monsef I, et al. High-dose chemotherapy followed by autologous stem cell transplantation for patients with relapsed or refractory Hodgkin lymphoma: a systematic review with meta-analysis. Crit Rev Oncol Hematol 2014;44(8):771–8.
29. Carella AM, Carlier P, Congiu A, et al. Autologous bone marrow transplantation as adjuvant treatment for high-risk Hodgkin's disease in first complete remission after MOPP/ABVD protocol. Bone Marrow Transplant 1991;8(2):99–103.
30. Carella AM, Bellei M, Brice P, et al. High-dose therapy and autologous stem cell transplantation versus conventional therapy for patients with advanced Hodgkin's lymphoma responding to front-line therapy: long-term results. Haematologica 2009;94(1):146–8.
31. Arakelyan N, Berthou C, Desablens B, et al. Early versus late intensification for patients with high-risk Hodgkin lymphoma—3 cycles of intensive chemotherapy plus low-dose lymph node radiation therapy versus 4 cycles of combined doxorubicin, bleomycin, vinblastine, and dacarbazine plus myeloablative chemotherapy with autologous stem cell transplantation: five-year results of a randomized trial on behalf of the GOELAMS Group. Cancer 2008;113(12): 3323–30.
32. Federico M, Bellei M, Brice P, et al. High-dose therapy and autologous stem-cell transplantation versus conventional therapy for patients with advanced Hodgkin's lymphoma responding to front-line therapy. J Clin Oncol 2003;21(12): 2320–5.
33. Reece DE, Sureda A. High dose therapy and autologous stem cell transplant does not improve survival compared with continued combination chemotherapy in people at high risk of relapse after initial treatment of advanced Hodgkin's lymphoma. Cancer Treat Rev 2003;29(6):555–9.
34. Viviani S, Zinzani PL, Rambaldi A, et al. ABVD versus BEACOPP for Hodgkin's lymphoma when high-dose salvage is planned. N Engl J Med 2011;365(3): 203–12.

35. Lavoie JC, Connors JM, Phillips GL, et al. High-dose chemotherapy and autologous stem cell transplantation for primary refractory or relapsed Hodgkin lymphoma: long-term outcome in the first 100 patients treated in Vancouver. Blood 2005;106(4):1473–8.
36. Tarella C, Cuttica A, Vitolo U, et al. High-dose sequential chemotherapy and peripheral blood progenitor cell autografting in patients with refractory and/or recurrent Hodgkin lymphoma: a multicenter study of the intergruppo Italiano Linfomi showing prolonged disease free survival in patients treated at first recurrence. Cancer 2003;97(11):2748–59.
37. Vigouroux S, Milpied N, Andrieu JM, et al. Front-line high-dose therapy with autologous stem cell transplantation for high risk Hodgkin's disease: comparison with combined-modality therapy. Bone Marrow Transplant 2002;29(10):833–42.
38. Czyz J, Szydlo R, Knopinska-Posluszny W, et al. Treatment for primary refractory Hodgkin's disease: a comparison of high-dose chemotherapy followed by ASCT with conventional therapy. Bone Marrow Transplant 2004;33(12):1225–9.
39. Anderlini P, Champlin RE. Reduced intensity conditioning for allogeneic stem cell transplantation in relapsed and refractory Hodgkin lymphoma: where do we stand? Biol Blood Marrow Transplant 2006;12(6):599–602.
40. Sureda A, Domenech E, Schmitz N, et al. The role of allogeneic stem cell transplantation in Hodgkin's lymphoma. Curr Treat Options Oncol 2014;15(2):238–47.
41. Anderson JE, Litzow MR, Appelbaum FR, et al. Allogeneic, syngeneic, and autologous marrow transplantation for Hodgkin's disease: the 21-year Seattle experience. J Clin Oncol 1993;11(12):2342–50.
42. Milpied N, Fielding AK, Pearce RM, et al. Allogeneic bone marrow transplant is not better than autologous transplant for patients with relapsed Hodgkin's disease. European Group for Blood and Bone Marrow Transplantation. J Clin Oncol 1996;14(4):1291–6.
43. Gajewski JL, Phillips GL, Sobocinski KA, et al. Bone marrow transplants from HLA-identical siblings in advanced Hodgkin's disease. J Clin Oncol 1996;14(2):572–8.
44. Akpek G, Ambinder RF, Piantadosi S, et al. Long-term results of blood and marrow transplantation for Hodgkin's lymphoma. J Clin Oncol 2001;19(23):4314–21.
45. Peniket AJ, Ruiz de Elvira MC, Taghipour G, et al. An EBMT registry matched study of allogeneic stem cell transplants for lymphoma: allogeneic transplantation is associated with a lower relapse rate but a higher procedure-related mortality rate than autologous transplantation. Bone Marrow Transplant 2003;31(8):667–78.
46. Jones RJ, Piantadosi S, Mann RB, et al. High-dose cytotoxic therapy and bone marrow transplantation for relapsed Hodgkin's disease. J Clin Oncol 1990;8(3):527–37.
47. Sureda A, Robinson S, Canals C, et al. Reduced-intensity conditioning compared with conventional allogeneic stem-cell transplantation in relapsed or refractory Hodgkin's lymphoma: an analysis from the Lymphoma Working Party of the European Group for Blood and Marrow Transplantation. J Clin Oncol 2008;26(3):455–62.
48. Robinson SP, Sureda A, Canals C, et al. Reduced intensity conditioning allogeneic stem cell transplantation for Hodgkin's lymphoma: identification of prognostic factors predicting outcome. Haematologica 2009;94(2):230–8.

49. Burroughs LM, O'Donnell PV, Sandmaier BM, et al. Comparison of outcomes of HLA-matched related, unrelated, or HLA-haploidentical related hematopoietic cell transplantation following nonmyeloablative conditioning for relapsed or refractory Hodgkin lymphoma. Biol Blood Marrow Transplant 2008;14(11):1279–87.
50. Peggs KS, Hunter A, Chopra R, et al. Clinical evidence of a graft-versus-Hodgkin's-lymphoma effect after reduced-intensity allogeneic transplantation. Lancet 2005;365(9475):1934–41.
51. Carella AM, Cavaliere M, Lerma E, et al. Autografting followed by nonmyeloablative immunosuppressive chemotherapy and allogeneic peripheral-blood hematopoietic stem-cell transplantation as treatment of resistant Hodgkin's disease and non-Hodgkin's lymphoma. J Clin Oncol 2000;18(23):3918–24.
52. Anderlini P, Saliba R, Acholonu S, et al. Reduced-intensity allogeneic stem cell transplantation in relapsed and refractory Hodgkin's disease: low transplant-related mortality and impact of intensity of conditioning regimen. Bone Marrow Transplant 2005;35(10):943–51.
53. Alvarez I, Sureda A, Caballero MD, et al. Nonmyeloablative stem cell transplantation is an effective therapy for refractory or relapsed Hodgkin lymphoma: results of a Spanish prospective cooperative protocol. Biol Blood Marrow Transplant 2006;12(2):172–83.
54. Devetten MP, Hari PN, Carreras J, et al. Unrelated donor reduced-intensity allogeneic hematopoietic stem cell transplantation for relapsed and refractory Hodgkin lymphoma. Biol Blood Marrow Transplant 2009;15(1):109–17.
55. Messer M, Steinzen A, Vervolgyi E, et al. Unrelated and alternative donor allogeneic stem cell transplant in patients with relapsed or refractory Hodgkin lymphoma: a systematic review. Leuk Lymphoma 2014;55(2):296–306.
56. Peggs KS, Kayani I, Edwards N, et al. Donor lymphocyte infusions modulate relapse risk in mixed chimeras and induce durable salvage in relapsed patients after T-cell-depleted allogeneic transplantation for Hodgkin's lymphoma. J Clin Oncol 2011;29(8):971–8.
57. Sureda A, Canals C, Arranz R, et al. Allogeneic stem cell transplantation after reduced intensity conditioning in patients with relapsed or refractory Hodgkin's lymphoma. Results of the HDR-ALLO study—a prospective clinical trial by the Grupo Espanol de Linfomas/Trasplante de Medula Osea (GEL/TAMO) and the Lymphoma Working Party of the European Group for Blood and Marrow Transplantation. Haematologica 2012;97(2):310–7.
58. Greaves P, Wilson A, Matthews J, et al. Early relapse and refractory disease remain risk factors in the anthracycline and autologous transplant era for patients with relapsed/refractory classical Hodgkin lymphoma: a single centre intention-to-treat analysis. Br J Haematol 2012;157(2):201–4.
59. Engelhardt BG, Holland DW, Brandt SJ, et al. High-dose chemotherapy followed by autologous stem cell transplantation for relapsed or refractory Hodgkin lymphoma: prognostic features and outcomes. Leuk Lymphoma 2007;48(9):1728–35.
60. Brice P, Bastion Y, Divine M, et al. Analysis of prognostic factors after the first relapse of Hodgkin's disease in 187 patients. Cancer 1996;78(6):1293–9.
61. Popat U, Hosing C, Saliba RM, et al. Prognostic factors for disease progression after high-dose chemotherapy and autologous hematopoietic stem cell transplantation for recurrent or refractory Hodgkin's lymphoma. Bone Marrow Transplant 2004;33(10):1015–23.
62. Sureda A, Arranz R, Iriondo A, et al. Autologous stem-cell transplantation for Hodgkin's disease: results and prognostic factors in 494 patients from the

Grupo Espanol de Linfomas/Transplante Autologo de Medula Osea Spanish Cooperative Group. J Clin Oncol 2001;19(5):1395–404.
63. Czyz J, Dziadziuszko R, Knopinska-Postuszuy W, et al. Outcome and prognostic factors in advanced Hodgkin's disease treated with high-dose chemotherapy and autologous stem cell transplantation: a study of 341 patients. Ann Oncol 2004;15(8):1222–30.
64. Martinez C, Canals C, Sarina B, et al. Identification of prognostic factors predicting outcome in Hodgkin's lymphoma patients relapsing after autologous stem cell transplantation. Ann Oncol 2013;24(9):2430–4.
65. Akhtar S, El Weshi A, Abdelsalam M, et al. Primary refractory Hodgkin's lymphoma: outcome after high-dose chemotherapy and autologous SCT and impact of various prognostic factors on overall and event-free survival. A single institution result of 66 patients. Bone Marrow Transplant 2007;40(7):651–8.
66. Pingali SR, Jewell SW, Havlat L, et al. Limited utility of routine surveillance imaging for classical Hodgkin lymphoma patients in first complete remission. Cancer 2014;120(14):2122–9.
67. Moskowitz AJ, Perales MA, Kewalramani T, et al. Outcomes for patients who fail high dose chemoradiotherapy and autologous stem cell rescue for relapsed and primary refractory Hodgkin lymphoma. Br J Haematol 2009; 146(2):158–63.
68. Younes A, Gopal AK, Smith SE, et al. Results of a pivotal phase II study of brentuximab vedotin for patients with relapsed or refractory Hodgkin's lymphoma. J Clin Oncol 2012;30(18):2183–9.
69. Chen R, Palmer JM, Thomas SH, et al. Brentuximab vedotin enables successful reduced-intensity allogeneic hematopoietic cell transplantation in patients with relapsed or refractory Hodgkin lymphoma. Blood 2012;119(26):6379–81.
70. Gopal AK, Ramchandren R, O'Connor OA, et al. Safety and efficacy of brentuximab vedotin for Hodgkin lymphoma recurring after allogeneic stem cell transplantation. Blood 2012;120(3):560–8.
71. Moskowitz AJ, Hamlin PA Jr, Perales MA, et al. Phase II study of bendamustine in relapsed and refractory Hodgkin lymphoma. J Clin Oncol 2013;31(4):456–60.
72. Younes A, Sureda A, Ben-Yehuda D, et al. Panobinostat in patients with relapsed/refractory hodgkin's lymphoma after autologous stem-cell transplantation: results of a phase II study. J Clin Oncol 2012;30(18):2197–203.
73. Witzig TE, Tang H, Micallef IN, et al. Multi-institutional phase 2 study of the farnesyltransferase inhibitor tipifarnib (R115777) in patients with relapsed and refractory lymphomas. Blood 2011;118(18):4882–9.
74. Fehniger TA, Larson S, Trinkaus K, et al. A phase 2 multicenter study of lenalidomide in relapsed or refractory classical Hodgkin lymphoma. Blood 2011; 118(19):5119–25.
75. Green MR, Monti S, Rodig SJ, et al. Integrative analysis reveals selective 9p24.1 amplification, increased PD-1 ligand expression, and further induction via JAK2 in nodular sclerosing Hodgkin lymphoma and primary mediastinal large B-cell lymphoma. Blood 2010;116(17):3268–77.
76. Green MR, Rodig S, Juszczynski P, et al. Constitutive AP-1 activity and EBV infection induce PD-L1 in Hodgkin lymphomas and posttransplant lymphoproliferative disorders: implications for targeted therapy. Clin Cancer Res 2012; 18(6):1611–8.
77. Hoppe RT, Advani RH, Ai WZ, et al. Hodgkin lymphoma, version 2.2012 featured updates to the NCCN guidelines. J Natl Compr Canc Netw 2012; 10(5):589–97.

78. van Eggermond AM, Schaapveld M, Lugtenburg PJ, et al. Risk of multiple primary malignancies following treatment of Hodgkin lymphoma. Blood 2014;124(3):319–27.
79. Swerdlow AJ, Higgins CD, Smith P, et al. Second cancer risk after chemotherapy for Hodgkin's lymphoma: a collaborative British cohort study. J Clin Oncol 2011;29(31):4096–104.
80. Franklin J, Pluetschow A, Paus M, et al. Second malignancy risk associated with treatment of Hodgkin's lymphoma: meta-analysis of the randomised trials. Ann Oncol 2006;17(12):1749–60.
81. Engert A, Diehl V, Franklin J, et al. Escalated-dose BEACOPP in the treatment of patients with advanced-stage Hodgkin's lymphoma: 10 years of follow-up of the GHSG HD9 study. J Clin Oncol 2009;27(27):4548–54.
82. Behringer K, Mueller H, Goergen H, et al. Gonadal function and fertility in survivors after Hodgkin lymphoma treatment within the German Hodgkin Study Group HD13 to HD15 trials. J Clin Oncol 2013;31(2):231–9.
83. Greaves P, Sarker SJ, Chowdhury K, et al. Fertility and sexual function in long-term survivors of haematological malignancy: using patient-reported outcome measures to assess a neglected area of need in the late effects clinic. Br J Haematol 2014;164(4):526–35.
84. Heidenreich PA, Hancock SL, Lee BK, et al. Asymptomatic cardiac disease following mediastinal irradiation. J Am Coll Cardiol 2003;42(4):743–9.
85. Adams MJ, Lipsitz SR, Colan SD, et al. Cardiovascular status in long-term survivors of Hodgkin's disease treated with chest radiotherapy. J Clin Oncol 2004;22(15):3139–48.
86. Aleman BM, van den Belt-Dusebout AW, De Bruin ML, et al. Late cardiotoxicity after treatment for Hodgkin lymphoma. Blood 2007;109(5):1878–86.

Multiple Myeloma

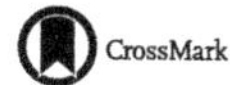

Sarah A. Holstein, MD, PhD, Hong Liu, MD, PhD,
Philip L. McCarthy, MD*

KEYWORDS

- Immunomodulatory agents • Proteasome inhibitors • Maintenance therapy
- Reduced-intensity conditioning

KEY POINTS

- Patients eligible for high-dose therapy typically undergo induction therapy followed by upfront autologous stem cell transplant. Whether transplant can be delayed until time of first relapse with equivalent long-term outcomes is currently under study.
- Single-agent high-dose melphalan remains the standard of care for the high-dose regimen for autologous stem cell transplant.
- Reduced-intensity conditioning regimens for allogeneic transplant have improved transplant-related mortality rates, but disease relapse, graft-versus-host disease, and treatment-related mortality remain significant problems.
- Salvage autologous stem cell transplant is feasible and seems to be most effective for patients who have relapse at least 18 months or later from their initial transplant.
- The therapeutic landscape for myeloma is evolving rapidly, impacting both pre- and post-transplant treatment strategies.

INTRODUCTION

Induction therapy followed by consolidation with high-dose melphalan and autologous stem cell transplant (ASCT) has been considered the standard of care for transplant-eligible myeloma patients for several decades. The role of allogeneic stem cell transplant (AlloSCT) has been less clear, as both myeloablative and reduced-intensity approaches have been fraught with transplant-related mortality, graft versus host disease (GvHD), and disease relapse. In today's era of novel agents, which include the immunomodulatory agents (thalidomide, lenalidomide, pomalidomide) and proteasome inhibitors (bortezomib and carfilzomib), several unanswered questions remain regarding the role of transplant. These unresolved issues include the timing of initial transplant (upfront after induction therapy vs delayed until time of first relapse or later), the incorporation of novel agents into the high-dose regimen, the optimal maintenance regimen after transplant, the role of novel agents versus salvage (second) transplant after relapse from the first transplant, and the role of AlloSCT. In this article we provide an overview of transplantation for myeloma and discuss the areas that remain under active investigation.

Department of Medicine, Roswell Park Cancer Institute, Elm and Carlton Streets, Buffalo, NY 14263, USA
* Corresponding author.
E-mail address: philip.mccarthy@roswellpark.org

Hematol Oncol Clin N Am 28 (2014) 1113–1129
http://dx.doi.org/10.1016/j.hoc.2014.08.010 **hemonc.theclinics.com**
0889-8588/14/$ – see front matter

PATIENT EVALUATION OVERVIEW

As denoted in **Table 1**, the standard pretransplant evaluation includes assessment of organ function, infectious disease status, psychosocial status, and myeloma restaging. Human leukocyte antigen (HLA) typing is performed for patients being considered for AlloSCT and possibly for younger patients being considered for autologous stem cell transplant who could potentially be offered AlloSCT in the future.

INDICATIONS FOR TRANSPLANT

Traditionally, all patients younger than 65 years with adequate organ function and performance status and who have achieved disease control have been considered candidates for ASCT. Most transplant centers in the United States, however, will perform transplants on patients up to the age 75, and some centers have no age limit but instead rely on performance status and adequate organ function. Multiple studies have shown the feasibility and efficacy of performing ASCT in elderly patients.[1–5] The role of AlloSCT in myeloma continues to be debated.[6] Outside of a clinical trial, it is most often considered for younger patients with high-risk disease in either the upfront setting or after an early relapse after ASCT (**Box 1**, **Fig. 1**).

Table 1
Pretransplant evaluation

Test	Notes
Renal function	Creatinine clearance <50 mL/min may result in a dose modification of the high-dose melphalan
Hepatic function	Direct bilirubin, alkaline phosphatase, AST/ALT <3× normal
Myeloma restaging	Quantitative immunoglobulins, serum immunofixation electrophoresis (IFE), serum protein electrophoresis, urine IFE, urine protein electrophoresis, serum free light chains, skeletal survey, bone marrow aspirate/biopsy with standard karyotyping and FISH panel of CD138-selected cells, flow cytometry
PET/CT scan	Considered for patients with plasmacytoma
Pulmonary function tests	DLCO or DLVA ≥50% predicted; DLCO to be corrected for hemoglobin and/or alveolar ventilation
Cardiac function: ECG and echocardiogram/MUGA	Left ventricular ejection fraction (LVEF) ≥50% or cardiology consult if LVEF <50%
Osteoporosis evaluation	DEXA, vitamin D
Infectious disease testing	CMV immunoglobulin G/immunoglobulin M, hepatitis B/C, HIV, HTLV, Treponemal pallidum
HLA typing	If AlloSCT to be considered
Psychosocial evaluation	Social work evaluation, patient and caregiver orientation, family meeting
Dental consult	To evaluate for osteonecrosis of the jaw or severe dental problems that could complicate bisphosphonate use
Physical therapy consult	Maintaining strength after transplant
Dietary consult	Consideration for nutritional supplementation such as total parenteral nutrition following transplant

Abbreviations: AST, aspartate aminotransferase; ALT, alanine aminotransferase; CMV, cytomegalovirus; DEXA, dual-energy x-ray absorptiometry; DLCO, diffusing capacity of carbon monoxide; DLVA, DLCO adjusted for volume; ECG, electrocardiogram; FISH, fluorescence in situ hybridization; HIV, human immunodeficiency virus; HTLV, human T-lymphotropic virus; IFE, immunofixation electrophoresis; LVEF, left ventricular ejection fraction; MUGA, multigated acquisition; PET, positron emission tomography.

Box 1
Indications for transplant

Autologous

- Upfront: patients ≤75 (or older?) years of age who have achieved best response after induction therapy
- Delayed: patients ≤75 (or older?) years of age who have relapsed after initial therapy and who have achieved disease control. Stem cells are usually collected after initial best response but may also be collected after treatment of first relapse
- Salvage: patients ≤75 (or older?) years of age who have relapsed after initial autologous transplant (preferably after a minimum of 18 months of disease control from the initial transplant) and who have again achieved disease control

Allogeneic

- Upfront: patients ≤40–50 years of age with high-risk disease features (young age; del 17p, t[4;14], t[14;16]; plasma cell leukemia; high lactate dehydrogenase level, and high-risk gene expression profile [GEP70 in USA, EMC 92 in Europe]) who have achieved best response after induction therapy
- Salvage: patients ≤65 years of age with high-risk disease (young age; del 17p, t[4;14], t[14;16]; plasma cell leukemia, high lactate dehydrogenase level, high-risk gene expression profile) features who have relapsed after initial autologous stem cell transplant

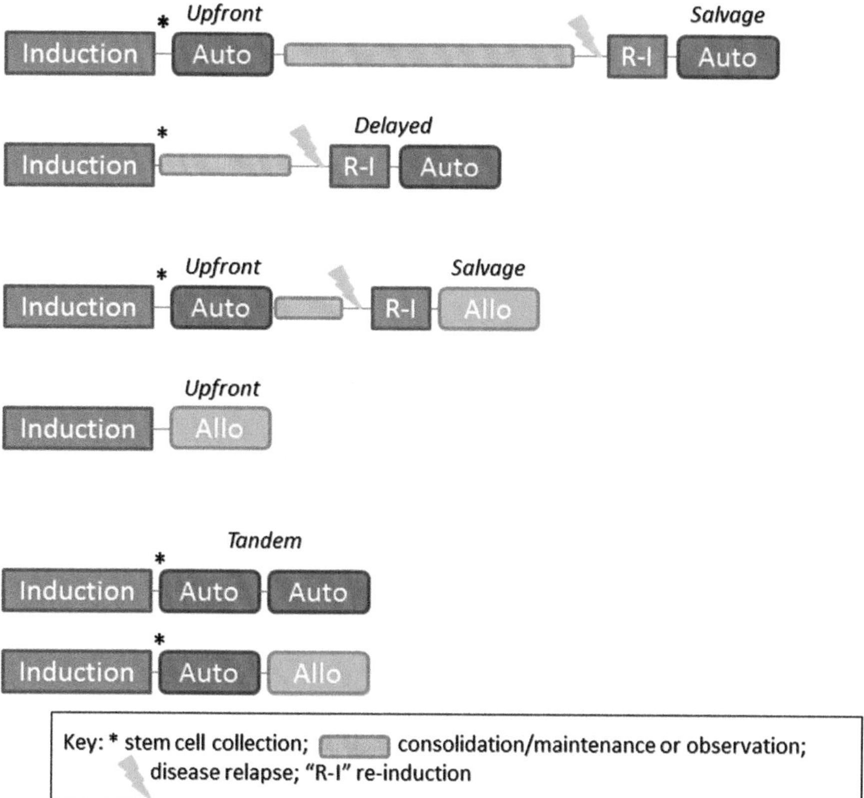

Fig. 1. Timing of transplants and subsequent therapies in myeloma.

AUTOLOGOUS STEM CELL TRANSPLANT

The most widely used high-dose regimen is single-agent melphalan at a dose of 200 mg/m^2 (MEL200). As shown in the text box below, MEL200 has been compared with lower doses of melphalan, melphalan in combination with total body irradiation (TBI), melphalan in combination with other agents, and non–melphalan-containing regimens. In aggregate, the toxicity profiles and disease-related outcomes have favored MEL200. It should be noted that there is variation among the studies with respect to timing of melphalan and stem cell infusion and whether melphalan is given over 1 day or 2 days. In general, melphalan is dose reduced to 140 mg/m^2 (MEL140) for patients with renal insufficiency (generally creatinine clearance <40) although there are limited data to support this practice.[7,8] MEL140 is also considered for patients older than 70 years.[9]

More recently, there has been interest in adding bortezomib to high-dose melphalan. While only small, nonrandomized studies have been conducted, these studies do demonstrate tolerability of this approach.[10–16] The number of doses and timing of bortezomib administration with respect to melphalan administration and stem cell infusion has not yet been fully established (**Box 2**).

Box 2
Summary of MEL200 versus alternative conditioning regimens for autologous transplant for myeloma

- MEL200 versus MEL140 + TBI[17]
  - MEL200 associated with faster hematologic recovery, fewer transfusions, shorter hospitalization, and less severe mucositis.
  - There was no difference in PFS and OS.
- MEL200 versus MEL100 (tandem transplants)[18]
  - MEL200 associated with more severe thrombocytopenia, mucositis, and gastrointestinal adverse events.
  - MEL200 associated with a statistically significant improvement in median PFS.
- MEL200 (over 2 days) versus thiotepa/busulfan/cyclophosphamide[19] (not randomized)
  - No differences in response rates, PFS, OS.
- MEL200 (over 2 days) versus MEL100 (over 2 days)/idarubicin/cyclophosphamide[20]
  - Study terminated because of a treatment-related mortality rate of 20% in the investigational arm compared with 0% in the standard melphalan arm.
  - No differences in response rates, PFS, OS.
- MEL200 versus MEL60 (over 3 day)/thiotepa/etoposide[21] (not randomized)
  - Combination arm associated with higher number of febrile days, more total parenteral nutrition.
  - Median PFS and OS higher in the combination arm.
- MEL200 (over 1 or 2 days) versus MEL140/busulfan (BUMEL)[22] (not randomized)
  - First 225 patients received BUMEL, but interim analysis showed high incidence of veno-occlusive disease (8%). Remaining patients received MEL200.
  - No differences in response rates or OS but 5-year PFS better with BUMEL.

ALLOGENEIC STEM CELL TRANSPLANTATION

The initial studies that were performed using AlloSCT with myeloablative regimens were associated with unacceptably high early mortality rates ranging from 16% to 50%.[23–26] Thus, the field has moved away from myeloablative regimens and is instead focusing on reduced-intensity conditioning or nonmyeloablative approaches. Several phase II studies with reduced-intensity conditioning allografts have been performed.[27–32] The conditioning regimens have primarily consisted of fludarabine plus melphalan with or without antithymocyte globulin (ATG) or TBI. Rates of chronic graft-versus-host disease (GVHD) and transplant-related mortality have ranged from 27% to 58% and 15% to 40%, respectively. There are data to support graft versus myeloma effect, as there is improved progression-free survival (PFS) and overall survival (OS) for patients with chronic GVHD as opposed to those without, and donor lymphocyte infusions are associated with antimyeloma activity.[33–36]

TIMING FOR TRANSPLANTATION

The possible scenarios for sequencing and timing of transplants are shown in **Fig. 1**. Historically, ASCT has been performed in the upfront setting after induction therapy. In today's era of active novel agents, which can induce deep responses, it is unknown whether ASCT can be delayed until the time of first relapse. A summary of recent and ongoing trials addressing this question is shown in **Box 3**. In all of these trials, stem cells are collected after induction therapy.

TANDEM AUTOLOGOUS VERSUS SINGLE AUTOLOGOUS TRANSPLANTATION

Once the benefit of ASCT was established in myeloma, several groups explored the approach of performing back-to-back, or tandem, ASCTs. The first randomized trial performed by Attal and colleagues[39] found improved event-free survival (EFS) and OS with tandem transplant. However, subsequent studies did not uniformly show benefit of tandem transplant over a single transplant.[40,41] A meta-analysis of 6 randomized clinical trials concluded that tandem transplant was associated with a statistically significant better response rate but at the cost of an increased transplant-related mortality rate.[42] There was no difference in EFS or OS. Currently, most transplant centers in the United States do not routinely perform tandem autologous transplants outside of a clinical trial. Both the BMT CTN 0702 and EMN 02 trials are addressing the question of whether single or tandem ASCT is superior along with the role of consolidation.

TANDEM AUTOLOGOUS VERSUS AUTOLOGOUS-ALLOGENEIC TRANSPLANTATION

Several studies comparing upfront tandem ASCT with ASCT followed by AlloSCT have been performed and are summarized in **Box 4**. Several of these studies used a biologic assignment approach in which patients who had an HLA-identical sibling donor received the autologous-allogeneic transplantation, whereas patients who did not have a sibling match underwent double ASCT. In aggregate, these studies do not show a significant benefit for tandem autologous-allogeneic transplant,[43] and this approach is not routinely recommended outside of a clinical trial.

POSTTRANSPLANTATION MONITORING

The standard day-100 evaluations include restaging studies assessing for monoclonal protein as well as a bone marrow aspirate and biopsy (**Table 2**). There is increasing

Box 3
Summary of delayed versus Upfront ASCT trials

- IFM/DFCI 2009 DETERMINATION (ongoing)
  - Lenalidomide/bortezomib/dexamethasone (RVD) × 3 induction followed by randomization to either (1) MEL200-ASCT with RVD × 2 consolidation and lenalidomide maintenance or (2) RVD × 5 and lenalidomide maintenance
- EMN02 (ongoing)
  - Bortezomib/cyclophosphamide/dexamethasone induction followed by randomization to either (1) bortezomib/melphalan/prednisone × 4 or (2) single or tandem MEL200-ASCT. Second randomization to either (1) lenalidomide maintenance or (2) RVD × 2 consolidation followed by lenalidomide maintenance
- MPR versus Mel200[37]
  - Lenalidomide/dexamethasone × 4 induction followed by randomization to either (1) melphalan/prednisone/lenalidomide (MPR) × 6 or (2) tandem MEL200-ASCT. Second randomization to either (1) lenalidomide maintenance or (2) no maintenance.
  - Median PFS of 22.4 months (MPR) versus 43 months (MEL200) (P<0.001) with no statistical difference in 4-year OS.
  - Median PFS and 3-year OS of 41.9 months and 88% (R maintenance) versus 21.6 months and 79.2% (no maintenance) (P<.001 and P = .14).
- CRD versus MEL200[38]
  - Lenalidomide/dexamethasone × 4 induction followed by randomization to either (1) cyclophosphamide/lenalidomide/dexamethasone (CRD) × 6 or (2) MEL200-ASCT. Second randomization to maintenance with either lenalidomide/prednisone (RP) or lenalidomide (R) maintenance.
  - With a median follow-up of 31 months, the median PFS was not reached in the MEL200-ASCT arm and was 28 months in the CRD arm. No difference in OS has been noted thus far. The 2-year PFS from starting maintenance was 73% for RP and 56% for R (P = .03).

Box 4
Summary of double autologous versus autologous/allogeneic tandem transplant trials

- IFM99-03/IFM99-04[44,45]
  - No difference in EFS and trend toward improved OS in double auto arm
- PETHEMA[46]
  - Higher complete response (CR) rates after autologous/allogeneic but no difference in EFS or OS
- Italian study[47]
  - Higher CR rates and improved PFS and OS in allogeneic arm
- BMT CTN[48]
  - No difference in PFS or OS
- HOVON-50/54[49]
  - No difference in CR rate, PFS, or OS
- German DSMM[50]
  - Higher CR rate in autologous/allogeneic but no difference in OS
- EBMT-NMAM200[51] (compared autologous/allogeneic with single or double ASCT)
  - Higher PFS, OS, and nonrelapse mortality rates in autologous/allogeneic

Table 2
Posttransplant evaluation at day 100

Test	Notes
Myeloma restaging	Quantitative immunoglobulins, serum and urine IFE, serum and urine protein electrophoresis, serum free light chains, skeletal survey, bone marrow aspirate/biopsy with standard karyotyping and FISH panel of CD138-selected cells, flow cytometry
PET/CT scan	Considered for patients with plasmacytoma
Osteoporosis evaluation	DEXA, vitamin D

Abbreviations: DEXA, dual-energy x-ray absorptiometry; FISH, fluorescence in situ hybridization; IFE, immunofixation electrophoresis; PET, positron emission tomography.

interest in the detection of minimal residual disease (MRD) as patients who achieve MRD-negative status seem to have improved outcomes compared with those who are MRD positive.[52–55] Two major techniques under investigation are multiparameter flow cytometry and allele-specific oligonucleotide polymerase chain reaction (ASO PCR), which have sensitivities in the 10^{-4} to 10^{-5} range.[56,57] Consensus guidelines regarding the use of multi-parameter flow cytometry will be forthcoming. The routine use of ASO-PCR has been limited by the requirement to make patient-specific primers.

MAINTENANCE THERAPY AFTER TRANSPLANT

Because nearly all patients have relapse after ASCT and because relapse after AlloSCT continues to be a problem, there has been significant interest in the use of posttransplant maintenance therapy to delay, and potentially prevent, disease relapse. Below is a summary of the major maintenance strategies used to date after ASCT (**Box 5**).

Thus far, initial studies investigating the use of lenalidomide in the post-AlloSCT setting have been small, and prolonged administration of lenalidomide has been limited by possible worsening of acute GVHD and disease progression despite lenalidomide maintenance.[78–80] Larger studies are needed to define the role of lenalidomide alone or in combination with other therapies in this setting.

Many of the ongoing studies in the post-ASCT setting are lenalidomide based and involve the addition of other agents to lenalidomide, including ixazomib (an oral proteasome inhibitor), vorinostat (HDAC inhibitor), clarithromycin/dexamethasone, or minocycline. Several bortezomib-based studies are also underway, including bortezomib plus vorinostat. Pomalidomide is currently being studied in the context of maintenance after salvage ASCT, and it may be assumed that it eventually will be explored as a maintenance strategy after initial ASCT.

MANAGEMENT OF RELAPSED DISEASE AFTER TRANSPLANTATION

As shown in **Fig. 2**, the options after relapse after initial ASCT include (1) salvage ASCT, (2) salvage AlloSCT, or (3) multiple lines of salvage therapies (**Box 6**). Currently, there are no data to definitively support one approach over another, and prospective randomized studies comparing novel agents with salvage transplant are needed.

Salvage ASCTs have been reported to be feasible by multiple groups.[81–87] In general, the PFS after the second transplant is approximately half of the PFS from the first transplant, and patients who relapsed early after the initial transplant have worse outcomes.[84–86,88] Analysis by the Center for International Blood and Marrow Transplant Research of 187 patients who underwent salvage ASCT found that those patients

Box 5
Maintenance strategies after autologous stem cell transplantation

- Interferon alpha
  - Studies were mixed as to whether maintenance therapy improved PFS or OS.[58–63]
  - The unfavorable side-effect profile of interferon and the advent of immunomodulatory drugs (IMiDs) led to abandonment of this strategy.
- Thalidomide
  - Eight randomized studies, some of which included thalidomide in combination with corticosteroid.[48,64–70] Not all of these studies were able to demonstrate an OS benefit, and there is some evidence that thalidomide maintenance does not improve outcomes for patients with adverse cytogenetics.[71]
  - Prolonged thalidomide therapy is problematic because of toxicity, particularly neurotoxicity, and the use of thalidomide in the posttransplant setting has largely stopped in the United States.
- Lenalidomide
  - Three randomized studies have assessed the use of lenalidomide after transplant. All 3 show significant improvements in PFS[72–74] with 2 of 3 studies showing improvement in OS.[72,74]
  - In the United States, lenalidomide maintenance until progression is currently considered by many to be the standard of care.
- Bortezomib
  - There have been no randomized studies that directly compare bortezomib maintenance with placebo in the posttransplant setting.
  - The HOVON-65/GMMG-HD4 trial compared VAD (vincristine, doxorubicin, dexamethasone)/transplant/thalidomide maintenance with PAD (bortezomib, doxorubicin, dexamethasone)/transplant/bortezomib maintenance.[75] Patients in renal failure at presentation or with 17p abnormalities had improved OS on the bortezomib arm. Patients with del13 and t(4;14) did not benefit from bortezomib maintenance when compared with thalidomide maintenance.
  - In the absence of a clinical trial, bortezomib is commonly given in an every-other-week dosing schedule
- Lenalidomide/bortezomib/dexamethasone (RVD)
  - Nooka and colleagues[76] assessed patients with high-risk disease who received up to 3 years of RVD posttransplant therapy followed by maintenance lenalidomide. The 3-year OS rate was 93%.
  - Arkansas's 2006-66 trial included 3 years of posttransplant RVD therapy.[77] When compared with Total Therapy 3, which had 3 years of VTD therapy, there were no substantial differences in the outcomes of patients with high-risk disease based on gene expression profiling.

who had relapse 36 months or more after the first transplant derived greater benefit from the second transplant (longer PFS and OS) than those who relapsed early.[89] Recently, the results of a multicenter, randomized, phase 3 study comparing salvage autologous transplant with cyclophosphamide (400 mg/m^2/wk × 12 weeks) were reported.[90] This study enrolled patients who required treatment for progressive/relapsed disease at least 18 months after first transplant and treated them with bortezomib/doxorubicin/dexamethasone followed by either transplant or cyclophosphamide. The median time to progression was longer in the ASCT arm (19 vs 11 months, *P*<.0001), although OS did not differ. Prospective randomized trials

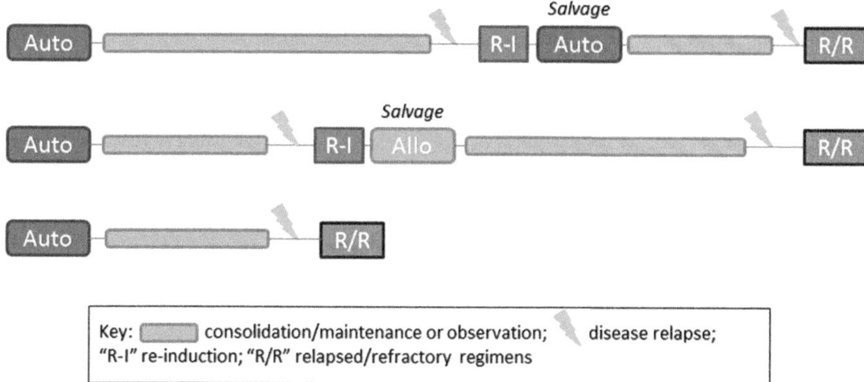

Fig. 2. Treatment options after relapse after initial ASCT.

comparing more modern salvage regimens (eg, pomalidomide/carfilzomib/dexamethasone) to salvage ASCT are needed to better define the role of salvage ASCT.

A recent analysis by the Center for International Blood and Marrow Transplant Research compared a cohort of 137 patients who received a second ASCT with a cohort of 152 patients who received a nonmyeloablative or reduced-intensity conditioning AlloSCT in patients relapsing after ASCT.[91] Notably, the nonrelapse mortality

Box 6
Regimens for relapsed/refractory myeloma

- Lenalidomide + dexamethasone
- Bortezomib + dexamethasone
- Lenalidomide + bortezomib + dexamethasone
- Lenalidomide + cyclophosphamide + dexamethasone (or prednisone)
- Bortezomib + thalidomide + dexamethasone
- Bortezomib + cyclophosphamide + dexamethasone
- Bortezomib + liposomal doxorubicin + dexamethasone
- Pomalidomide + dexamethasone
- Pomalidomide + bortezomib + dexamethasone
- Pomalidomide + carfilzomib + dexamethasone
- Pomalidomide + cyclophosphamide + dexamethasone (or prednisone)
- Carfilzomib + dexamethasone
- Carfilzomib + cyclophosphamide + dexamethasone
- Carfilzomib + lenalidomide + dexamethasone
- D-PACE (dexamethasone plus infusional cisplatin, doxorubicin, cyclophosphamide, etoposide)
- DCEP (dexamethasone, cyclophosphamide, etoposide, cisplatin)
- Bendamustine
- Clinical trial

Box 7
Novel agents under investigation for myeloma

- Proteasome inhibitors (ixazomib, marizomib, oprozomib)
- Monoclonal antibodies
  - Anti-CD38 (daratumumab, SAR650984)
  - Anti-CD138 (indatuximab ravtansine [BT062])
  - Anti-CS1 (elotuzumab)
  - Anti-CD40 (dacetuzumab, lucatumumab)
  - Anti-CD56 (lorvotuzumab)
  - Anti-BAFF (tabalumab)
  - Anti-IL6 (siltuximab)
- Histone deacetylase inhibitors (vorinostat, panobinostat, romidepsin)
- Cell cycle inhibitors (seliciclib, MLN8237, ARRY-520, dinaciclib)
- Kinase/growth factor inhibitors (masitinib, dasatinib, enzastaurin, GSK2110183, selumetinib)
- HSP90 inhibitors (tanespimycin, ganetespib)
- mTORC inhibitors (MLN0128, INK128, everolimus, temsirolimus)
- Nuclear export inhibitor (KPT330)
- PARP1/2 inhibitor (veliparib)
- Bcl-2 inhibitor (ABT199)

at 1 year after transplant was higher in the AlloSCT group (13% vs 2%, $P = .001$), and the OS was superior in the ASCT group at both 1 and 3 years.

NOVEL THERAPIES AND THEIR INTEGRATION WITH TRANSPLANTATION

The therapeutic landscape for myeloma is rapidly changing. As shown below, as of 2014, more than 30 novel agents are under investigation.[92] Although many are being tested either alone or in combination with standard therapies in the relapsed/refractory setting, it is to be expected that some may eventually be incorporated into induction regimens, conditioning regimens for transplant, and in the maintenance setting after transplant (**Box 7**).

SUMMARY

Despite notable advances in myeloma therapeutics, which are leading to significantly improved response rates after induction therapy and improved survival in the relapsed/refractory setting, ASCT remains an integral part of the treatment strategy for most myeloma patients. The optimal timing of ASCT, which has traditionally been used in the upfront setting, is an area of active investigation. The role of AlloSCT, particularly in young patients with high-risk disease, continues to be defined. There is increasing evidence that posttransplant maintenance therapy, particularly with lenalidomide, can significantly improve outcomes, and ongoing studies are evaluating whether alternative maintenance strategies might yield even better results. It is predicted that with more routine use of cytogenetic and gene expression profiling in the future, we will be better able to identify those subgroups of patients who are expected to benefit most from early versus late versus no ASCT as well as those who will benefit from AlloSCT. The rapidly expanding armamentarium of myeloma therapeutics ensures that the pretransplant, transplant, and posttransplant treatment strategies will continue to evolve.

REFERENCES

1. Jantunen E, Kuittinen T, Penttila K, et al. High-dose melphalan (200 mg/m2) supported by autologous stem cell transplantation is safe and effective in elderly (>or=65 years) myeloma patients: comparison with younger patients treated on the same protocol. Bone Marrow Transplant 2006;37:917–22.
2. Bashir Q, Shah N, Parmar S, et al. Feasibility of autologous hematopoietic stem cell transplant in patients aged >/=70 years with multiple myeloma. Leuk Lymphoma 2012;53:118–22.
3. Kumar SK, Dingli D, Lacy MQ, et al. Autologous stem cell transplantation in patients of 70 years and older with multiple myeloma: results from a matched pair analysis. Am J Hematol 2008;83:614–7.
4. Sirohi B, Powles R, Treleaven J, et al. The role of autologous transplantation in patients with multiple myeloma aged 65 years and over. Bone Marrow Transplant 2000;25:533–9.
5. Siegel DS, Desikan KR, Mehta J, et al. Age is not a prognostic variable with autotransplants for multiple myeloma. Blood 1999;93:51–4.
6. Lokhorst H, Einsele H, Vesole D, et al. International Myeloma Working Group consensus statement regarding the current status of allogeneic stem-cell transplantation for multiple myeloma. J Clin Oncol 2010;28:4521–30.
7. Badros A, Barlogie B, Siegel E, et al. Results of autologous stem cell transplant in multiple myeloma patients with renal failure. Br J Haematol 2001;114:822–9.
8. Parikh GC, Amjad AI, Saliba RM, et al. Autologous hematopoietic stem cell transplantation may reverse renal failure in patients with multiple myeloma. Biol Blood Marrow Transplant 2009;15:812–6.
9. Badros A, Barlogie B, Siegel E, et al. Autologous stem cell transplantation in elderly multiple myeloma patients over the age of 70 years. Br J Haematol 2001;114:600–7.
10. Miyamoto T, Yoshimoto G, Kamimura T, et al. Combination of high-dose melphalan and bortezomib as conditioning regimen for autologous peripheral blood stem cell transplantation in multiple myeloma. Int J Hematol 2013;98:337–45.
11. Nishihori T, Alekshun TJ, Shain K, et al. Bortezomib salvage followed by a Phase I/II study of bortezomib plus high-dose melphalan and tandem autologous transplantation for patients with primary resistant myeloma. Br J Haematol 2012;157:553–63.
12. Roussel M, Moreau P, Huynh A, et al. Bortezomib and high-dose melphalan as conditioning regimen before autologous stem cell transplantation in patients with de novo multiple myeloma: a phase 2 study of the Intergroupe Francophone du Myelome (IFM). Blood 2010;115:32–7.
13. Thompson PA, Prince HM, Seymour JF, et al. Bortezomib added to high-dose melphalan as pre-transplant conditioning is safe in patients with heavily pretreated multiple myeloma. Bone Marrow Transplant 2011;46:764–5.
14. Lee SR, Kim SJ, Park Y, et al. Bortezomib and melphalan as a conditioning regimen for autologous stem cell transplantation in multiple myeloma. Korean J Hematol 2010;45:183–7.

15. Lonial S, Kaufman J, Tighiouart M, et al. A phase I/II trial combining high-dose melphalan and autologous transplant with bortezomib for multiple myeloma: a dose- and schedule-finding study. Clin Cancer Res 2010;16:5079–86.
16. Doo NW, Thompson PA, Prince HM, et al. Bortezomib with high dose melphalan conditioning for autologous transplant is safe and effective in patients with heavily pretreated and high risk multiple myeloma. Leuk Lymphoma 2013;54: 1465–72.
17. Moreau P, Facon T, Attal M, et al. Comparison of 200 mg/m(2) melphalan and 8 Gy total body irradiation plus 140 mg/m(2) melphalan as conditioning regimens for peripheral blood stem cell transplantation in patients with newly diagnosed multiple myeloma: final analysis of the Intergroupe Francophone du Myelome 9502 randomized trial. Blood 2002;99:731–5.
18. Palumbo A, Bringhen S, Bruno B, et al. Melphalan 200 mg/m(2) versus melphalan 100 mg/m(2) in newly diagnosed myeloma patients: a prospective, multicenter phase 3 study. Blood 2010;115:1873–9.
19. Anagnostopoulos A, Aleman A, Ayers G, et al. Comparison of high-dose melphalan with a more intensive regimen of thiotepa, busulfan, and cyclophosphamide for patients with multiple myeloma. Cancer 2004;100:2607–12.
20. Fenk R, Schneider P, Kropff M, et al. High-dose idarubicin, cyclophosphamide and melphalan as conditioning for autologous stem cell transplantation increases treatment-related mortality in patients with multiple myeloma: results of a randomised study. Br J Haematol 2005;130:588–94.
21. Abu Zaid B, Abdul-Hai A, Grotto I, et al. Autologous transplant in multiple myeloma with an augmented conditioning protocol. Leuk Lymphoma 2013;54: 2480–4.
22. Lahuerta JJ, Mateos MV, Martinez-Lopez J, et al. Busulfan 12 mg/kg plus melphalan 140 mg/m2 versus melphalan 200 mg/m2 as conditioning regimens for autologous transplantation in newly diagnosed multiple myeloma patients included in the PETHEMA/GEM2000 study. Haematologica 2010; 95:1913–20.
23. Bensinger WI, Buckner CD, Anasetti C, et al. Allogeneic marrow transplantation for multiple myeloma: an analysis of risk factors on outcome. Blood 1996;88: 2787–93.
24. Gahrton G, Svensson H, Cavo M, et al. Progress in allogenic bone marrow and peripheral blood stem cell transplantation for multiple myeloma: a comparison between transplants performed 1983–93 and 1994–8 at European Group for Blood and Marrow Transplantation centres. Br J Haematol 2001; 113:209–16.
25. Alyea E, Weller E, Schlossman R, et al. Outcome after autologous and allogeneic stem cell transplantation for patients with multiple myeloma: impact of graft-versus-myeloma effect. Bone Marrow Transplant 2003;32:1145–51.
26. Kroger N, Einsele H, Wolff D, et al. Myeloablative intensified conditioning regimen with in vivo T-cell depletion (ATG) followed by allografting in patients with advanced multiple myeloma. A phase I/II study of the German Study-group Multiple Myeloma (DSMM). Bone Marrow Transplant 2003;31:973–9.
27. Giralt S, Aleman A, Anagnostopoulos A, et al. Fludarabine/melphalan conditioning for allogeneic transplantation in patients with multiple myeloma. Bone Marrow Transplant 2002;30:367–73.
28. Badros A, Barlogie B, Siegel E, et al. Improved outcome of allogeneic transplantation in high-risk multiple myeloma patients after nonmyeloablative conditioning. J Clin Oncol 2002;20:1295–303.

29. Kroger N, Sayer HG, Schwerdtfeger R, et al. Unrelated stem cell transplantation in multiple myeloma after a reduced-intensity conditioning with pretransplantation antithymocyte globulin is highly effective with low transplantation-related mortality. Blood 2002;100:3919–24.
30. Perez-Simon JA, Martino R, Alegre A, et al. Chronic but not acute graft-versus-host disease improves outcome in multiple myeloma patients after non-myeloablative allogeneic transplantation. Br J Haematol 2003;121:104–8.
31. Maloney DG, Molina AJ, Sahebi F, et al. Allografting with nonmyeloablative conditioning following cytoreductive autografts for the treatment of patients with multiple myeloma. Blood 2003;102:3447–54.
32. Bashir Q, Khan H, Thall PF, et al. A randomized phase II trial of fludarabine/melphalan 100 versus fludarabine/melphalan 140 followed by allogeneic hematopoietic stem cell transplantation for patients with multiple myeloma. Biol Blood Marrow Transplant 2013;19:1453–8.
33. Mohty M, Boiron JM, Damaj G, et al. Graft-versus-myeloma effect following antithymocyte globulin-based reduced intensity conditioning allogeneic stem cell transplantation. Bone Marrow Transplant 2004;34:77–84.
34. Lokhorst HM, Schattenberg A, Cornelissen JJ, et al. Donor lymphocyte infusions for relapsed multiple myeloma after allogeneic stem-cell transplantation: predictive factors for response and long-term outcome. J Clin Oncol 2000;18:3031–7.
35. Salama M, Nevill T, Marcellus D, et al. Donor leukocyte infusions for multiple myeloma. Bone Marrow Transplant 2000;26:1179–84.
36. Lokhorst HM, Wu K, Verdonck LF, et al. The occurrence of graft-versus-host disease is the major predictive factor for response to donor lymphocyte infusions in multiple myeloma. Blood 2004;103:4362–4.
37. Palumbo A, Cavallo F, Gay F, et al. Autologous transplantation and maintenance therapy in multiple myeloma. N Engl J Med 2014;371:895–905.
38. Palumbo A, Gay F, Spencer A, et al. A phase III study of ASCT vs cyclophosphamide-lenalidomide-dexamethasone and lenalidomide-prednisone maintenance vs lenalidomide alone in newly diagnosed myeloma patients. Blood 2013;122:763.
39. Attal M, Harousseau JL, Facon T, et al. Single versus double autologous stem-cell transplantation for multiple myeloma. N Engl J Med 2003;349:2495–502.
40. Cavo M, Tosi P, Zamagni E, et al. Prospective, randomized study of single compared with double autologous stem-cell transplantation for multiple myeloma: Bologna 96 clinical study. J Clin Oncol 2007;25:2434–41.
41. Abdelkefi A, Ladeb S, Torjman L, et al. Single autologous stem-cell transplantation followed by maintenance therapy with thalidomide is superior to double autologous transplantation in multiple myeloma: results of a multicenter randomized clinical trial. Blood 2008;111:1805–10.
42. Kumar A, Kharfan-Dabaja MA, Glasmacher A, et al. Tandem versus single autologous hematopoietic cell transplantation for the treatment of multiple myeloma: a systematic review and meta-analysis. J Natl Cancer Inst 2009;101:100–6.
43. Armeson KE, Hill EG, Costa LJ. Tandem autologous vs autologous plus reduced intensity allogeneic transplantation in the upfront management of multiple myeloma: meta-analysis of trials with biological assignment. Bone Marrow Transplant 2013;48:562–7.
44. Garban F, Attal M, Michallet M, et al. Prospective comparison of autologous stem cell transplantation followed by dose-reduced allograft (IFM99-03 trial) with tandem autologous stem cell transplantation (IFM99-04 trial) in high-risk de novo multiple myeloma. Blood 2006;107:3474–80.

45. Moreau P, Garban F, Attal M, et al. Long-term follow-up results of IFM99-03 and IFM99-04 trials comparing nonmyeloablative allotransplantation with autologous transplantation in high-risk de novo multiple myeloma. Blood 2008;112: 3914–5.
46. Rosinol L, Perez-Simon JA, Sureda A, et al. A prospective PETHEMA study of tandem autologous transplantation versus autograft followed by reduced-intensity conditioning allogeneic transplantation in newly diagnosed multiple myeloma. Blood 2008;112:3591–3.
47. Bruno B, Rotta M, Patriarca F, et al. A comparison of allografting with autografting for newly diagnosed myeloma. N Engl J Med 2007;356:1110–20.
48. Krishnan A, Pasquini MC, Logan B, et al. Autologous haemopoietic stem-cell transplantation followed by allogeneic or autologous haemopoietic stem-cell transplantation in patients with multiple myeloma (BMT CTN 0102): a phase 3 biological assignment trial. Lancet Oncol 2011;12:1195–203.
49. Lokhorst HM, van der Holt B, Cornelissen JJ, et al. Donor versus no-donor comparison of newly diagnosed myeloma patients included in the HOVON-50 multiple myeloma study. Blood 2012;119:6219–25 [quiz: 399].
50. Knop S, Liebisch P, Hebart H, et al. Allogeneic stem cell transplant versus tandem high-dose melphalan for front-line treatment of deletion 13q14 myeloma - an interim analysis of the German DSMM V Trial. ASH Annual Meeting Abstracts 2009;114:51.
51. Gahrton G, Iacobelli S, Bjorkstrand B, et al. Autologous/reduced-intensity allogeneic stem cell transplantation vs autologous transplantation in multiple myeloma: long-term results of the EBMT-NMAM2000 study. Blood 2013;121:5055–63.
52. Puig N, Sarasquete ME, Balanzategui A, et al. Critical evaluation of ASO RQ-PCR for minimal residual disease evaluation in multiple myeloma. A comparative analysis with flow cytometry. Leukemia 2014;28:391–7.
53. Paiva B, Vidriales MB, Cervero J, et al. Multiparameter flow cytometric remission is the most relevant prognostic factor for multiple myeloma patients who undergo autologous stem cell transplantation. Blood 2008;112:4017–23.
54. Rawstron AC, Child JA, de Tute RM, et al. Minimal residual disease assessed by multiparameter flow cytometry in multiple myeloma: impact on outcome in the Medical Research Council Myeloma IX Study. J Clin Oncol 2013;31:2540–7.
55. Martinez-Lopez J, Lahuerta JJ, Pepin F, et al. Prognostic value of deep sequencing method for minimal residual disease detection in multiple myeloma. Blood 2014;123:3073–9.
56. Rawstron AC, Davies FE, DasGupta R, et al. Flow cytometric disease monitoring in multiple myeloma: the relationship between normal and neoplastic plasma cells predicts outcome after transplantation. Blood 2002;100:3095–100.
57. van der Velden VH, Cazzaniga G, Schrauder A, et al. Analysis of minimal residual disease by Ig/TCR gene rearrangements: guidelines for interpretation of real-time quantitative PCR data. Leukemia 2007;21:604–11.
58. Harousseau JL, Attal M, Divine M, et al. Autologous stem cell transplantation after first remission induction treatment in multiple myeloma. A report of the French Registry on Autologous Transplantation in Multiple Myeloma. Stem Cells 1995;13(Suppl 2):132–9.
59. Alegre A, Diaz-Mediavilla J, San-Miguel J, et al. Autologous peripheral blood stem cell transplantation for multiple myeloma: a report of 259 cases from the Spanish Registry. Spanish Registry for Transplant in MM (Grupo Espanol de Trasplante Hematopoyetico-GETH) and PETHEMA. Bone Marrow Transplant 1998;21:133–40.

60. Bjorkstrand B, Svensson H, Goldschmidt H, et al. Alpha-interferon maintenance treatment is associated with improved survival after high-dose treatment and autologous stem cell transplantation in patients with multiple myeloma: a retrospective registry study from the European Group for Blood and Marrow Transplantation (EBMT). Bone Marrow Transplant 2001;27:511–5.
61. Powles R, Raje N, Cunningham D, et al. Maintenance therapy for remission in myeloma with Intron A following high-dose melphalan and either an autologous bone marrow transplantation or peripheral stem cell rescue. Stem Cells 1995; 13(Suppl 2):114–7.
62. Cunningham D, Powles R, Malpas J, et al. A randomized trial of maintenance interferon following high-dose chemotherapy in multiple myeloma: long-term follow-up results. Br J Haematol 1998;102:495–502.
63. Krejci M, Hajek R, Scudla V, et al. Autologous transplantation of peripheral hematopoietic cells and subsequent maintenance therapy with interferon alpha or interferon alpha and dexamethasone in patients with multiple myeloma–results from the 4W randomized clinical trial of the Czech Myeloma Group. Vnitr Lek 2001;47(Suppl 1):40–7 [in Czech].
64. Attal M, Harousseau JL, Leyvraz S, et al. Maintenance therapy with thalidomide improves survival in patients with multiple myeloma. Blood 2006;108: 3289–94.
65. Barlogie B, Tricot G, Anaissie E, et al. Thalidomide and hematopoietic-cell transplantation for multiple myeloma. N Engl J Med 2006;354:1021–30.
66. Spencer A, Prince HM, Roberts AW, et al. Consolidation therapy with low-dose thalidomide and prednisolone prolongs the survival of multiple myeloma patients undergoing a single autologous stem-cell transplantation procedure. J Clin Oncol 2009;27:1788–93.
67. Stewart AK, Trudel S, Bahlis NJ, et al. A randomized phase 3 trial of thalidomide and prednisone as maintenance therapy after ASCT in patients with MM with a quality-of-life assessment: the National Cancer Institute of Canada Clinicals Trials Group Myeloma 10 Trial. Blood 2013;121:1517–23.
68. Morgan GJ, Gregory WM, Davies FE, et al. The role of maintenance thalidomide therapy in multiple myeloma: MRC Myeloma IX results and meta-analysis. Blood 2012;119:7–15.
69. Maiolino A, Hungria VT, Garnica M, et al. Thalidomide plus dexamethasone as a maintenance therapy after autologous hematopoietic stem cell transplantation improves progression-free survival in multiple myeloma. Am J Hematol 2012; 87:948–52.
70. Lokhorst HM, van der Holt B, Zweegman S, et al. A randomized phase 3 study on the effect of thalidomide combined with adriamycin, dexamethasone, and high-dose melphalan, followed by thalidomide maintenance in patients with multiple myeloma. Blood 2010;115:1113–20.
71. Morgan GJ, Davies FE, Gregory WM, et al. Long-term follow-up of MRC Myeloma IX trial: survival outcomes with bisphosphonate and thalidomide treatment. Clin Cancer Res 2013;19:6030–8.
72. McCarthy PL, Owzar K, Hofmeister CC, et al. Lenalidomide after stem-cell transplantation for multiple myeloma. N Engl J Med 2012;366:1770–81.
73. Attal M, Lauwers-Cances V, Marit G, et al. Lenalidomide maintenance after stem-cell transplantation for multiple myeloma. N Engl J Med 2012;366:1782–91.
74. Gay F, Cavallo F, Caravita T, et al. Maintenance therapy with lenalidomide significantly improved survival of yong newly diagnosed multiple myeloma patients. Blood 2013;122:2089.

75. Sonneveld P, Schmidt-Wolf IG, van der Holt B, et al. Bortezomib induction and maintenance treatment in patients with newly diagnosed multiple myeloma: results of the randomized phase III HOVON-65/GMMG-HD4 trial. J Clin Oncol 2012;30:2946–55.
76. Nooka AK, Kaufman JL, Muppidi S, et al. Consolidation and maintenance therapy with lenalidomide, bortezomib and dexamethasone (RVD) in high-risk myeloma patients. Leukemia 2014;28:690–3.
77. Nair B, van Rhee F, Shaughnessy JD Jr, et al. Superior results of Total Therapy 3 (2003-33) in gene expression profiling-defined low-risk multiple myeloma confirmed in subsequent trial 2006-66 with VRD maintenance. Blood 2010; 115:4168–73.
78. Kneppers E, van der Holt B, Kersten MJ, et al. Lenalidomide maintenance after nonmyeloablative allogeneic stem cell transplantation in multiple myeloma is not feasible: results of the HOVON 76 Trial. Blood 2011;118:2413–9.
79. Alsina M, Becker PS, Zhong X, et al. Lenalidomide maintenance for high-risk multiple myeloma after allogeneic hematopoietic cell transplantation. Biol Blood Marrow Transplant 2014;20(8):1183–9.
80. Wolschke C, Stubig T, Hegenbart U, et al. Postallograft lenalidomide induces strong NK cell-mediated antimyeloma activity and risk for T cell-mediated GvHD: results from a phase I/II dose-finding study. Exp Hematol 2013;41: 134–42.e3.
81. Krivanova A, Hajek R, Krejci M, et al. Second autologous transplantation for multiple myeloma patients relapsing after the first autograft – a pilot study for the evaluation of experimental maintenance therapies. Report of the prospective non-randomized pilot study of the Czech Myeloma Group. Onkologie 2004;27: 275–9.
82. Elice F, Raimondi R, Tosetto A, et al. Prolonged overall survival with second on-demand autologous transplant in multiple myeloma. Am J Hematol 2006;81: 426–31.
83. Burzynski JA, Toro JJ, Patel RC, et al. Toxicity of a second autologous peripheral blood stem cell transplant in patients with relapsed or recurrent multiple myeloma. Leuk Lymphoma 2009;50:1442–7.
84. Fenk R, Liese V, Neubauer F, et al. Predictive factors for successful salvage high-dose therapy in patients with multiple myeloma relapsing after autologous blood stem cell transplantation. Leuk Lymphoma 2011;52:1455–62.
85. Jimenez-Zepeda VH, Mikhael J, Winter A, et al. Second autologous stem cell transplantation as salvage therapy for multiple myeloma: impact on progression-free and overall survival. Biol Blood Marrow Transplant 2012;18: 773–9.
86. Shah N, Ahmed F, Bashir Q, et al. Durable remission with salvage second autotransplants in patients with multiple myeloma. Cancer 2012;118:3549–55.
87. Gonsalves WI, Gertz MA, Lacy MQ, et al. Second auto-SCT for treatment of relapsed multiple myeloma. Bone Marrow Transplant 2013;48:568–73.
88. Cook G, Liakopoulou E, Pearce R, et al. Factors influencing the outcome of a second autologous stem cell transplant (ASCT) in relapsed multiple myeloma: a study from the British Society of Blood and Marrow Transplantation Registry. Biol Blood Marrow Transplant 2011;17:1638–45.
89. Michaelis LC, Saad A, Zhong X, et al. Salvage second hematopoietic cell transplantation in myeloma. Biol Blood Marrow Transplant 2013;19:760–6.
90. Cook G, Williams C, Brown JM, et al. High-dose chemotherapy plus autologous stem-cell transplantation as consolidation therapy in patients with relapsed

multiple myeloma after previous autologous stem-cell transplantation (NCRI Myeloma X Relapse [Intensive trial]): a randomised, open-label, phase 3 trial. Lancet Oncol 2014;15(8):874–85.
91. Freytes CO, Vesole DH, Lerademacher J, et al. Second transplants for multiple myeloma relapsing after a previous autotransplant-reduced-intensity allogeneic vs autologous transplantation. Bone Marrow Transplant 2014;49:416–21.
92. Ocio EM, Richardson PG, Rajkumar SV, et al. New drugs and novel mechanisms of action in multiple myeloma in 2013: a report from the International Myeloma Working Group (IMWG). Leukemia 2014;28:525–42.

High Dose Melphalan and Autologous Peripheral Blood Stem Cell Transplantation in AL Amyloidosis

Vaishali Sanchorawala, MD

KEYWORDS

• AL amyloidosis • Stem cell transplantation • Melphalan • Supportive care
• Treatment-related mortality • Patient selection

KEY POINTS

- High-dose melphalan (HDM) and autologous peripheral blood stem cell transplantation (SCT) can lead to durable remissions and long-term survival in AL amyloidosis.
- The morbidity and mortality of HDM-SCT in AL amyloidosis patients can be minimized with careful patient selection and center experience.
- Survival strongly depends on achievement of a hematologic complete response and patients with less organ involvement and absence of cardiac involvement do better.
- Continued efforts to refine patient selection and management, and incorporate novel anti-plasma cell agents in combination or sequentially, should further improve prognosis in AL amyloidosis.

INTRODUCTION

The amyloidoses are a group of diseases that share a common feature of extracellular deposition of pathologic, insoluble, fibrils in many tissues and organs. These fibrils have a characteristic beta-pleated sheet configuration that stains with the Congo red dye, producing apple green birefringence under polarized light microscopy.[1] Classification of the amyloidoses is based on the precursor protein that forms the amyloid fibrils, and the distribution of amyloid deposition (systemic or localized).[2]

AL amyloidosis (ie, immunoglobulin light chain amyloidosis) is the most common form of systemic amyloidosis in the United States and Europe. Although AL amyloidosis is considered an uncommon disease, it has an incidence similar to

Conflicts of interest: The author declares no competing financial interests.
Stem Cell Transplantation Program, Section of Hematology and Oncology, Amyloidosis Center, Boston Medical Center, 820 Harrison Avenue, FGH-1007, Boston, MA 02118, USA
E-mail address: vaishali.sanchorawala@bmc.org

Hematol Oncol Clin N Am 28 (2014) 1131–1144
http://dx.doi.org/10.1016/j.hoc.2014.08.013 **hemonc.theclinics.com**
0889-8588/14/$ – see front matter

Hodgkin lymphoma or chronic myelogenous leukemia.[3] It affects 5 to 12 persons per million per year, although autopsy studies suggest that the actual incidence might be higher. The annual incidence of AL amyloidosis in Olmstead County, Minnesota, is 8 in a million patients.[4] The amyloidogenic precursor protein in AL amyloidosis is an immunoglobulin light chain or a fragment of light chain, usually the variable region, produced by the clonal plasma cell population in the bone marrow. The plasma cell burden in this disorder is usually low (5%–10%), although AL amyloidosis can be associated with multiple myeloma in 10% to 15% of cases.[5]

TREATMENT TARGETS

A detailed elaboration of the pathogenesis of AL amyloidosis is beyond the scope of this article. However, each of the steps in the pathogenesis of amyloidosis, from the production of the precursor protein to formation of amyloid deposits, is a potential target for treatment.[6] Preclinical and clinical studies are being designed or are ongoing for several of these targets. Reducing the amyloidogenic precursor protein (ie, light chains produced by the clonal plasma cell dyscrasia) with chemotherapeutic agents has been used for the past several decades. Several interventions aimed at facilitating degradation of the amyloid deposits have been reported in AL amyloidosis. A detailed description of all the treatment options is beyond the scope of this article, which is focused on targeting the clonal plasma cell dyscrasia.

TREATMENT: GENERAL PRINCIPLES

The keys to effective treatment of AL amyloidosis are early diagnosis and correct typing. Ideally, treatment should be started before irreversible organ damage has occurred. Once the diagnosis of AL has been firmly established, the design of the therapeutic strategy depends on a fine balance between the efficacy of the chosen regimen and the individual patient's expected ability to tolerate the toxicity of the treatment regimen, especially in the setting of cardiac involvement with amyloidosis. The current therapeutic approach to systemic AL amyloidosis is based on the observation that organ function is restored if the synthesis of the amyloidogenic protein precursor is shut down. Therefore, the aim of therapy is to rapidly reduce the supply of misfolded amyloid-forming monoclonal free light chains by suppressing the underlying plasma cell dyscrasia while using supportive measures to preserve target organ functions.

MONITORING THE THERAPEUTIC EFFECT

The criteria for hematologic and organ responses have been unified, formalized, and recently updated at the XIIth International Symposium on Amyloidosis.[7,8] Hematologic response usually translates into clinically improved organ function and is associated with a substantial survival advantage and improved quality of life. However, if the organ damage is advanced, it may be irreversible despite hematologic remission. Most patients with a hematologic response show a clinical response after 3 to 6 months, although late responses have been observed. Even though partial hematologic responses can be beneficial, it seems that significant reductions in free light chain levels are associated with the best clinical responses.[9,10] However, the rate of clinical response is higher in patients with a complete hematologic response than in those with a partial one.

INITIAL PILOT STUDIES OF HIGH-DOSE CHEMOTHERAPY AND STEM CELL TRANSPLANTATION IN AL AMYLOIDOSIS

Intravenous high-dose melphalan (HDM) chemotherapy and autologous peripheral blood stem cell transplantation (SCT) has been successful in inducing complete hematologic remissions and prolonging survival in multiple myeloma.[11,12] Therefore, it was logical to apply this approach to the treatment of AL amyloidosis. The Amyloid Research and Treatment Program, now called the Amyloidosis Center, at Boston University School of Medicine, has a long-standing investigative interest in the pathophysiology and treatment of the various forms of systemic amyloidoses. In 1994, a multidisciplinary clinical group was formed at Boston University Medical Center to develop high-dose chemotherapy protocols for AL amyloidosis. This group was made up of clinicians allied with the Amyloid Research and Treatment Program, representing the disciplines of cardiology, nephrology, pulmonology, neurology, gastroenterology, and rheumatology, together with hematologists in the Stem Cell Transplant Program of the Section of Hematology and Oncology and clinical pathologists from the Apheresis and Blood Bank.

The initial experience with HDM-SCT in 5 subjects with AL amyloidosis was reported in 1996.[13] This pilot study showed that AL amyloidosis subjects with significant systemic disease could be successfully treated with HDM-SCT. Furthermore, 3 of the 5 subjects achieved a complete hematologic response (CR), with disappearance of their underlying clonal plasma cell disorder following treatment. Moreover, all 5 subjects experienced reversal of amyloid-related organ dysfunction.

CUMULATIVE EXPERIENCE OF HIGH-DOSE MELPHALAN AND STEM CELL TRANSPLANTATION AT A SINGLE CENTER

An expanded series with 312 subjects was conducted by the Amyloidosis Center in 2004.[14] Hematologic complete response (CR) occurred in 40% of evaluable subjects and 66% of the subjects achieved improvement in at least 1 organ function with a hematologic CR. Moreover, the median survival was 4.6 years for this cohort.

The long-term follow-up of 80 subjects treated in the first 3 years of the program (1994–1997) was reviewed.[15] The early death rate, within 100 days of SCT, was 14%. Hematologic CR was achieved by 51% (32 of 63) and the median survival was 4.75 years. The median survival exceeded 10 years for subjects achieving a CR after HDM-SCT, compared with 50 months for those not achieving a CR. The long-term survival beyond 10 years was achieved in 23.5% (95% CI, 15% and 33%) of subjects with AL amyloidosis treated with HDM-SCT. Hematologic relapses occurred in 34% (n = 11/32) subjects at a median time of 2.5 years (range 2–8).

Recently, the outcomes of 421 subjects treated with HDM-SCT from July 1994 to December 2008 were analyzed.[16] Treatment-related mortality was 11% overall and decreased to 6% in the last 5 years. For this group, the median event-free survival (EFS) and overall survival (OS) were 2.6 and 6.3 years, respectively. Of 340 subjects evaluable at 1 year beyond HDM-SCT, 43% achieved a CR and 78% of them experienced an organ response. For CR subjects, median EFS and OS were 8.3 and 13.2 years, respectively. Among the 195 subjects who did not obtain CR, 52% reached an organ response, and the median EFS and OS were 2 and 5.9 years, respectively. A subgroup of 26% of the non-CR subjects remained clinically stable at 5 years of follow-up. Hematologic relapses occurred in 40 subjects (28%) at a median time of 3.7 years (range, 1.5–12.7).

Most recently, long-term outcomes of 607 subjects with AL amyloidosis undergoing HDM-SCT from July 1994 to Aug 2013 were analyzed. The median age was 57 years.

Of these, 53% had cardiac involvement and 41% had multiorgan involvement. Treatment-related mortality was 9% and 80% of the deaths were associated with cardiac involvement. Hematologic CR was achieved by 34% by an intention-to-treat analysis. Hematologic CR was 45% for those who received 200 mg/m^2 of melphalan compared to 33% for those who received 100 to 140 mg/m^2 melphalan ($P = .02$). The median OS was 6.7 years. The median OS was significantly better for those who achieved a hematologic CR, for those without cardiac involvement, and for those with less than 2 organ systems involvement (**Figs. 1–3**). Hematologic relapses occurred in 20% of subjects with hematologic CR at a median of 4 years (range 1.6–12.4 years).

ELIGIBILITY CRITERIA FOR HIGH-DOSE MELPHALAN AND STEM CELL TRANSPLANTATION

The Amyloidosis Center eligibility criteria for treatment with HDM-SCT are a confirmed tissue diagnosis of amyloidosis, clear evidence of a clonal plasma cell dyscrasia, age greater than 18 years, and minimum measures of performance status (Southwest Oncology Group [SWOG] 0–2), cardiac function (left ventricular ejection fraction >40%), pulmonary function (oxygen saturation >95% on room air), and hemodynamic stability (baseline systolic blood pressure >90 mm Hg). Patients on hemodialysis or peritoneal dialysis for renal failure are not excluded if other eligibility criteria are met.[14] The dose of melphalan can vary from 100 to 200 mg/m^2 based on the risk-adapted approach, described by Comenzo and Gertz,[17] to reduce treatment-related morbidity and mortality associated with HDM-SCT. The patients can be stratified into 3 risk categories: (1) good-risk patients are of any age and have 1 to 2 organs involved, no cardiac involvement, and creatinine clearance greater than 50 mL/min; (2) intermediate-risk patients

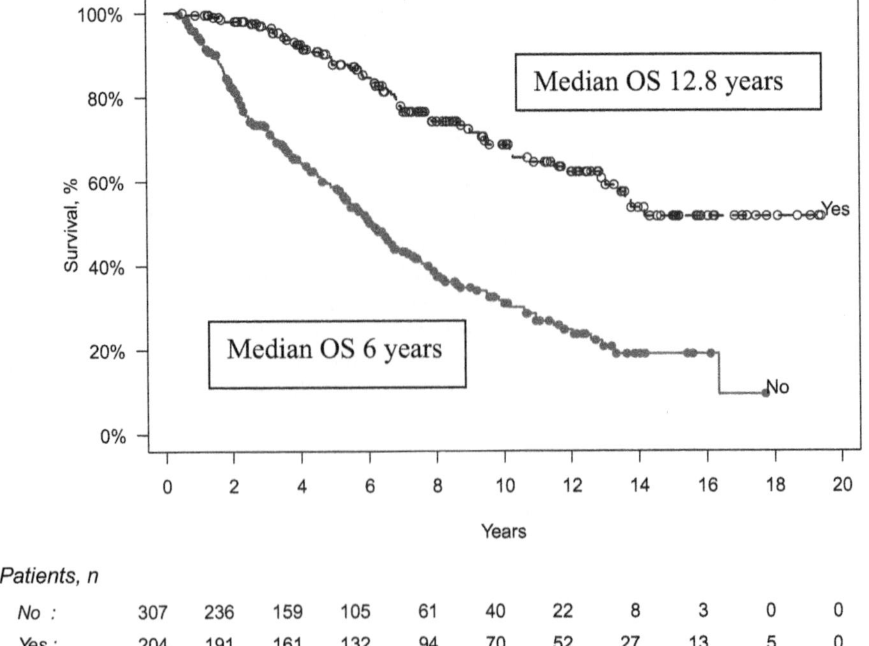

Fig. 1. OS of patients with and without hematologic CR.

Log–Rank P–value<.0001
Median OS 8.8 years
Median OS 4 years
No
Yes
Survival, %
100%
80%
60%
40%
20%
0%
0
2
4
6
8
10
12
14
16
18
20
Years

287	236	194	146	92	68	48	23	9	1	0
320	194	128	93	65	43	26	12	7	4	0

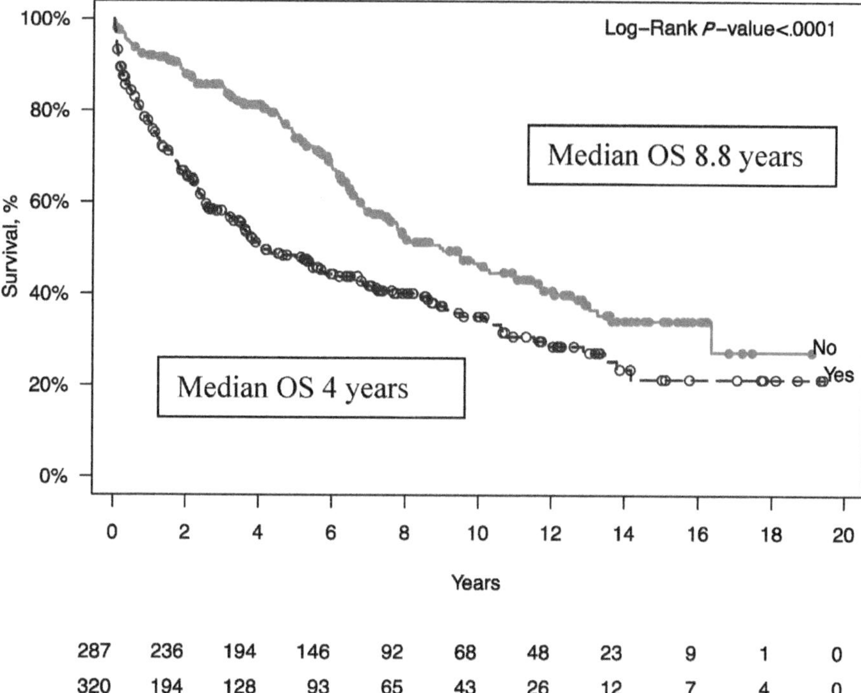

Fig. 2. OS of patients with presence and absence of cardiac involvement.

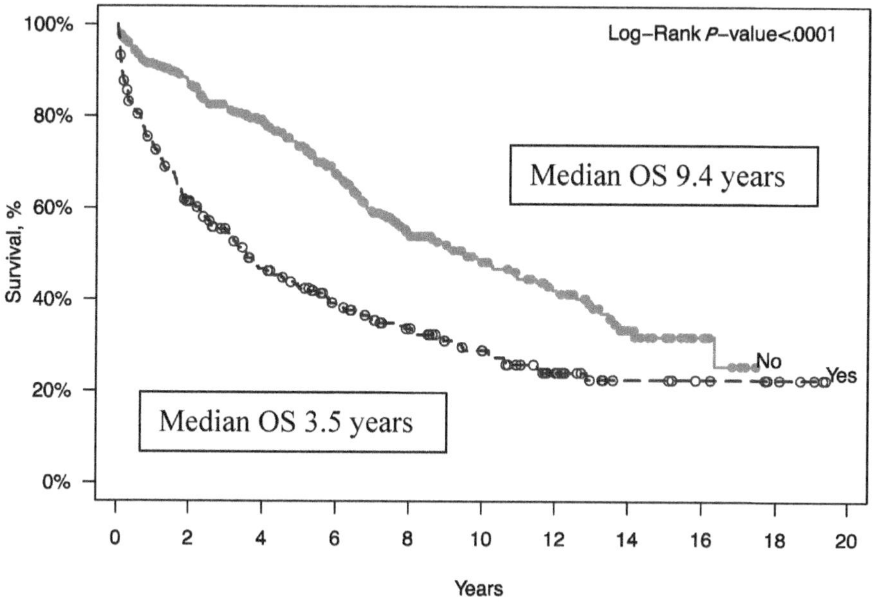

Log–Rank P–value<.0001
Median OS 9.4 years
Median OS 3.5 years
No
Yes
Survival, %
100%
80%
60%
40%
20%
0%
0
2
4
6
8
10
12
14
16
18
20
Years

356	285	222	165	102	71	50	24	8	0	0
251	145	100	74	55	40	24	11	8	5	0

Fig. 3. OS of patients with less than or equal to 2 or greater than 2 organ system involvement.

are less than 71 years old and have 1 to 2 organs involved, 1 of which must include cardiac or renal with creatinine clearance less than 51 mL/min; and (3) poor-risk patients have either 3 organs involved or advanced cardiac involvement. The cardiac biomarker staging system can also define risk of treatment-related complications while undergoing HDM-SCT.[18,19] Elevated cardiac troponin T levels are associated with poor survival while undergoing HDM-SCT.[20]

INDUCTION REGIMENS, CHOICE, AND DURATION

Because the burden of clonal plasma cells is modest in most patients with AL amyloidosis, induction with a cytoreductive regimen before HDM-SCT, as is done in multiple myeloma, seems unnecessary, although possible benefits from infusional vincristine, adriamycin and dexamethasone (VAD) treatment before SCT have been reported.[21] Evidence from a randomized clinical trial indicates that the delay associated with pretransplant cytoreduction, using oral melphalan and prednisone, can allow disease progression and can lead to survival disadvantage in patients with cardiac involvement.[22] Induction therapy with novel agents before HDM-SCT, specifically bortezomib and dexamethasone, is being explored in the setting of a clinical trial and data seem promising. However, induction therapy should be used with caution so that it does not cause delay of more definitive treatment or deterioration of organ function.

STEM CELL MOBILIZATION AND COLLECTION

Previous exposure to alkylating agents impairs hematopoietic stem cell collection. A total dose of oral melphalan exceeding 200 mg may significantly reduce the ability to mobilize CD34+ cells. Contrary to the common experience in multiple myeloma, deaths have been reported during mobilization and leukapheresis of patients with AL amyloidosis who have cardiac or multiorgan involvement.[14] Overall, the incidence of major complications during stem cell mobilization and collection is approximately 15%. To minimize the risk of toxicity, it is recommended that only granulocyte colony-stimulating factor (G-CSF) be used for mobilization because its use in combination with cyclophosphamide is associated with increased cardiac morbidity, a significantly higher number of aphereses required for CD34 harvesting, greater need of hospitalization, and increased toxicity. However, cyclophosphamide may have a role in stem cell mobilization in patients with AL amyloidosis and multiple myeloma. The recommended dosage of G-CSF is 10 to 16 mcg/kg/d, either as a single dose or in 2 divided doses, 3 days before stem cell collection. The recommended optimal dose of CD34+ cells in AL patients is at least 5×10^6 CD34+ cells/kg.[23] Contamination of the apheresis product with clonotypic plasma cells has been demonstrated but CD34 selection is not presently recommended.[24] Plerixafor, CXCR4 receptor antagonist, as a stem cell mobilization regimen has not been studied in subjects with AL amyloidosis in a well-designed clinical trial[25]; however, it can be beneficial in patients with fluid overload to reduce the dose of G-CSF, reduce the risk of capillary leak syndrome, and reduce the number of leukapheresis sessions needed for optimal stem cell collection yield.[26]

CONDITIONING REGIMENS BEFORE STEM CELL TRANSPLANTATION

Total body irradiation (550 cGy) before SCT was investigated in a small feasibility study; however, it is not used in current regimens because of cardiac toxicity and what seems to be greater overall morbidity and mortality. Thus, conditioning is usually performed with intravenous melphalan alone, using a risk-adapted dose-modification schema. Tandem cycles of HDM have shown to improve the proportion of subjects who ultimately achieve a hematologic CR in 31% of subjects, leading to overall CR rate of 67%.[27] A pilot study of incorporation of bortezomib with HDM in the treatment of AL amyloidosis has shown promising results with high hematologic response rates.[28]

CLINICAL RESPONSES TO HIGH-DOSE MELPHALAN AND STEM CELL TRANSPLANTATION

The initial report of renal responses following HDM-SCT was published in 2001. In this report, 36% of patients had a renal response at 12 months defined as a 50% reduction in 24-hour urinary protein excretion in the absence of a 25% or greater reduction in creatinine clearance.[29] There was a striking difference in renal response rate among those with a complete hematologic response (71%) and those with persistence of the plasma cell dyscrasia (11%). Since then, reports of improvements in quality of life,[30] hepatic responses,[31] and cardiac responses[32] have been published. Similar to renal response, clinical responses in other organ systems are more evident with hematologic responses and can take up to 6 to 12 months or longer to occur.

SPECIAL PROBLEMS ASSOCIATED WITH HIGH-DOSE MELPHALAN AND STEM CELL TRANSPLANTATION IN AL AMYLOIDOSIS

Patients with AL amyloidosis typically have organ impairment that predisposes them to increased peritransplant morbidity and mortality. Unique clinical challenges with AL amyloidosis patients that warrant special mention relate to the management of nutrition, macroglossia, orthostatic hypotension, volume status, and cardiac arrhythmias. Pretransplant assessment of gastrointestinal function and mucosal integrity is essential. The Amyloidosis Center has found that appropriate assessment includes a detailed review of gastrointestinal signs and symptoms, serial stool examinations for occult blood loss, endoscopic studies to define pathologic condition if indicated, and a complete assessment of coagulation status. Patients with poor nutrition because of gastrointestinal dysfunction and dysmotility, anorexia, or dysgeusia have generally required oral or parenteral nutrition supplements in the pretransplant and posttransplant period. Nephrotic syndrome associated with renal amyloidosis has been observed not uncommonly to lead to severe hypoalbuminemia and peripheral edema or anasarca. In patients with anasarca and serum albumin levels less than 2.0 g/dL, the Amyloidosis Center has found that albumin infusions to raise the serum albumin followed by loop diuretics are effective. Hypoalbuminemia, autonomic insufficiency, hypoadrenalism, and cardiac disease can all lead to severe orthostatic hypotension. Behavioral modifications, avoidance of dehydration, use of thigh-high fitted stockings to improve venous return, and use of midodrine (an alpha adrenergic agonist) with careful monitoring of urinary retention can be helpful in alleviation of postural hypotension from autonomic neuropathy. Cardiac disease has been observed to predispose patients to atrial and ventricular arrhythmias as well as to symptoms and signs of restrictive cardiomyopathy.[33] Management of such patients in coordination with an experienced cardiologist has proven to be critical. Amiodarone is often an effective antiarrhythmic, whereas beta blockers, calcium channel blockers, and digoxin have often been poorly tolerated by these patients. Deficiency of factor X, along with the poor endothelial and connective tissue integrity from amyloid deposition, is associated with an increased risk of cutaneous and mucosal bleeding, including pathognomonic raccoon-eye periorbital ecchymoses. Patients with factor X deficiency are at particularly high risk of bleeding complications during periods of thrombocytopenia.[34] Hence, the Amyloidosis Center has found that screening for factor X deficiency must be done before treatment. Neither fresh frozen plasma nor cryoprecipitate are abundant sources of factor X; significant bleeding due to factor X deficiency is best treated with factor IX complex or recombinant factor VIIa. Additional unusual problems that may be encountered in these patients include difficulties with emergent endotracheal intubation in patients with macroglossia, spontaneous splenic,[35] esophageal and hepatic rupture,[36] and hypercoagulability in association with nephrotic syndrome.

EXPERIENCE OF HIGH-DOSE MELPHALAN AND STEM CELL TRANSPLANTATION IN THE TREATMENT OF AL AMYLOIDOSIS AT OTHER CENTERS

HDM-SCT is an effective treatment for AL amyloidosis. The results of single-center and multicenter studies are detailed in **Table 1**. Encouraging hematologic and clinical responses have been reported in these studies, though treatment-related mortality is substantially higher (15%–40%) than in multiple myeloma (<5%). A case-matched control study has suggested the superiority of HDM-SCT compared with conventional chemotherapy regimens[37]; however, the only randomized phase III study by the French group in the literature failed to show a survival benefit for HDM-SCT.[38] However, in this study, many of the subjects randomized to the HDM-SCT arm were not actually transplanted, the toxicity on the transplant arm was excessive, and follow-up was short. Thus, the question of optimal therapy remains open, particularly as transplant techniques are refined and nontransplant regimens are improved. However, it is clear that patients should be carefully selected for transplant because advanced cardiac disease, involvement of more than 2 organs, hypotension, and poor performance status are poor prognostic factors for the outcome of HDM-SCT.

Table 1
Results of single center and multicenter studies of high-dose melphalan and stem cell transplantation in AL amyloidosis

	Number of Patients	Treatment-Related Mortality	Hematologic CR	Organ Response
Single Center				
Gertz et al,[49] 2007	270	11%	33%	NR
Mollee et al,[50] 2004	20	35%	28%	Renal 46%, cardiac 25%, liver 50%
Schonland et al,[51] 2005	41	7%	50%	40%
Skinner et al,[14] 2004	277	13%	40%	44%
Chow et al,[52] 2005	15	0%	67%	27%
Multicenter				
Moreau et al,[53] 1998	21	43%	25%	83%
Gertz et al,[54] 2004	28	14%	NA	75%
Goodman et al,[55] 2006	92	23%	83% (CR+PR)	48%
Vesole et al,[56] 2006	114	18%	36%	Renal 46%, liver 58%, cardiac 47%

Abbreviations: NA, Not available; NR, Not reported; PR, Partial response.

HIGH-DOSE MELPHALAN AND STEM CELL TRANSPLANTATION FOLLOWING HEART TRANSPLANTATION

In patients with end-stage heart failure, heart transplantation may be required as a life-saving procedure. Because of the high likelihood of amyloid recurrence in the transplanted organ, as well as progression in other organs, heart transplantation must be followed by antiplasma cell therapy. Although the long-term survival is statistically inferior to that of patients with nonamyloid heart disease, the actuarial 5-year survival seems to be 65% with treatment of the underlying plasma cell dyscrasia. Thus, carefully selected patients, without other significant organ involvement, can benefit from heart transplantation followed by aggressive antiplasma cell treatment.[39–41]

SUPPORTIVE THERAPY

Supportive treatment aimed at improving or palliating organ function, maintaining quality of life, and prolonging survival while antiplasma cell therapy has time to take effect has an important impact on survival. Supportive care should be considered a fundamental part of an integrated treatment approach with these patients and requires the coordinated expertise of several specialists who are familiar with this disease. Treatment of amyloid cardiomyopathy is highly specialized because agents used for other cardiomyopathies can be dangerous in amyloidosis.[42] The mainstay of treatment is salt restriction and careful administration of diuretics, such as furosemide, scrupulously avoiding aggravation of intravascular volume contraction (due to concomitant nephrotic syndrome), and postural hypotension. If furosemide becomes ineffective in controlling edema, the addition of metolazone or spironolactone can be beneficial. Angiotensin-converting enzyme inhibitors should not be used routinely because of the high risk of precipitating hypotension in the setting of diastolic and autonomic dysfunction; however, a few patients with reduced stroke volume can benefit from these agents when used with great caution. Digoxin can be toxic because of binding to amyloid in the heart but is occasionally useful in patients with atrial fibrillation and rapid ventricular response. Calcium channel blockers can aggravate congestive heart failure. Patients with recurrent syncope may require permanent pacemaker implantation. Patients with ventricular arrhythmias may benefit from treatment with amiodarone or the use of artificial implantable cardiac defibrillators, though this has not been rigorously proven. In patients with end-stage heart failure, heart transplantation is the only life-saving procedure, which may allow subsequent treatment to control the amyloidogenic clone. Orthostatic hypotension is challenging to manage. Midodrine can be helpful in some patients. Urinary retention and piloerection are the main side effects because supine hypertension is rare in these patients. The use of waist-high, fitted elastic stockings is helpful. In the Amyloidosis Center experience, fludrocortisone is poorly tolerated because of aggravation of fluid retention. Continuous noradrenalin infusion has been reported to be a successful treatment of severe hypotension refractory to conventional treatment. Therapy for renal amyloidosis is limited to the control of the edema by diuretics. The main damaging mechanism is progressive tubular injury caused by glomerular protein loss. The use of angiotensin-converting enzyme inhibitors, in an attempt to reduce proteinuria, is reasonable, although their efficacy has not been proven. Treatment of hyperlipidemia should be considered. Hypercoagulable state is rarely, if ever, seen in these nephrotic patients and prophylactic anticoagulation is not recommended. End-stage renal failure is treated by dialysis. Both peritoneal dialysis and hemodialysis are equally effective. If the disease is not controlled by chemotherapy, extrarenal progression of amyloidosis is the main cause of death. Renal transplantation should be offered on a case-by-case basis to patients without symptomatic extrarenal involvement.[43] Diarrhea is a common problem and can be incapacitating. Octreotide decreases diarrhea both in its short-acting form and its long-acting depository form. Chronic intestinal pseudoobstruction is usually refractory to treatment. Adequate oral or intravenous feeding is essential in patients with significant undernourishment. Patients who present with severe liver failure may be considered for liver transplantation; cases of successful sequential liver and SCTs have been reported.[44] Neuropathic pain is difficult to control. Gabapentin, although well-tolerated, often fails to relieve pain. Duloxetine may be effective in controlling pain of neuropathy. Nonnephrotoxic analgesics may be used as adjuvant agents. Bleeding in AL amyloidosis is frequent and multifactorial. Factor X deficiency can improve following effective chemotherapy, including HDM-SCT,[34] or after splenectomy.

CURRENT RECOMMENDATIONS AND FUTURE DIRECTIONS

The data from the Amyloidosis Center and that from other centers indicate that, despite multisystem organ dysfunction, selected patients with AL amyloidosis can tolerate HDM and autologous SCT. Moreover, high-dose chemotherapy can induce complete hematologic responses in a substantial proportion of patients who complete treatment. Furthermore, complete hematologic responses in AL amyloidosis are associated with reversal of amyloid-related organ dysfunction and may lead to prolonged survival in this disease, which is typically fatal within 2 years when managed with standard oral chemotherapy regimens of oral cyclic melphalan and prednisone.

During the past 20 years, a large number of AL amyloidosis patients with HDM-SCT have been treated, including patients older than 65 years old,[45] patients on dialysis,[46] and patients with cardiac disease.[47,48] Although patient selection remains important in achieving an acceptable outcome, the author believes it is in part attributable to the multidisciplinary approach to patient management. A team of subspecialists who are familiar with the manifestations and treatment of amyloidosis evaluate each patient. These subspecialists remain available to the transplant physicians throughout therapy and the amyloid clinical team meets regularly to review each patient's progress during treatment. The Amyloidosis Center encourages other transplant centers undertaking treatment of these complicated patients to adopt a similar multidisciplinary management approach.

SUMMARY

Promising treatments, other than HDM-SCT, are available for patients with AL amyloidosis. Although these treatment regimens are not discussed here, the availability of new regimens for treatment of AL amyloidosis may, in the future, provide additional options for patients who are not eligible for HDM-SCT. Timing and sequencing of regimens containing these agents, and comparison with or combination with HDM-SCT, will be determined in future trials.

Prompt diagnosis of amyloidosis and appropriate referral has great potential to improve outcome for these patients. AL amyloidosis should be considered in the differential diagnosis of patients being evaluated for a variety of syndromes, including nephrotic range proteinuria, unexplained nonischemic cardiomyopathy, nondiabetic peripheral or autonomic neuropathy, and unexplained hepatomegaly. It is essential to recognize AL amyloidosis as the cause of macroglossia and periorbital ecchymoses. All patients presenting with monoclonal gammopathy or smoldering myeloma should be screened for nephropathy and cardiomyopathy on presentation and periodically afterward. Despite improvements in the diagnosis and treatment of AL amyloidosis, continued basic and clinical research is needed to continue to improve the outcome for these patients.

ACKNOWLEDGMENTS

I gratefully acknowledge my colleagues in the Amyloidosis Center, Clinical Trials Office, and the staff of the Solomont Center for Cancer and Blood Disorders at Boston Medical Center who assisted with the multidisciplinary evaluation and treatment of the patients.

REFERENCES

1. Merlini G, Bellotti V. Molecular mechanisms of amyloidosis. N Engl J Med 2003; 349:583–96.
2. Sipe JD, Benson MD, Buxbaum JN, et al. Amyloid fibril protein nomenclature: 2012 recommendations from the Nomenclature Committee of the International Society of Amyloidosis. Amyloid 2012;19:167–70.
3. Gertz MA, Lacy M, Dispenzieri A. Amyloidosis. Hematol Oncol Clin North Am 1999;13:1211–20.
4. Kyle RA, Linos A, Beard CM, et al. Incidence and natural history of primary systemic amyloidosis in Olmsted County, Minnesota, 1950 through 1989. Blood 1992;79:1817–22.
5. Kyle RA, Gertz MA. Primary systemic amyloidosis: clinical and laboratory features in 474 cases. Semin Hematol 1995;32:45–59.
6. Dember LM. Emerging treatment approaches for the systemic amyloidoses. Kidney Int 2005;68:1377–90.
7. Palladini G, Dispenzieri A, Gertz MA, et al. New criteria for response to treatment in immunoglobulin light chain amyloidosis based on free light chain measurement and cardiac biomarkers: impact on survival outcomes. J Clin Oncol 2012;30:4541–9.
8. Girnius S, Seldin DC, Cibeira MT, et al. New hematologic response criteria predict survival in patients with immunoglobulin light chain amyloidosis treated with high-dose melphalan and autologous stem-cell transplantation. J Clin Oncol 2013;31:2749–50.
9. Sanchorawala V, Seldin DC, Magnani B, et al. Serum free light-chain responses after high-dose intravenous melphalan and autologous stem cell transplantation for AL (primary) amyloidosis. Bone Marrow Transplant 2005; 36:597–600.
10. Lachmann HJ, Gallimore R, Gillmore JD, et al. Outcome in systemic AL amyloidosis in relation to changes in concentration of circulating free immunoglobulin light chains following chemotherapy. Br J Haematol 2003;122:78–84.
11. Attal M, Harousseau JL, Stoppa AM, et al. A prospective, randomized trial of autologous bone marrow transplantation and chemotherapy in multiple myeloma. Intergroupe Francais du Myelome. N Engl J Med 1996;335:91–7.
12. Child JA, Morgan GJ, Davies FE, et al. High-dose chemotherapy with hematopoietic stem-cell rescue for multiple myeloma. N Engl J Med 2003;348:1875–83.
13. Comenzo RL, Vosburgh E, Simms RW, et al. Dose-intensive melphalan with blood stem cell support for the treatment of AL amyloidosis: one-year follow-up in five patients. Blood 1996;88:2801–6.
14. Skinner M, Sanchorawala V, Seldin DC, et al. High-dose melphalan and autologous stem-cell transplantation in patients with AL amyloidosis: an 8-year study. Ann Intern Med 2004;140:85–93.

15. Sanchorawala V, Skinner M, Quillen K, et al. Long-term outcome of patients with AL amyloidosis treated with high-dose melphalan and stem-cell transplantation. Blood 2007;110:3561–3.
16. Cibeira MT, Sanchorawala V, Seldin DC, et al. Outcome of AL amyloidosis after high-dose melphalan and autologous stem cell transplantation: long-term results in a series of 421 patients. Blood 2011;118:4346–52.
17. Comenzo RL, Gertz MA. Autologous stem cell transplantation for primary systemic amyloidosis. Blood 2002;99:4276–82.
18. Dispenzieri A, Gertz MA, Kyle RA, et al. Serum cardiac troponins and N-terminal pro-brain natriuretic peptide: a staging system for primary systemic amyloidosis. J Clin Oncol 2004;22:3751–7.
19. Palladini G, Campana C, Klersy C, et al. Serum N-terminal pro-brain natriuretic peptide is a sensitive marker of myocardial dysfunction in AL amyloidosis. Circulation 2003;107:2440–5.
20. Gertz M, Lacy M, Dispenzieri A, et al. Troponin T level as an exclusion criterion for stem cell transplantation in light-chain amyloidosis. Leuk Lymphoma 2008;49:36–41.
21. Perz JB, Schonland SO, Hundemer M, et al. High-dose melphalan with autologous stem cell transplantation after VAD induction chemotherapy for treatment of amyloid light chain amyloidosis: a single centre prospective phase II study. Br J Haematol 2004;127:543–51.
22. Sanchorawala V, Wright DG, Seldin DC, et al. High-dose intravenous melphalan and autologous stem cell transplantation as initial therapy or following two cycles of oral chemotherapy for the treatment of AL amyloidosis: results of a prospective randomized trial. Bone Marrow Transplant 2004;33:381–8.
23. Oran B, Malek K, Sanchorawala V, et al. Predictive factors for hematopoietic engraftment after autologous peripheral blood stem cell transplantation for AL amyloidosis. Bone Marrow Transplant 2005;35:567–75.
24. Comenzo RL, Michelle D, LeBlanc M, et al. Mobilized CD34+ cells selected as autografts in patients with primary light-chain amyloidosis: rationale and application. Transfusion 1998;38:60–9.
25. DiPersio JF, Stadtmauer EA, Nademanee A, et al. Plerixafor and G-CSF versus placebo and G-CSF to mobilize hematopoietic stem cells for autologous stem cell transplantation in patients with multiple myeloma. Blood 2009;113:5720–6.
26. Lee SY, Sanchorawala V, Seldin DC, et al. Plerixafor-augmented peripheral blood stem cell mobilization in AL amyloidosis with cardiac involvement: a case series. Amyloid 2014;21:149–53.
27. Sanchorawala V, Wright DG, Quillen K, et al. Tandem cycles of high-dose melphalan and autologous stem cell transplantation increases the response rate in AL amyloidosis. Bone Marrow Transplant 2007;40:557–62.
28. Sanchorawala V, Quillen K, Sloan JM, et al. Bortezomib and high-dose melphalan conditioning for stem cell transplantation for AL amyloidosis: a pilot study. Haematologica 2011;96:1890–2.
29. Dember LM, Sanchorawala V, Seldin DC, et al. Effect of dose-intensive intravenous melphalan and autologous blood stem-cell transplantation on al amyloidosis-associated renal disease. Ann Intern Med 2001;134:746–53.
30. Seldin DC, Anderson JJ, Sanchorawala V, et al. Improvement in quality of life of patients with AL amyloidosis treated with high-dose melphalan and autologous stem cell transplantation. Blood 2004;104:1888–93.
31. Girnius S, Seldin DC, Skinner M, et al. Hepatic response after high-dose melphalan and stem cell transplantation in patients with AL amyloidosis associated liver disease. Haematologica 2009;94:1029–32.

32. Meier-Ewert HK, Sanchorawala V, Berk J, et al. Regression of cardiac wall thickness following chemotherapy and stem cell transplantation for light chain (AL) amyloidosis. Amyloid 2011;18(Suppl 1):125–6.
33. Meier-Ewert HK, Sanchorawala V, Berk JL, et al. Cardiac amyloidosis: evolving approach to diagnosis and management. Curr Treat Options Cardiovasc Med 2011;13:528–42.
34. Choufani EB, Sanchorawala V, Ernst T, et al. Acquired factor X deficiency in patients with amyloid light-chain amyloidosis: incidence, bleeding manifestations, and response to high-dose chemotherapy. Blood 2001;97:1885–7.
35. Oran B, Wright DG, Seldin DC, et al. Spontaneous rupture of the spleen in AL amyloidosis. Am J Hematol 2003;74:131–5.
36. Tam M, Seldin DC, Forbes BM, et al. Spontaneous rupture of the liver in a patient with systemic AL amyloidosis undergoing treatment with high-dose melphalan and autologous stem cell transplantation: a case report with literature review. Amyloid 2009;16:103–7.
37. Dispenzieri A, Kyle RA, Lacy MQ, et al. Superior survival in primary systemic amyloidosis patients undergoing peripheral blood stem cell transplantation: a case-control study. Blood 2004;103:3960–3.
38. Jaccard A, Moreau P, Leblond V, et al. High-dose melphalan versus melphalan plus dexamethasone for AL amyloidosis. N Engl J Med 2007;357:1083–93.
39. Dey BR, Chung SS, Spitzer TR, et al. Cardiac transplantation followed by dose-intensive melphalan and autologous stem-cell transplantation for light chain amyloidosis and heart failure. Transplantation 2010;90:905–11.
40. Gillmore JD, Goodman HJ, Lachmann HJ, et al. Sequential heart and autologous stem cell transplantation for systemic AL amyloidosis. Blood 2006;107:1227–9.
41. Lacy MQ, Dispenzieri A, Hayman SR, et al. Autologous stem cell transplant after heart transplant for light chain (Al) amyloid cardiomyopathy. J Heart Lung Transplant 2008;27:823–9.
42. Seldin DC, Berk JL, Sam F, et al. Amyloidotic cardiomyopathy: multidisciplinary approach to diagnosis and treatment. Heart Fail Clin 2011;7:385–93.
43. Sattianayagam PT, Gibbs SD, Pinney JH, et al. Solid organ transplantation in AL amyloidosis. Am J Transplant 2010;10:2124–31.
44. Binotto G, Cillo U, Trentin L, et al. Double autologous bone marrow transplantation and orthotopic liver transplantation in a patient with primary light chain (AL) amyloidosis. Amyloid 2011;18(Suppl 1):127–9.
45. Seldin DC, Anderson JJ, Skinner M, et al. Successful treatment of AL amyloidosis with high-dose melphalan and autologous stem cell transplantation in patients over age 65. Blood 2006;108:3945–7.
46. Casserly LF, Fadia A, Sanchorawala V, et al. High-dose intravenous melphalan with autologous stem cell transplantation in AL amyloidosis-associated end-stage renal disease. Kidney Int 2003;63:1051–7.
47. Girnius S, Seldin DC, Meier-Ewert HK, et al. Safety and efficacy of high-dose melphalan and auto-SCT in patients with AL amyloidosis and cardiac involvement. Bone Marrow Transplant 2014;49:434–9.
48. Madan S, Kumar SK, Dispenzieri A, et al. High-dose melphalan and peripheral blood stem cell transplantation for light-chain amyloidosis with cardiac involvement. Blood 2012;119:1117–22.
49. Gertz MA, Lacy MQ, Dispenzieri A, et al. Transplantation for amyloidosis. Curr Opin Oncol 2007;19:136–41.

50. Mollee PN, Wechalekar AD, Pereira DL, et al. Autologous stem cell transplantation in primary systemic amyloidosis: the impact of selection criteria on outcome. Bone Marrow Transplant 2004;33:271–7.
51. Schonland SO, Perz JB, Hundemer M, et al. Indications for high-dose chemotherapy with autologous stem cell support in patients with systemic amyloid light chain amyloidosis. Transplantation 2005;80:S160–163.
52. Chow LQ, Bahlis N, Russell J, et al. Autologous transplantation for primary systemic AL amyloidosis is feasible outside a major amyloidosis referral centre: the Calgary BMT Program experience. Bone Marrow Transplant 2005;36:591–6.
53. Moreau P, Leblond V, Bourquelot P, et al. Prognostic factors for survival and response after high-dose therapy and autologous stem cell transplantation in systemic AL amyloidosis: a report on 21 patients. Br J Haematol 1998;101:766–9.
54. Gertz MA, Blood E, Vesole DH, et al. A multicenter phase 2 trial of stem cell transplantation for immunoglobulin light-chain amyloidosis (E4A97): an Eastern Cooperative Oncology Group Study. Bone Marrow Transplant 2004;34:149–54.
55. Goodman HJ, Gillmore JD, Lachmann HJ, et al. Outcome of autologous stem cell transplantation for AL amyloidosis in the UK. Br J Haematol 2006;134:417–25.
56. Vesole DH, Perez WS, Akasheh M, et al. High-dose therapy and autologous hematopoietic stem cell transplantation for patients with primary systemic amyloidosis: a Center for International Blood and Marrow Transplant Research Study. Mayo Clin Proc 2006;81:880–8.

Bone Marrow Transplantation for Acquired Severe Aplastic Anemia

Andrea Bacigalupo, MD

KEYWORDS

- Acquired severe aplastic anemia • Bone marrow transplantation • Unrelated donors
- Graft-versus-host disease

KEY POINTS

- Stem cell transplantation for acquired aplastic anemia has made significant progress over the past decade, and this is true especially for alternative donor transplants, including unrelated, cord blood, and haploidentical grafts.
- Significant predictors of survival remain the age of the patient and the interval between diagnosis and transplants: young patients with a short interval have the best survival.
- Early referral to experienced centers is thus mandatory for this rare disease.
- Graft-versus-host disease prophylaxis should include either antithymocyte globulin or alemtuzumab, and the stem cell source should be bone marrow.
- Exceptions to this recommendation would be recent protocols using haploidentical family donors.
- Haploidentical and cord blood transplants remain an experimental procedure, whereas HLA-identical donors and a well-matched (8/8) unrelated donor can be considered standard of care.

HUMAN LEUKOCYTE ANTIGEN–IDENTICAL SIBLING TRANSPLANTS

Who Is a Candidate

Patients with acquired severe aplastic anemia (SAA) should be typed for human leukocyte antigen (HLA) at diagnosis, together with their siblings: if an HLA-identical sibling is identified, and if the patient is younger than 50 years, an allogeneic bone marrow transplant (BMT) is currently the recommended first-line treatment.[1] Usually in patients older than 50 years, immunosuppressive therapy (IST) is given up front, because mortality increases with increasing age of patients.[2] In a study conducted by the European Group for Blood and Marrow Transplantation (EBMT), a 5-year survival advantage was seen for young patients with very low neutrophil counts ($<0.2 \times 10^9$/L) undergoing first-line BMT[3]; the opposite was true for a 50-year-old patient with a neutrophil count greater than 0.5×10^9/L, in whom the survival advantage was seen for first-line IST.[3]

Division of Hematology and Bone Marrow Transplant Unit, IRCCS San Martino, Pzza R Bensi 1, Genova 16132, Italy
E-mail address: andrea.bacigalupo@hsanmartino.it

Hematol Oncol Clin N Am 28 (2014) 1145–1155
http://dx.doi.org/10.1016/j.hoc.2014.08.004 hemonc.theclinics.com
0889-8588/14/$ – see front matter

- Young patients with low neutrophil counts are best candidates for a first-line allogeneic transplant if an HLA-identical sibling is available. Above the age of 40, one course of immunosuppressive therapy with antithymocyte globulin (ATG) and cyclosporine may be given, also in the presence of an identical sibling.

Human Leukocyte Antigen–Identical Sibling Transplants and Stem Cell Source

Bone marrow (BM) was the only source of stem cells in the early 1970s.[4] Cord blood (CB) and peripheral blood (PB) arrived in the late 1980s and early 1990s.[5,6] PB in particular has become very popular, owing to the common belief that PB grafts are safer on the donor side and improve survival, by preventing relapse, on the patient side. Both these ideas are incorrect: from the donor's perspective, the largest study in the literature (51,024 donations)[7] shows significantly greater risk of severe adverse events (SAE) for PB donations (25 vs 12 for BM, $P<.05$), and a higher risk (though not significant) of death, with 4 deaths in 23,254 PB donations and 1 death in 27,770 BM donations.[7] Regarding leukemia relapse, a recent randomized study[8] has shown no difference in relapse in patients with leukemia receiving BM or PB. In addition, PB grafts increase significantly the risk of extensive chronic graft-versus-host disease (cGvHD),[8] and cGvHD after PB transplants is less responsive to treatment.[9] Despite these data, PB grafts also have been largely used in patients with acquired SAA in whom leukemia relapse is not an issue, mainly with the hypothesis that PB grafts would solve the problem of rejection, especially in sensitized patients.[10] In the period 2001 through 2010 the proportion of patients in the EBMT Registry receiving PB was 40% in siblings and 48% in unrelated donor grafts (Bacigalupo A, 2014, unpublished data), and it was therefore important to assess the outcome of BM versus PB.

A first combined EBMT/Center for International Blood and Marrow Transplant Research (CIBMTR) analysis[11] has shown a significant survival advantage for BM grafts in young patients (<20 years of age) but not in older patients (≥20 years of age): this study also confirmed the increased risk of cGvHD for recipients of PB grafts.[11] In 2012 The EBMT published a second analysis on a much larger number of patients (N = 1886) who received a first matched sibling transplant between 1999 and 2009, with BM (n = 1163) or PB (n = 723) as a stem cell source.[12] The conclusions of this study were unequivocal: PB grafts from HLA-identical siblings, when compared with BM grafts, were associated with a greater risk of acute grade II to IV graft-versus-host disease (GvHD) (17% vs 11%, $P<.001$) and a greater risk of cGvHD (22% vs 11, $P<.001$).[12] The survival disadvantage for PB in comparison with BM was significant in patients aged 1 to 19 years (76% vs 90%, $P<.00001$) and in those 20 years and older (64% vs 74%, $P = .001$); this was true also for those older than 50 years (39% for PB vs 69% for BM, $P = .01$).

In an additional study comparing 3 different stem cell sources, namely BM, PB, and granulocyte colony–stimulating factor (G-CSF)–mobilized BM,[13] acute and chronic GvHD were again higher in PB graft recipients, and there was no advantage for G-CSF–mobilized BM in terms of engraftment and survival.

- BM should therefore be the stem source of choice for HLA-identical stem cell transplants in patients with acquired aplastic anemia. The use of PB is associated with worse survival and more cGvHD.

Conditioning Regimen

Cyclophosphamide

The standard of care for sibling BMT remains the original Seattle protocol, with cyclophosphamide (CY) 50 mg/kg/d on each of 4 days, and ATG (CY-ATG).[4] Results of this conditioning regimen are well established, with current survival ranging from 65% to 95%, according to patient age.[1,4] This conditioning regimen is associated with a very low incidence of second tumors[14] and preservation of fertility.[15]

Fludarabine

In some centers the CY200 regimen is considered too weak for highly sensitized patients, namely patients who are refractory to platelet transfusions: in one study 38 sensitized SAA patients, with a median age of 20 years (range 14–36 years), underwent BMT with a conditioning regimen including fludarabine (FLU) 30 mg/m^2/d for 3 days (days −9, −8, and −7) and CY 50 mg/kg/d for 4 days (days −5, −4, −3, and −2).[16] GvHD prophylaxis consisted of cyclosporine A and short-course methotrexate (CyA-MTX).[16] Engraftment was observed in all patients after transplantation: 25 of the 27 patients with available chimeric studies at day 180 maintained donor chimerism. The risk of grade II to IV acute GvHD was 11% and of extensive cGvHD, 25%. Graft rejection with relapse of aplasia was observed in 1 patient. The overall survival (OS) for the whole group was 79%.[16] In this particular case, the combination CY-ATG was changed to CY-FLU, with the same large dose of CY, which delivered good results in terms of engraftment.

An additional problem to patient sensitization is the strong effect of age seen with the CY-ATG conditioning.[2,17] For this reason, FLU-based regimens have been also introduced in older adults.[18–20] In a retrospective EBMT study,[21] patients older than 30 receiving FLU-based regimens were compared with a matched paired group of patients conditioned with CY 200 mg/kg over the same period of time (1998–2007): patients conditioned with FLU had a higher probability of OS than the control group (P = .04) when adjusting for recipient's age, possibly related to a trend toward a reduced incidence of graft failure in patients receiving FLU (0% vs 11%, P = .09), whereas no difference was observed regarding incidence of GvHD.[21] In a more recent analysis of the EBMT (Bacigalupo A, 2014, unpublished data), the effect of age was combined with conditioning regimen in transplants from HLA-identical siblings, in the period 2001 through 2010 (**Fig. 1**): survival of patients aged 1 to 20 years was 89% (group A, n = 935); survival of those aged 21 to 40 was 76% (group B, n = 770); survival of patients older than 40 receiving a FLU-based regimen and ATG or alemtuzumab (CAMP) in the conditioning regimen was 74% (group C, n = 51); survival of patients older than 40 receiving a FLU-based regimen, but no ATG and no CAMP, was 64% (group D, n = 57); and survival of those older than 40, not receiving a FLU-based regimen, and no ATG and no CAMP, was 54% (group E, n = 238). This study suggests that survival can improve in patients older than 40 years if appropriate modifications are made in the conditioning regimen.

Irradiation

Irradiation, in the form of either total lymphoid irradiation (TLI) or total body irradiation (TBI), is currently rarely used in patients receiving an HLA sibling transplant: the high risk of malignancies in SAA patients exposed to radiation during conditioning[14] has discouraged centers from adopting this policy, although exceptions still exist.[22,23]

Antithymocyte globulin and alemtuzumab

The role of in vivo T-cell depletion with ATG or CAMP for BMT in HLA-identical siblings has been disputed: a randomized trial failed to show a survival advantage for patients receiving ATG in the conditioning regimen when compared with controls.[24] The EBMT retrospective study, on much larger number of patients,[12] has shown a clear advantage for ATG-treated patients. A recent United Kingdom study has compared the use of ATG with the use of CAMP for in vivo T-cell depletion.[25] One hundred patients

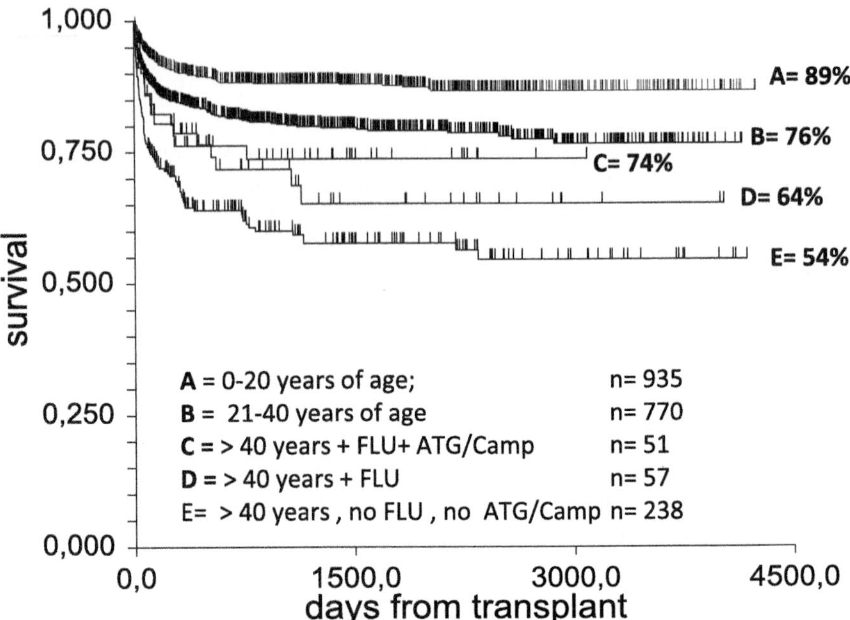

Fig. 1. Actuarial survival of patients with severe aplastic anemia, grafted from HLA-identical siblings in the period 2001 to 2010, stratified by age and conditioning regimens. The best outcome is seen in patients aged 0 to 20 years (group A). Survival of patients aged 21 to 40 (group B) compares with survival of older patients, only if the conditioning regimen is fludarabine (FLU)-based, and contains antithymocyte globulin (ATG) or alemtuzumab (Camp) (group C). When older patients (>40 years) are grafted without ATG/Camp (group D) or without ATG/Camp and without FLU (group E), survival is inferior (64% and 540025, respectively).

received CAMP and 55 patients ATG-based regimens; the donor was a matched sibling in 56%, a matched unrelated donor in 39%, and other related or mismatched unrelated donor in 5% of patients. Engraftment failure occurred in 9% of the CAMP group and 11% of the ATG group. The outcome was similar for sibling BMT using CAMP or ATG (91% vs 85%, respectively; $P = .562$). A lower risk of cGvHD was observed in the CAMP group (11% vs 26%, $P = .031$). Also in this study the use of BM as stem cell source was associated with better OS and event-free survival, and less acute GvHD and cGvHD.[24]

An additional way is to use "CAMP in the bag," producing ex vivo T-cell depletion: the method is probably not widespread, but may lead to significant protection against chronic and acute GvHD.

- The standard conditioning regimen for patients with acquired SAA undergoing an HLA-identical sibling transplant remains CY200 + ATG or CAMP. In vivo T-cell depletion with ATG or CAMP seems particularly important in patients older than 40 years. FLU-based regimens may be used in older patients. Irradiation should probably be avoided in HLA-identical sibling transplants.

Engraftment and Donor Chimerism

Engraftment and graft failure have been a major issue in HLA-identical sibling transplants for acquired SAA. The use of chimerism studies, using short tandem repeat

(STR) polymerase, has been a major advance in our understanding of how donor/recipient myeloid and lymphoid cells interact.[26] In a study on 94 SAA transplants, patients were classified as (1) complete donor chimeras (n = 43%), (2) transient mixed chimeras (n = 16%), (3) stable mixed chimeras (n = 20%), (4) progressive mixed chimeras (n = 15%), and (5) early graft rejection (5%).[27] This study showed that mixed chimerism occurs in a large proportion of patients and that the kinetics of sequential chimerism is a predictor of outcome. Treatment of mixed chimerism has not been standardized: mixed chimerism associated with declining PB counts may be treated with low doses of donor lymphocyte infusions (DLI) while maintaining GvHD prophylaxis with cyclosporine. Unfortunately there are no reports on this approach, and the use of DLI for mixed chimerism continues on a patient-to-patient basis. The author's group has treated 9 SAA patients, with a total of 42 DLI for mixed chimerism: 6 patients achieved complete donor chimerism (100%) on BM cells and 4 on $CD3^+$ cells; 2 patients died, 1 of rejection and 1 of GvHD; and 7 patients survive 3 to 10 years after DLI.

- Serial tests of donor/recipient chimerism by STR technology should be performed after transplantation in SAA, on unfractionated BM cells and possibly on selected $CD3^+$ PB T cells. DLI, given together with cyclosporine, is effective in converting most of these patients to complete donor chimerism. Caution must be exercised with DLI dosing because of the potential risk of lethal GvHD.

The Age Effect

Determining the upper age limit for eligibility to transplant in aplastic anemia is a difficult conundrum. A strong age effect has always been reported, and still remains a major predictor of survival.[17] As already shown herein, modifications of conditioning regimens and GvHD prophylaxis with either ATG or CAMP may improve survival in the older patient population. It would seem reasonable to restrict transplantation from identical siblings to SAA patients who are younger than 60 years. There are always exceptions to the rule, but one may wish to consider that mortality in SAA is high in older patients, probably more so than in leukemia patients of the same age.

UNRELATED DONOR TRANSPLANTS

Transplant-related mortality (TRM) has been greatly reduced over the past decade in patients with acquired SAA undergoing an unrelated donor (UD) transplant, as shown in a report by the French Cooperative Transplant Group (SFGM).[28] Factors contributing to improved outcome include modifications of the conditioning regimen with the introduction of low-dose TBI,[29,30] and more stringent criteria of HLA compatibility for donor selection. Despite these changes, mortality can still be significant, as shown in a pediatric study of 195 SAA children undergoing UD transplants: mortality was 43% for 8 of 8 matched donors and 61% for less than 8 of 8 matched donors.[31]

Conditioning Regimen

Fludarabine, cyclophosphamide, and low-dose total body irradiation

The combination of FLU, CY, and low-dose TBI is being used internationally by several centers[29–32] in both children and adults: a high mortality with larger doses of TBI from Registry data[31] has led to the development of programs with TBI of 2 to 3 Gy.[29,30] The EBMT has reported 100 patients who received a FLU-CY-ATG regimen with (FCA-TBI) or without (FCA) low-dose (2 Gy) TBI[32]: the regimen without TBI was given mainly to children younger than 14 years and the TBI regimen to adults. The 5-year survival was 73% for FCA and 79% for FCA-TBI[32]; acute GvHD grade III to IV was seen in 18% and 7%, respectively. Graft failure was seen in 17% in patients receiving either

FCA or FCA-TBI, although 9 of 17 survived long term. The most significant predictor of survival was the interval between diagnosis and transplant, with a 5-year survival of 87% and 55% for patients grafted within or beyond 2 years from diagnosis. Major causes of death were graft failure (n = 7), posttransplant lymphoproliferative disease (n = 4), and GvHD (n = 4).[32]

Fludarabine, cyclophosphamide, and alemtuzumab

Another interesting study has recently been published by a British group, using a combination of FLU-CY and CAMP (FCC)[24]: the protocol is radiation free, and of course this has strong added value for a nonmalignant disease. Results were extremely good for both related and UDs. The FCC program should be seriously considered for SAA patients undergoing a UD transplant. The issues of mixed chimerism, already discussed for HLA-identical siblings, come into the equation also for UD grafts, and need to be addressed appropriately. It is probable that CAMP should be used in centers experienced in using this agent.

Cyclophosphamide dose

The optimal dose of CY to be combined with FLU is unclear. In a de-escalation study for BM transplantation from UDs in patients with SAA, all patients received fixed doses of ATG, FLU, and low-dose TBI.[33] The starting dose of CY was 150 mg/kg, with de-escalation to 100 mg/kg, 50 mg/kg, or 0 mg/kg. A CY dose level of 0 mg/kg was closed because of graft failure in 3 of 3 patients. The 150 mg/kg CY dose level was closed because of excessive organ toxicity or viral pneumonia, resulting in 50% mortality. CY dose levels of 50 and 100 mg/kg remain open. Thus, the dose of CY to be combined with FLU should range between 50 and 100 mg/kg.[33]

- The most common conditioning regimen for patients with acquired SAA undergoing a UD transplant is the combination of FLU, CY, ATG, and low-dose TBI (2–3 Gy). The dose of CY should be less than 150 mg/kg. The FLU-CY-CAMP combination also seems interesting. ATG or CAMP should be part of the GvHD prophylaxis regimen in UD transplants for acquired SAA, together with cyclosporine and methotrexate.
- A short interval between diagnosis and transplantation remains a strong predictor of survival.

Stem Cell Source

A study of the CIBMTR has compared BM and PB in UD transplants for acquired SAA[34]: 296 patients received either BM (n = 225) or PB (n = 71) from unrelated donors, matched at HLA-A, -B, -C, and -DRB1. Hematopoietic recovery was similar after PB and BM transplantation. Acute grade II to IV GvHD was more frequent in PB than in BM ($P = .02$; 48% vs 31%). cGvHD risks were not significantly different after adjusting for age at transplantation (hazard ratio = 1.39, $P = .14$). Mortality, independent of age, was higher after PB compared with BM transplantation (76% vs 61%, $P = .04$). The investigators concluded that in UD transplants, similarly to HLA-identical siblings, BM is the preferred graft source in SAA.

Having ascertained that marrow is the best stem cell source, the question concerns the optimal dose of cells. Previous studies have shown a strong effect of BM cell dose, with best results in patients receiving more than 4.2×10^8 cells/kg.[35] Whether this is still true could be questioned, because higher doses of marrow cells also mean higher doses of T cells, especially in patients receiving UD grafts: a marrow cell dose ranging between 3 and 4 $\times$ 10^8/kg seems to allow optimal outcome (personal data, unpublished).

- BM remains the stem cell source of choice for patients with acquired aplastic anemia undergoing a UD transplant.

CORD BLOOD TRANSPLANTS

Results of unrelated CB transplants in acquired SAA are limited to a small number of cases, owing to the propensity of SAA patients to reject a graft and to the high rate of graft failure in general after CB transplants. The EBMT has summarized the outcome of 71 SAA patients undergoing an unrelated CB graft[36]: the median age was 13 years and most patients (69%) received a reduced-intensity conditioning, mostly FLU-based. A total nucleated cell dose greater than 3.9×10^7/kg had a significant positive impact on engraftment and survival. Based on this result, a prospective study has been designed to include only patients undergoing an unrelated CB transplant containing greater than 4.0×10^7/kg total nucleated cells.[36]

HUMAN LEUKOCYTE ANTIGEN–HAPLOIDENTICAL RELATED TRANSPLANTS

As with CB transplants, grafts from HLA-haploidentical family donors also are restricted to only a few patients, and have been recently reviewed.[37] Although results can be satisfactory in children, this procedure has been considered highly experimental in adults, and is recommended to be performed only in experienced centers.[37]

However, things may have changed recently, and encouraging results have been reported with modifications of the transplant protocol, including the use mesenchymal stem cells (MSC),[38] the combination of marrow and PB,[39] and high-dose cyclophosphamide after transplantation (PT-CY).[40]

The study with combined BM + PB[39] is based on a nonmyeloablative conditioning regimen (FCA) intensive growth factor therapy (G-CSF + thrombopoietin mimetics), GvHD prophylaxis with methotrexate, mycophenolate mofetil, and cyclosporine A, intensive fungal prophylaxis with micafungin, and high-dose immunoglobulin 0.4 g/kg weekly[39]: although it is unclear which of these components are crucial for the protocol, results are exceptionally good, with an overall 5-year survival exceeding 80% in patients with an average age of 25 years.[39] The addition of CB MSC to this protocol does not seem to improve OS further.[38]

A recent study reports initial findings with haploidentical hematopoietic stem cell transplantation (haplo-HSCT) using a reduced-intensity conditioning with PT-CY in 8 patients with refractory SAA.[40] Six of 8 patients were engrafted. Graft failure was associated with donor-directed HLA antibodies, despite intensive pre-HSCT desensitization with plasma exchange and rituximab.[40] There was only 1 case of grade II skin GvHD.

- Haploidentical transplants should be considered experimental, with a high risk of failure, and should be offered to patients not responding to immunosuppressive therapy. Recent advances with modified transplant protocols may change these recommendations in the near future.

SUMMARY

Stem cell transplantation for acquired aplastic anemia has made significant progress over the past decade; this is true especially for alternative donor transplants, including unrelated, CB, and haploidentical grafts. Significant predictors of survival remain patient age and the interval between diagnosis and transplantation: young patients with a short interval have the best survival. Early referral to experienced centers is thus mandatory for this rare disease. GvHD prophylaxis should include either ATG or

CAMP, and the stem cell source should be BM. Exceptions to this recommendation would be recent protocols using haploidentical family donors. Haploidentical and CB transplants remain an experimental procedure, whereas HLA-identical donors and a well-matched (8/8) UD can be considered the standard of care.

REFERENCES

1. Aljurf M, Zahrani HA, Van Lint MT, et al. Standard treatment of acquires severe aplastic anemia, in adult patients 18-40 years old, with an HLA identical sibling. Bone Marrow Transplant 2013;48:178–9.
2. Locasciulli A, Oneto R, Bacigalupo A, et al, Severe Aplastic Anemia Working Party of the European Blood and Marrow Transplant Group. Outcome of patients with acquired aplastic anemia given first line bone marrow transplantation or immunosuppressive treatment in the last decade: a report from the European Group for Blood and Marrow Transplantation (EBMT). Haematologica 2007;92:11–8.
3. Bacigalupo A, Brand R, Oneto R, et al. Treatment of acquired severe aplastic anemia: bone marrow transplantation compared with immunosuppressive therapy – The European Group for Blood and Marrow Transplantation Experience. Semin Hematol 2000;37:69–80.
4. Storb R, Leisenring W, Anasetti C, et al. Long-term follow-up of allogeneic marrow transplants in patients with aplastic anemia conditioned by cyclophosphamide combined with antithymocyte globulin. Blood 1997;89:3890–1.
5. Gluckman E, Broxmeyer HA, Auerbach AD, et al. Hematopoietic reconstitution in a patient with Fanconi's anemia by means of umbilical-cord blood from an HLA-identical sibling. N Engl J Med 1989;321(17):1174–8.
6. Bensinger WI, Weaver CH, Appelbaum FR, et al. Transplantation of allogeneic peripheral blood stem cells mobilized by recombinant human granulocyte colony-stimulating factor. Blood 1995;85(6):1655–8.
7. Halter J, Kodera Y, Ispizua AU, et al. Severe events in donors after allogeneic hematopoietic stem cell donation. Haematologica 2009;94(1):94–101.
8. Anasetti C, Logan BR, Lee SJ, et al, Clinical Trials Network. Peripheral-blood stem cells versus bone marrow from unrelated donors. N Engl J Med 2012;367(16): 1487–96.
9. Flowers ME, Parker PM, Johnston LJ, et al. Comparison of chronic graft-versus-host disease after transplantation of peripheral blood stem cells versus bone marrow in allogeneic recipients: long-term follow-up of a randomized trial. Blood 2002;100(2):415–9. PubMed PMID: 12091330.Flowers PB and cGvHD.
10. Seth T, Kanga U, Sood P, et al. Audit of peripheral stem cell transplantation for aplastic anemia in multitransfused infected patients. Transplant Proc 2012; 44(4):922–4.
11. Schrezenmeier H, Passweg JR, Marsh JC, et al. Worse outcome and more chronic GVHD with peripheral blood progenitor cells than bone marrow in HLA-matched sibling donor transplants for young patients with severe acquired aplastic anemia: a report from the European Group for Blood and Marrow Transplantation and the Center for International Blood and Marrow Transplant Research. Blood 2007;110(4):1397–400.
12. Bacigalupo A, Socié G, Schrezenmeier H, et al, Aplastic Anemia Working Party of the European Group for Blood and Marrow Transplantation (WPSAA-EBMT). Bone marrow versus peripheral blood as the stem cell source for sibling transplants in acquired aplastic anemia: survival advantage for bone marrow in all age groups. Haematologica 2012;97(8):1142–8.

13. Chu R, Brazauskas R, Kan F, et al. Comparison of outcomes after transplantation of G-CSF-stimulated bone marrow grafts versus bone marrow or peripheral blood grafts from HLA-matched sibling donors for patients with severe aplastic anemia. Biol Blood Marrow Transplant 2011;17(7):1018–24.
14. Socié G, Henry-Amar M, Bacigalupo A, et al. Malignant tumors occurring after treatment of aplastic anemia. N Engl J Med 1993;329:1152–7.
15. Hinterberger-Fischer M, Kier P, Kalhs P, et al. Fertility, pregnancies and offspring complications after bone marrow transplantation. Bone Marrow Transplant 1991; 7(1):5–9. PubMed PMID: 1904290.
16. Al-Zahrani H, Nassar A, Al-Mohareb F, et al. Fludarabine-based conditioning chemotherapy for allogeneic hematopoietic stem cell transplantation in acquired severe aplastic anemia. Biol Blood Marrow Transplant 2011;17(5):717–22.
17. Gupta V, Eapen M, Brazauskas R, et al. Impact of age on outcomes after bone marrow transplantation for acquired aplastic anemia using HLA-matched sibling donors. Haematologica 2010;95(12):2119–25.
18. George B, Methews V, Viswabandya A, et al. Fludarabine and cyclophosphamide based reduced intensity conditioning (RIC) regimens reduce rejection and improve outcome in Indian patients undergoing allogeneic stem cell transplantation for severe aplastic anemia. Bone Marrow Transplant 2007;40(1):13–8.
19. Maury S, Aljurf M. Management of adult patients older than 40 years refractory to at least one immunosuppressive course: HLA-identical sibling HSCT using fludarabine-based conditioning. Bone Marrow Transplant 2013;48(2):196–7. http://dx.doi.org/10.1038/bmt.2012.251.
20. Srinivasan R, Takahashi Y, McCoy JP, et al. Overcoming graft rejection in heavily transfused and allo-immunised patients with bone marrow failure syndromes using fludarabine-based haematopoietic cell transplantation. Br J Haematol 2006; 133(3):305–14.
21. Maury S, Bacigalupo A, Anderlini P, et al, Severe Aplastic Anemia Working Party, European Group for Blood and Marrow Transplantation (EBMT-SAAWP). Improved outcome of patients older than 30 years receiving HLA-identical sibling hematopoietic stem cell transplantation for severe acquired aplastic anemia using fludarabine-based conditioning: a comparison with conventional conditioning regimen. Haematologica 2009;94(9):1312–5. http://dx.doi.org/10.3324/haematol.2009.006916.
22. Inamoto Y, Suzuki R, Kuwatsuka Y, et al. Long-term outcome after bone marrow transplantation for aplastic anemia using cyclophosphamide and total lymphoid irradiation as conditioning regimen. Biol Blood Marrow Transplant 2008;14(1): 43–9.
23. Champlin RE, Perez WS, Passweg JR, et al. Bone marrow transplantation for severe aplastic anemia: a randomized controlled study of conditioning regimens. Blood 2007;109:4582–5.
24. Marsh JC, Pearce RM, Koh MB, et al, British Society for Blood and Marrow Transplantation, Clinical Trials Committee. Retrospective study of alemtuzumab vs ATG-based conditioning without irradiation for unrelated and matched sibling donor transplants in acquired severe aplastic anemia: a study from the British Society for Blood and Marrow Transplantation. Bone Marrow Transplant 2014;49(1): 42–8. http://dx.doi.org/10.1038/bmt.2013.115.
25. Hoelle W, Beck JF, Dueckers G, et al. Clinical relevance of serial quantitative analysis of hematopoietic chimerism after allogeneic stem cell transplantation in children for severe aplastic anemia. Bone Marrow Transplant 2004;33(2): 219–23.

26. Socie G, Lawler M, Gluckman E, et al. Studies on hemopoietic chimerism following allogeneic bone marrow transplantation in the molecular biology era. Leuk Res 1995;19(8):497–504.
27. Lawler M, McCann SR, Marsh JC, et al, Severe Aplastic Anaemia Working Party of the European Blood and Marrow Transplant Group. Serial chimerism analyses indicate that mixed haemopoietic chimerism influences the probability of graft rejection and disease recurrence following allogeneic stem cell transplantation (SCT) for severe aplastic anaemia (SAA): indication for routine assessment of chimerism post SCT for SAA. Br J Haematol 2009;144:933–45.
28. Maury S, Balere-Appert ML, Chir Z, et al, French Society of Bone Marrow Transplantation and Cellular Therapy (SFGM-TC). Unrelated stem cell transplantation for severe acquired aplastic anemia: improved outcome in the era of high-resolution HLA matching between donor and recipient. Haematologica 2007; 92:589–96.
29. Deeg HJ, Amylon ID, Harris RE, et al. Marrow transplants from unrelated donors for patients with aplastic anemia: minimum effective dose of total body irradiation. Biol Blood Marrow Transplant 2001;7:208–15.
30. Kojima S, Matsuyama T, Kato S, et al. Outcome of 154 patients with severe aplastic anemia who received transplants from unrelated donors: the Japan Marrow Donor Program. Blood 2002;100:799–803.
31. Perez-Albuerne ED, Eapen M, Klein J, et al. Outcome of unrelated donor stem cell transplantation for children with severe aplastic anemia. Br J Haematol 2008; 141(2):216–23.
32. Bacigalupo A, Socié G, Lanino E, et al, Severe Aplastic Anemia Working Party of the European Group for Blood and Marrow Transplantation. Fludarabine, cyclophosphamide, antithymocyte globulin, with or without low dose total body irradiation, for alternative donor transplants, in acquired severe aplastic anemia: a retrospective study from the EBMT-SAA working party. Haematologica 2010; 95(6):976–82.
33. Tolar J, Deeg HJ, Arai S, et al. Fludarabine-based conditioning for marrow transplantation from unrelated donors in severe aplastic anemia: early results of a cyclophosphamide dose deescalation study show life-threatening adverse events at predefined cyclophosphamide dose levels. Biol Blood Marrow Transplant 2012;18(7):1007–11. http://dx.doi.org/10.1016/j.bbmt.2012.04.014.
34. Eapen M, Le Rademacher J, Antin JH, et al. Effect of stem cell source on outcomes after unrelated donor transplantation in severe aplastic anemia. Blood 2011;118(9):2618–21.
35. Niederwieser D, Pepe M, Storb R, et al. Improvement in rejection, engraftment rate and survival without increase in graft-versus-host disease by high marrow cell dose in patients transplanted for aplastic anaemia. Br J Haematol 1988;69: 23–8.
36. Peffault de la Tour R, Rocha V, Socie G. Cod blood transplants in aplastic anemia. Bone Marrow Transplant 2013;48:201–2.
37. Ciceri F, Lupo Stanghellini MT, Korthof E. Haploidentical transplantation in patients with acquired aplastic anemia. Bone Marrow Transplant 2013;48:183–5.
38. Li XH, Gao CJ, Da WM, et al. Reduced intensity conditioning, combined transplantation of haploidentical hematopoietic stem cells and mesenchymal stem cells in patients with severe aplastic anemia. PLoS One 2014;9(3):e89666. http://dx.doi.org/10.1371/journal.pone.0089666.
39. Gao L, Li Y, Zhang Y, et al. Long-term outcome of HLA-haploidentical hematopoietic SCT without in vitro T-cell depletion for adult severe aplastic anemia after

modified conditioning and supportive therapy. Bone Marrow Transplant 2014; 49(4):519–24.
40. Clay J, Kulasekararaj AG, Potter V, et al. Nonmyeloablative peripheral blood haploidentical stem cell transplantation for refractory severe aplastic anemia. Biol Blood Marrow Transplant 2014. http://dx.doi.org/10.1016/j.bbmt.2014.06.028.

Hematopoietic Stem Cell Transplantation for Primary Immunodeficiencies

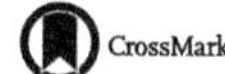

Elizabeth Kang, MD[a,*], Andrew Gennery, MD[b]

KEYWORDS

- Immunodeficiency • Immune reconstitution • Infection • Immunosuppression
- Inflammation

KEY POINTS

- Transplantation is curative for many types of immunodeficiency.
- Conditioning regimens should vary depending on the disease and patient condition.
- Full donor engraftment may not be required for cure.
- Outcomes improve with earlier transplant before infection and/or end-organ damage.

INTRODUCTION

The first hematopoietic stem cell transplants (HSCT) for patients with primary immunodeficiencies (PIDS), specifically severe combined immunodeficiency (SCID) and Wiskott-Aldrich syndrome (WAS), were performed in 1968.[1,2] Since then, HSCT has been regularly used to treat a growing spectrum of immunodeficiencies. A recent Primary Immune Deficiency Treatment Consortium (PIDTC) survey reported more than 1000 patients transplanted in North America alone for SCID, WAS, or chronic granulomatous disease (CGD), which are the three most common types of PID.[3]

Further, more than 200 distinct immunodeficiencies have now been described and at least 10 new genetic forms of PIDS are described each year: many of these new diseases have successfully been treated by HSCT.[4] Thus transplantation is a major treatment option for patients with genetic mutations in cells of the hematopoietic system that lead to an impaired immune response. However, the rarity of these disorders and the unique aspects intrinsic to each disease make it difficult to define a universal

[a] Hematotherapeutics Unit, Laboratory of Host Defenses, National Institute of Allergy and Infectious Diseases, National Institutes of Health, 10-CRC Room 6-3752, 10 Centre Drive, Bethesda, MD 20892, USA; [b] Paediatric Immunology Department, Institute of Cellular Medicine, Great North Children's Hospital, c/o Ward 3, Queen Victoria Road, Newcastle upon Tyne NE1 4LP, UK

* Corresponding author.

E-mail address: ekang@niaid.nih.gov

Hematol Oncol Clin N Am 28 (2014) 1157–1170

http://dx.doi.org/10.1016/j.hoc.2014.08.006

0889-8588/14/$ – see front matter Published by Elsevier Inc.

hemonc.theclinics.com

transplant regimen. This article discusses those PIDs most commonly treated by HSCT and disease-specific issues regarding transplantation for these patients.

SEVERE COMBINED IMMUNODEFICIENCIES AND RELATED DISORDERS

SCID comprises several disorders mainly characterized by a lack of functional T cells caused by (1) a failure to produce cytokines necessary for T-cell maturation (interleukin [IL]-2 receptor common gamma chain, Jak3, and IL7RA deficiencies) (2) accumulation of toxic purine metabolites (Adenosine Deaminase [ADA]-SCID), (3) defective differentiation of a neutrophil/T-cell precursor (reticular dysgenesis), or (4) defective VDJ rearrangements (Rag2, Rag2, Artemis). SCID disorders can also be characterized by the presence or absence of natural killer (NK) or B cells.

Patients with these disorders usually do not survive beyond the first year of life. The only chance of long-term survival is immunologic reconstitution by normal T cells. The SCID genotype has significant implications on the need for conditioning and transplant outcome. Although immunosuppression is typically not required for these patients because the absence of T lymphocytes prevents graft rejection, there are some SCID variants in which immunosuppressive agents may be required to facilitate long-term immunoreconstitution.[5] Preexisting infections, particularly viral infections, such as cytomegalovirus (CMV) or adenovirus, may limit the ability to use myeloablative chemotherapy conditioning, although reduced intensity conditioning (RIC) may be tolerated.[6] In addition, maternal engraftment of leukocytes during pregnancy is common in some SCID genotypes because there are no autologous T cells to reject transplacental maternal T cells.[7] Maternal T lymphocytes do not provide effective immunity, but may cause maternofetal graft-versus-host disease (GvHD) manifesting as an eczematous rash, splenomegaly, and occasionally pneumonitis or other complications.[8] There is also the potential complication of a graft-versus-graft (GvG) reaction depending on the donor used. Infusion of unfractionated human leukocyte antigen (HLA)–identical sibling marrow can lead to rejection of the maternal T lymphocytes, with or without a clinical GvG reaction.[9] Using a maternal donor can result in rapid immune reconstitution with or without GvHD that is usually amenable to treatment with low-dose steroids.[10] In contrast, rejection of a paternal graft can occur either with or without a clinical GvG reaction.

The best donor is an HLA-matched sibling donor, with a 90% overall survival rate in the most favorable circumstances.[11] When a matched sibling or family donor is unavailable, an alternative donor is necessary. Given the lack of autologous T cells and the ready availability of a parental donor, haploidentical transplants are a common choice. Bone marrow grafts depleted of T cells were studied prospectively resulting in an 81% overall survival with 77 patients having received a haploidentical graft and 12 using an HLA-matched related donor. All grafts were infused without preconditioning (except for 2 receiving placental blood) or posttransplant GvHD prophylaxis and most deaths occurred within 12 months following transplantation, most from preexisting infection. Note that 68 of the 72 had normal T-cell function but 45 of the 72 survivors required intravenous immunoglobulin replacement.[12] Although this method means that patients without an HLA-identical sibling donor can be offered transplantation and cure, there is a significant, albeit diminishing, mortality risk associated with T lymphocyte–depleted transplants.[11,13]

The results from HSCT are superior when the procedure is performed early, before end-organ damage occurs from infection. Twenty-one infants diagnosed early because of a positive family history were transplanted within 28 days of birth, 16 of whom had IL-2 receptor gamma chain–deficient or JAK3-deficient SCID, and all received

T lymphocyte–depleted stem cells, without any conditioning or GvHD prophylaxis.[14] Twenty patients (95%) survived, with a maximum follow-up of 19 years. A 2-center study from the United Kingdom similarly compared outcomes of 48 probands and 60 older affected siblings with an overall survival in the early transplants of 90% versus 60% in the older siblings.[15] A recent report from the PIDTC on 240 children with SCID transplanted between 2000 and 2009 showed that survival in older patients was as good as in those transplanted at less than 3 months, as long as they were infection free or previous infection had cleared.[16] Initiatives to mandate testing for SCID at birth are therefore underway in many US states and Canadian provinces.[17–19]

Attempts to perform in utero transplantation have been made in patients with a positive family history of SCID.[20] However, confirming the diagnosis requires invasive procedures, which can lead to fetal loss, and T lymphocytopenia with diminished mitogen response has been reported after some procedures, leaving the patient at risk of opportunistic infection.[21,22] Furthermore, occult maternofetal T-lymphocyte engraftment may lead to graft rejection, and obtaining maternal stem cells to treat the patient is not feasible during pregnancy. GvHD is also undetectable in utero, and treatment via the mother and monitoring of the fetal responses are either not possible or impractical. Thus, for those patients with a positive family history, the preferred option is to confirm the diagnosis, initiate prophylactic antimicrobial treatment at birth, and search for a donor to perform a transplant as soon as possible.

More recently with high sequencing analysis of HLA, the results of matched unrelated donor transplantation using adult donors or umbilical cord blood (UCB) is gaining support as a viable alternative. HSCT using HLA-matched unrelated donors provides similar results to those of HLA-matched siblings.[11,23] UCB products that are already banked are more readily available, allowing early transplantation. Fernandes and colleagues[24] compared the results of UCB transplant with mismatched related donor transplant in a retrospective study involving 249 transplants (74 UCB vs 174 mismatched related donor). Most UCB transplants were done with a myeloablative conditioning regimen and recipients had a higher frequency of complete donor chimerism and faster lymphocyte count recovery, but there was a trend toward more severe acute GvHD and more chronic GvHD. The 5-year survival rates were similar at 62% for mismatched related donor transplant versus 57% for UCB.

In addition, the role of conditioning remains undetermined. Although comprehensive studies are lacking, certain tenets apply and considerations for pretransplant conditioning include the presence of infection or end-organ damage, the molecular diagnosis, the type of donor available, the likelihood of full immune reconstitution, and the risk of short-term and long-term side effects. In a multicenter study between the United States and Europe of 103 patients with SCID, infusion of stem cells from an unrelated donor restored T-lymphocyte immune reconstitution, although the risk of GvHD was significantly higher than when a matched related donor was used.[25] A study of 77 patients with SCID in the United Kingdom, who received stem cell infusions, showed a 90% survival in matched sibling donor/matched family donor transplants but only 60% when alternative donors were used. Infants with NK^-SCID were more likely to survive and had high-level donor T-cell chimerism with superior long-term recovery of CD4 T-cell immunity than NK^+ recipients. A third of patients with NK^+SCID required additional transplant procedures.[26]

In a series of 98 patients with SCID, 32% received pretransplant chemotherapy conditioning: the rate of engraftment was significantly higher in these patients than in non-conditioned patients, but overall survival was less, mainly because of infection-related deaths.[13] More recently, European centers have described the outcome of transplantation for 699 patients with SCID, of whom 25% had a T-B- phenotype, and of whom

42% received conditioning. There was no survival advantage for the nonconditioned patients.[11] A small single-center study of 24 patients, of whom at least half had T-B- SCID, showed more favorable outcomes for patients who received conditioning and, in a multicenter study of 178 patients with SCID, the molecular diagnosis significantly affected outcome.[27] Patients with T-B- SCID had worse survival, with diminished rates of stem cell engraftment, and slower T and B lymphocyte immune reconstitution, but there a better overall rate of cure of disease in patients who had received conditioning.[28] These findings were replicated in the most recent European report.[11]

In NK-SCID (IL-2, Jak3, IL7RA, ADA-SCID), prethymic and early intrathymic stromal niches are vacant and thus available for donor T-lymphocyte precursor engraftment, leading to sustained donor-derived thymopoiesis in the absence of myelopoiesis.[29] In contrast, in NK+ SCID caused by VDJ recombination defects, later stages of T-lymphocyte differentiation are blocked; therefore, without conditioning, high numbers of DN2/DN3 cells compete with donor T-lymphocyte progenitors for thymic niches, resulting in a restricted T-cell repertoire and reliance on postthymic T-lymphocyte expansion.[30–32] Infusion of large doses of stem cells as well as other stromal factors aids engraftment of donor stem cells and improves immune reconstitution.[30,33] Myeloid engraftment, most often achieved following conditioning, facilitates engraftment of donor stem cells, permitting long-term thymopoiesis, even in NK- SCID phenotypes.[32,34]

Moreover, although restoration of T lymphocytes occurs following infusion of T-depleted stem cells, many patients with nonconditioned transplants fail to gain functional B lymphocytes, particularly patients with VDJ recombination defects.[12,30–32,35–37] Recipient B lymphocytes have reduced numbers of memory and isotype-switched B lymphocytes, and poor antibody responses to antigen stimulation, compared with donor-derived B lymphocytes.[38] In contrast, recipient B lymphocytes from patients with IL7RA-deficient SCID are able to function in the presence of donor T lymphocytes and produce antibody to appropriate antigen stimulation.[38,39] Also, patients with IL-2 receptor gamma chain–deficient or JAK3-deficient SCID without conditioning can develop B lymphocyte function, likely because of donor B-lymphocyte microchimerism. In contrast, not all conditioned transplants achieve donor B lymphocyte engraftment and independence from immunoglobulin replacement.

Patients with ADA-deficient SCID differ from those with other molecular defects because accumulation of toxic metabolites causes common lymphoid precursor toxicity leading to abnormalities of T, B, and NK lymphocyte development and function. In addition, patients often have preexisting inflammatory pneumonitis caused by the metabolic defect.[40,41] In a retrospective multicenter study of 106 infants with ADA-deficient SCID, outcomes were better for patients who had matched sibling and family donors than matched unrelated or T lymphocyte–depleted donors.[42] Superior survival was seen in patients who received nonconditioned transplants rather than myeloablative procedures. When using haploidentical donors without conditioning, nonengraftment was a major problem, although donor B-lymphocyte engraftment was achieved even after nonconditioned transplants.

In addition, the use of chemotherapeutic agents, even when beneficial, has long-term implications. Patients with Artemis-deficient SCID experience significant long-term sequelae following the use of alkylating agents, including significant growth failure, dental problems, and autoimmunity; findings that are not associated with nonconditioned transplants.[43,44] Impaired fertility is associated with many of the conditioning agents used, although detailed information from the SCID cohort is not available. Moreover, the long-term risk of malignancy may be increased, at least in some patients who receive irradiation as part of the preconditioning regimen, but the only data are anecdotal.[45] Therefore, more studies are needed to delineate specific long-term immunologic and general health outcomes in large cohorts of patients with the same molecular diagnoses, conditioning regimens, and donors. In addition, more data are needed on the use of nonmyeloablative regimens or RIC so that optimum treatment can be offered to appropriate patient groups.[46,47]

NON–SEVERE COMBINED IMMUNODEFICIENCIES

In general, patients with non-SCID disorders have at least some residual T lymphocyte–mediated immunity, thus requiring the use of at least some immunosuppression and/or conditioning to ensure engraftment of donor cells. In addition, there is often sufficient time to look for alternative nonfamily adult matched donors or cord blood stem cell units from national and international registries. Moreover, depending on the genetic defect, full donor chimerism may not be necessary to restore immune function. This aspect, combined with improvements in conditioning regimens, has resulted in the use of RIC with good outcomes.[6] In addition, T lymphocyte–depleted haploidentical donors were not used in these conditions because of the risk of nonengraftment or rejection. These patients are often older with preexisting viral infections, and T-lymphocyte depletion prolongs the time to reconstitution, thus increasing the risk of death from disseminated viral infection. However, several groups have been investigating modified grafts depleting specific T-cell subsets, while keeping others to maintain engraftment and antiviral activity, or using posttransplant cyclophosphamide to reduce reactive T cells after the graft infusion.[48,49]

Wiskott-Aldrich Syndrome

WAS protein (WASP) is expressed in hematologic cells and is necessary for cellular activation and production of cell synapses. Without WASP activation, cells have difficulty migrating and signaling appropriately, leading to recurrent infections as well as thrombocytopenia and autoimmunity.

The median life expectancy for patients with WAS is only 15 years without successful immune reconstitution following HSCT. Transplantation using related HLA-matched donors leads to survival rates of 71% to 80%.[50–53] As with all other PIDs, HLA-matched unrelated donors including UCB have also been used to treat patients with WAS. Patients transplanted at an earlier age, and those without infection-related damage, do better. Although there are data showing a significantly worse 5-year survival for patients who are transplanted after age 5 years, this may be more related to the presence of more end-organ damage in the older patients than actual age.[50,53,54] Transplants using T lymphocyte–depleted HSCT from HLA-mismatched family donors had previously been less satisfactory, with survival rates between 37% and 55%. However, a multicenter study of 194 patients showed comparable results for matched family or unrelated donors, and significant improvement in survival with T lymphocyte–depleted HLA-mismatched family donors, particularly in transplants performed since 2000.[53] Only a myeloablative conditioning regimen facilitates sufficient donor stem cell and stable multilineage engraftment fully correcting the hematological and immunologic defects, but 10% of patients still reject the graft, and more develop mixed or split donor cell chimerism.[55] Autoimmunity is common in long-term survivors after transplantation, particularly for those with persistent mixed or split donor chimerism after receiving stem cells from a matched unrelated donor.[53,55]

CD40 Ligand

CD40 ligand is expressed on activated T cells and is necessary for the proliferation and isotype switching of B cells in response to T-cell antigens. As a result, patients are unable to switch from making immunoglobulin (Ig) M to making IgG, IgA, or IgE and have a variable defect in T-lymphocyte and macrophage maturation. CD40 ligand–deficient patients are susceptible to infection from a wide variety of pathogens, including parasites like cryptosporidium, and are also at increased risk for developing autoimmune disorders and malignancies. Replacement gamma globulin is the standard treatment but the only curative option is HSCT.

To date, the largest reported series of transplants consists of 38 patients from 8 European countries.[56] The cohort was heterogenous in terms of age and physical condition at time of transplant, donor type, and conditioning regimen used. Of the 38, 21 had significant preexisting respiratory or hepatic disease. Overall survival was almost 70%, although 4 patients experienced autologous reconstitution. Cure of the disease was achieved in 58% of the cohort. The presence of lung disease, but not liver disease, as well as an HLA-mismatched donor correlated with poor survival. The outcome for patients with an HLA-matched unrelated donor was the same as for those with an HLA-matched sibling. There were too few patients included in the study to determine the optimum conditioning regimen.

Patients have also been successfully transplanted using RIC.[6,57] These regimens may reduce the risk of toxicity in sick patients, but there is a risk of rejection, which was a significant problem in the European series. Cryptosporidial infection can complicate the transplant procedure in these patients even when initial pretransplant testing of stool was negative by microscopy.[58] Patients with severe liver damage who are too sick to tolerate HSCT can receive an orthotopic liver graft before HSCT but once liver transplant has been achieved HSCT should proceed promptly to prevent cryptosporidial infection in the transplanted liver.[59] In addition, there is a report of 1 patient undergoing a successful transplant using a haploidentical donor with T-cell depletion and using T-cell add backs to establish full donor chimerism as well as to help clear a CMV reactivation.[60]

Chronic Granulomatous Disease

Mutations in one of the 6 genes responsible for the nicotinamide adenine dinucleotide phosphate (NADPH) oxidase complex results in a phagocyte disorder predisposing patients to risk from specific bacterial and fungal infections. Patients also have a higher incidence of autoimmune or inflammatory disorders, including pneumonitis or colitis as well as the development of granulomas, which can lead to luminal obstruction. Standard management includes use of prophylactic antibiotics; antifungals; immunosuppressants for the granuloma or autoinflammatory problems; and, in the United States, interferon gamma. At present, the only available cure is HSCT.

From 1973 until 2011 approximately 99 transplants (not including cord blood transplants) were performed for CGD, and 50 of those occurred in the last 10 years.[61] The first large multicenter study described the results in 27 patients using a myeloablative regimen except for 4 patients with RIC, 2 of whom lost their grafts. Thus the recommendation at that time was to use myeloablative conditioning regimens.[62] Investigators at the National Institutes of Health (NIH) showed the feasibility of using a nonmyeloablative regimen and HLA-matched sibling donors, particularly in high-risk patients, including those with an ongoing infection.[63]

As in other disorders, matched unrelated donor transplants are also being considered more frequently and the largest multicenter study to date reported results in 56 patients with CGD undergoing either related (21) or unrelated (35) donor transplantation. The nonmyeloablative conditioning regimen consisted of targeted-dose busulfan with fludarabine and serotherapy, and resulted in a 93% overall survival with 75% of the patients being categorized as high risk (presence of ongoing infection or active autoinflammatory process).[64]

UCB transplants have also been performed, first reported in 1999. An 8-year-old boy was conditioned with 10 Gy of total body irradiation (TBI), combined with antithymocyte globulin (ATG) and Cytoxan, but died at day 51 because of infection.[65] Since then a total of 11 reported patients have undergone cord blood transplantation from either related or unrelated donors. Several patients have required retransplantation because of graft failure, but all have done well with either autologous recovery or engraftment after a second transplant.[61] Given these results, it seems that a myeloablative regimen is necessary for UCB.

For many immunologists and pediatricians, the decision as to whom to refer for transplant is still not clear. This disorder is not fatal, and, although it is associated with a shortened life expectancy and significant morbidity, several patients have long infection-free periods and can have a good quality of life. Although the overall survival was the same between transplanted versus nontransplanted patients, quality of life seemed to be better in the transplanted group.[66] Moreover, investigators at NIH, using a cohort of more than 200 patients, correlated outcomes with the percentage of oxidase production, showing a significant increase in mortality with lower oxidase production.[67] This finding suggests that patients with lower oxidase production would benefit from transplantation and the PIDTC is now implementing a multicenter study to investigate the role of transplantation in the management of patients with CGD compared with standard medical therapy in cohorts with the same level of oxidase production.[3]

DNA Repair Disorders

Several disorders result from mutations in DNA double-strand break repair genes. The disorders give rise to a combination of immunodeficiency and a predisposition to leukemia or lymphoma; HSCT abolishes this risk, but coexistent multisystemic abnormalities including microcephaly and learning disability remain. The underlying DNA repair defect results in exquisite sensitivity to alkylating agents and radiotherapy, similar to patients with Fanconi anemia.[68,69]

In particular, patients with double-strand break repair disorders are generally intolerant of myeloablative or TBI-containing conditioning regimens. Patients with Nijmegen breakage syndrome have been successfully transplanted with RIC regimens[70] and there are a few reports of successful transplant for patients with DNA ligase 4 or cernunnos-XLF deficiency, with best results achieved when using RIC.[71–74] Outcome from transplant for dyskeratosis congenital was reported for a cohort of 34 patients. A range of donors, stem cell sources, and conditioning regimens was used, and there was a high incidence of GvHD and other transplant-related complications, with a 10-year survival of only 30%.[75] Conditioning regimen intensity and transplants from mismatched related or unrelated donors were associated with early mortality. A smaller cohort with shorter follow-up showed survival of 78% following HSCT using HLA-matched unrelated donors and RIC.[76] Similar to patients with Artemis-SCID, careful follow-up is required to determine whether problems are seen in the radiosensitive patient cohorts.

Hemophagocytic Syndromes

The familial hemophagocytic syndromes include diseases of disordered cytotoxicity, X-linked lymphoproliferative (XLP) disease, and X-linked inhibitor of apoptosis protein (XIAP) deficiency. Hemophagocytic lymphohistiocytosis (HLH) is characterized by multisystem inflammation resulting from prolonged and excessive activation of antigen-presenting cells (macrophages, histiocytes) and CD8+T lymphocytes. Initial treatment of HLH should be antiinflammatory, usually with steroids, etoposide, or ATG and cyclosporine, with prompt transition to HSCT once the disease is controlled.[77–79] Poor outcome is particularly associated with the use of T-depleted haploidentical grafts, and active disease at the time of transplantation but successful outcome leads to long-term remission, even with less than 50% donor chimerism.[80] In one single-center study, an RIC was associated with a better outcome with less acute GvHD experienced. Patients who had RIC required donor lymphocyte infusions more often than those receiving myeloablative chemotherapy, but 3-year survival was better at 92% versus 43%.[58] Forty-three patients transplanted for XLP showed a survival of 80%, but only 50% for those presenting with HLH, with no difference in survival between those receiving a myeloablative or RIC regimen in this study.[81] Patients with XIAP have poor outcomes after transplantation, particularly those receiving myeloablative conditioning, with most deaths caused by transplant-related toxicities. Best results are seen for those patients whose HLH was controlled and transplanted using RIC.[82] Antibody-based conditioning regimens may improve the outcome in these patients, even when HLH is uncontrolled.[46,81] Patients transplanted for HLH secondary to Griscelli syndrome type 2 or Chédiak-Higashi syndrome can be immunologically cured but neurologic disease may develop or progress, even with full donor chimerism.[83,84]

FOXP3

Mutations in the FOXP3 gene result in a rare disorder known as IPEX (immune, polyendocrinopathy, X-linked). FOXP3 is necessary for the generation of regulatory T-cells and their lack leads to multiorgan autoimmunity. Severe enteropathy is the predominant feature, although the manifestations can vary. Although symptoms can be ameliorated by immunosuppression, transplantation is curative and can prevent progression of the endocrinopathies. Transplant has an overall survival of 80% with either related or unrelated donors, including the use of cord blood and using myeloablative as well as nonmyeloablative regimens. The preferred donor source and conditioning regimen are undetermined given the small numbers to date.[85–87]

Dedicator of Cytokinesis-8

Mutations in the dedicator of cytokinesis-8 (DOCK8) were first described in 2009 by NIH investigators.[88] Although the exact role of this gene is unknown, patients have low absolute T-cell counts and often a decreased number of NK cells, along with a mild to moderate eosinophilia and high IgE levels. Patients with DOCK8 mutations are characterized by cutaneous and sinopulmonary infection with bacterial organisms as well as extensive cutaneous viral infections. Patients often die of squamous cell carcinomas or hematological malignancies as well as of infections.

To date, there are at least 9 reported patients who have undergone transplantation. Two patients were transplanted using a CD66 yttrium labeled antibody with fludarabine, melphalan, and ATG. Both are doing well 2 years or more after transplantation. In Boston, an 8-year-old girl received a sibling HLA-matched product after a myeloablative conditioning regimen but died of *Klebsiella pneumoniae* sepsis. Another patient underwent a fludarabine/busulfan-based transplant with 200 cGy radiation and has a normal posttransplant phenotype, but at 6 years has only 6% donor myeloid chimerism despite 98% lymphoid engraftment. Further, both haploidentical and unrelated donor transplants have been performed successfully for this disease.[89–95]

Investigators at the NIH have also performed several transplants using both related and unrelated HLA-matched donors and a nonmyeloablative conditioning regimen with promising results (Dennis Hickstein, personal communication, 2014). They are now looking to expand their transplant program, using haploidentical transplants with posttransplant cyclophosphamide immunotherapy.[48]

DISCUSSION

Transplantation is an effective treatment of patients with various immunodeficiencies. As transplant techniques improve, the risk/benefit ratio will continue to improve, warranting application to other diseases with less risk of adverse effects. Improvements in conditioning regimens to reduce toxicity and graft manipulations such as CD3 T cell receptor (TCR) alpha/beta depletion of haploidentical grafts will improve outcomes and increase donor availability for more patients. However, small numbers continue to make definitive statements difficult about the best candidates and type of transplant to use. More multicenter efforts such as the creation of the PIDTC and collaboration with other groups such as the inborn errors bone marrow transplant (IEBMT) working group will lead to better evaluation of results, allow tailoring of regimens and techniques, and improve recommendations for this diverse group of patients. In addition, gene therapy is becoming a viable alternative treatment of some conditions and will have to be considered in the decision making for these patients.

REFERENCES

1. Gatti RA, Meuwissen HJ, Allen HD, et al. Immunological reconstitution of sex-linked lymphopenic immunological deficiency. Lancet 1968;2:1366–9.
2. Bach FH, Albertini RJ, Joo P, et al. Bone-marrow transplantation in a patient with the Wiskott-Aldrich syndrome. Lancet 1968;2:1364–6.
3. Griffith LM, Cowan MJ, Kohn DB, et al. Allogeneic hematopoietic cell transplantation for primary immune deficiency diseases: current status and critical needs. J Allergy Clin Immunol 2008;122:1087–96.
4. Al-Herz W, Bousfiha A, Casanova JL, et al. Primary immunodeficiency diseases: an update on the classification from the international union of immunological societies expert committee for primary immunodeficiency. Front Immunol 2014;5:162.
5. Buckley RH. Molecular defects in human severe combined immunodeficiency and approaches to immune reconstitution. Annu Rev Immunol 2004;22:625–55.
6. Rao K, Amrolia PJ, Jones A, et al. Improved survival after unrelated donor bone marrow transplantation in children with primary immunodeficiency using a reduced-intensity conditioning regimen. Blood 2005;105:879–85.
7. Muller SM, Ege M, Pottharst A, et al. Transplacentally acquired maternal T lymphocytes in severe combined immunodeficiency: a study of 121 patients. Blood 2001;98:1847–51.
8. Palmer K, Green TD, Roberts JL, et al. Unusual clinical and immunologic manifestations of transplacentally acquired maternal T cells in severe combined immunodeficiency. J Allergy Clin Immunol 2007;120:423–8.
9. Friedman NJ, Shiff SE, Ward FE, et al. Graft versus graft and graft versus host reactions after HLA-identical bone marrow transplantation in a patient with severe combined immunodeficiency with transplacentally acquired lymphoid chimerism. Pediatr Allergy Immunol 1991;2:111–6.
10. Barrett MJ, Buckley RH, Schiff SE, et al. Accelerated development of immunity following transplantation of maternal marrow stem cells into infants with severe combined immunodeficiency and transplacentally acquired lymphoid chimerism. Clin Exp Immunol 1988;72:118–23.
11. Gennery AR, Slatter MA, Grandin L, et al. Transplantation of hematopoietic stem cells and long-term survival for primary immunodeficiencies in Europe:

entering a new century, do we do better? J Allergy Clin Immunol 2010;126: 602–10.e1–11.

12. Buckley RH, Schiff SE, Schiff RI, et al. Hematopoietic stem-cell transplantation for the treatment of severe combined immunodeficiency. N Engl J Med 1999; 340:508–16.
13. Fischer A, Griscelli C, Friedrich W, et al. Bone-marrow transplantation for immunodeficiencies and osteopetrosis: European survey, 1968-1985. Lancet 1986;2: 1080–4.
14. Myers LA, Patel DD, Puck JM, et al. Hematopoietic stem cell transplantation for severe combined immunodeficiency in the neonatal period leads to superior thymic output and improved survival. Blood 2002;99:872–8.
15. Brown L, Xu-Bayford J, Allwood Z, et al. Neonatal diagnosis of severe combined immunodeficiency leads to significantly improved survival outcome: the case for newborn screening. Blood 2011;117:3243–6.
16. Pai SY, Logan BR, Griffith LM, et al. Transplantation of 240 patients with severe combined immunodeficiency (SCID) from 2000-2009: a Primary Immune Deficiency Treatment Consortium report. N Engl J Med 2014;371:434–46.
17. Chan K, Puck JM. Development of population-based newborn screening for severe combined immunodeficiency. J Allergy Clin Immunol 2005;115:391–8.
18. Puck JM, SCID Newborn Screening Working Group. Group population-based newborn screening for severe combined immunodeficiency: steps toward implementation. J Allergy Clin Immunol 2007;120:760–8.
19. Buckley RH. The long quest for neonatal screening for severe combined immunodeficiency. J Allergy Clin Immunol 2012;129:597–604 [quiz: 605–6].
20. Flake AW, Zanjani ED. Treatment of severe combined immunodeficiency. N Engl J Med 1999;341:291–2.
21. Flake AW, Roncarolo MG, Puck JM, et al. Treatment of X-linked severe combined immunodeficiency by in utero transplantation of paternal bone marrow. N Engl J Med 1996;335:1806–10.
22. Wengler GS, Lanfranchi A, Frusca T, et al. In-utero transplantation of parental CD34 haematopoietic progenitor cells in a patient with X-linked severe combined immunodeficiency (SCIDXI). Lancet 1996;348:1484–7.
23. Grunebaum E, Mazzolari E, Porta F, et al. Bone marrow transplantation for severe combined immune deficiency. JAMA 2006;295:508–18.
24. Fernandes JF, Rocha V, Labopin M, et al. Transplantation in patients with SCID: mismatched related stem cells or unrelated cord blood? Blood 2012;119: 2949–55.
25. Dvorak C, Hassan A, Slatter M, et al. Comparison of outcomes of hematopoietic stem cell transplantation without chemotherapy conditioning by using matched sibling and unrelated donors for treatment of severe combined immunodeficiency. J Allergy Clin Immunol, in press.
26. Hassan A, Lee P, Maggina P, et al. Absence of host natural killer cells is associated with engraftment permissiveness following non-conditioned allogeneic haematopoietic stem cell transplant for sever combined immunodeficiency. J Allergy Clin Immunol 2014;133:1660–6.
27. Dror Y, Gallagher R, Wara DW, et al. Immune reconstitution in severe combined immunodeficiency disease after lectin-treated, T-cell-depleted haplocompatible bone marrow transplantation. Blood 1993;81:2021–30.
28. Bertrand G, Duprat E, Lefranc MP, et al. Characterization of human FCGR3B*02 (HNA-1b, NA2) cDNAs and IMGT standardized description of FCGR3B alleles. Tissue Antigens 2004;64:119–31.

29. Prockop SE, Petrie HT. Regulation of thymus size by competition for stromal niches among early T cell progenitors. J Immunol 2004;173:1604–11.
30. Slatter MA, Brigham K, Dickinson AM, et al. Long-term immune reconstitution after anti-CD52-treated or anti-CD34-treated hematopoietic stem cell transplantation for severe T-lymphocyte immunodeficiency. J Allergy Clin Immunol 2008; 121:361–7.
31. Borghans JA, Bredius RG, Hazenberg MD, et al. Early determinants of long-term T-cell reconstitution after hematopoietic stem cell transplantation for severe combined immunodeficiency. Blood 2006;108:763–9.
32. Cavazzana-Calvo M, Carlier F, Le Deist F, et al. Long-term T-cell reconstitution after hematopoietic stem-cell transplantation in primary T-cell-immunodeficient patients is associated with myeloid chimerism and possibly the primary disease phenotype. Blood 2007;109:4575–81.
33. Dvorak CC, Gilman AL, Horn B, et al. Haploidentical related-donor hematopoietic cell transplantation in children using megadoses of CliniMACs-selected CD34(+) cells and a fixed CD3(+) dose. Bone Marrow Transplant 2013;48:508–13.
34. Friedrich W, Honig M, Muller SM. Long-term follow-up in patients with severe combined immunodeficiency treated by bone marrow transplantation. Immunol Res 2007;38:165–73.
35. Haddad E, Landais P, Friedrich W, et al. Long-term immune reconstitution and outcome after HLA-nonidentical T-cell-depleted bone marrow transplantation for severe combined immunodeficiency: a European retrospective study of 116 patients. Blood 1998;91:3646–53.
36. Mazzolari E, Forino C, Guerci S, et al. Long-term immune reconstitution and clinical outcome after stem cell transplantation for severe T-cell immunodeficiency. J Allergy Clin Immunol 2007;120:892–9.
37. Teigland CL, Parrott RE, Buckley RH. Long-term outcome of non-ablative booster BMT in patients with SCID. Bone Marrow Transplant 2013;48:1050–5.
38. Recher M, Berglund LJ, Avery DT, et al. IL-21 is the primary common gamma chain-binding cytokine required for human B-cell differentiation in vivo. Blood 2011;118:6824–35.
39. Buckley RH, Win CM, Moser BK, et al. Post-transplantation B cell function in different molecular types of SCID. J Clin Immunol 2013;33:96–110.
40. Booth C, Algar VE, Xu-Bayford J, et al. Non-infectious lung disease in patients with adenosine deaminase deficient severe combined immunodeficiency. J Clin Immunol 2012;32:449–53.
41. Grunebaum E, Cutz E, Roifman CM. Pulmonary alveolar proteinosis in patients with adenosine deaminase deficiency. J Allergy Clin Immunol 2012;129: 1588–93.
42. Hassan A, Booth C, Brightwell A, et al. Outcome of hematopoietic stem cell transplantation for adenosine deaminase deficient severe combined immunodeficiency. Blood 2012;120:3615–24.
43. Schuetz C, Neven B, Dvorak CC, et al. SCID patients with ARTEMIS vs RAG deficiencies following HCT: increased risk of late toxicity in ARTEMIS-deficient SCID. Blood 2014;123:281–9.
44. O'Marcaigh AS, DeSantes K, Hu D, et al. Bone marrow transplantation for T-B- severe combined immunodeficiency disease in Athabascan-speaking native Americans. Bone Marrow Transplant 2001;27:703–9.
45. Grunebaum E, Daneman A, Murguia-Favela L, et al. Multiple osteochondromas following irradiation-containing conditioning in severe combined immunodeficiency. Br J Haematol 2013;161:446–8.

46. Straathof KC, Rao K, Eyrich M, et al. Haemopoietic stem-cell transplantation with antibody-based minimal-intensity conditioning: a phase 1/2 study. Lancet 2009; 374:912–20.
47. Schulz AS, Glatting G, Hoenig M, et al. Radioimmunotherapy-based conditioning for hematopoietic cell transplantation in children with malignant and nonmalignant diseases. Blood 2011;117:4642–50.
48. Brodsky RA, Luznik L, Bolanos-Meade J, et al. Reduced intensity HLA-haploidentical BMT with post transplantation cyclophosphamide in nonmalignant hematologic diseases. Bone Marrow Transplant 2008;42:523–7.
49. Bertaina A, Merli P, Rutella S, et al. HLA-haploidentical stem cell transplantation after removal of alphabeta+ T and B-cells in children with non-malignant disorders. Blood 2014;124:822–6.
50. Kobayashi R, Ariga T, Nonoyama S, et al. Outcome in patients with Wiskott-Aldrich syndrome following stem cell transplantation: an analysis of 57 patients in Japan. Br J Haematol 2006;135:362–6.
51. Pai SY, DeMartiis D, Forino C, et al. Stem cell transplantation for the Wiskott-Aldrich syndrome: a single-center experience confirms efficacy of matched unrelated donor transplantation. Bone Marrow Transplant 2006;38:671–9.
52. Friedrich W, Schutz C, Schulz A, et al. Results and long-term outcome in 39 patients with Wiskott-Aldrich syndrome transplanted from HLA-matched and -mismatched donors. Immunol Res 2009;44:18–24.
53. Moratto D, Giliani S, Bonfim C, et al. Long-term outcome and lineage-specific chimerism in 194 patients with Wiskott-Aldrich syndrome treated by hematopoietic cell transplantation in the period 1980-2009: an international collaborative study. Blood 2011;118:1675–84.
54. Filipovich AH, Stone JV, Tomany SC, et al. Impact of donor type on outcome of bone marrow transplantation for Wiskott-Aldrich syndrome: collaborative study of the International Bone Marrow Transplant Registry and the National Marrow Donor Program. Blood 2001;97:1598–603.
55. Ochs HD, Filipovich AH, Veys P, et al. Wiskott-Aldrich syndrome: diagnosis, clinical and laboratory manifestations, and treatment. Biol Blood Marrow Transplant 2009;15:84–90.
56. Gennery AR, Khawaja K, Veys P, et al. Treatment of CD40 ligand deficiency by hematopoietic stem cell transplantation: a survey of the European experience, 1993-2002. Blood 2004;103:1152–7.
57. Kikuta A, Ito M, Mochizuki K, et al. Nonmyeloablative stem cell transplantation for nonmalignant diseases in children with severe organ dysfunction. Bone Marrow Transplant 2006;38:665–9.
58. McLauchlin J, Amar CF, Pedraza-Diaz S, et al. Polymerase chain reaction-based diagnosis of infection with *Cryptosporidium* in children with primary immunodeficiencies. Pediatr Infect Dis J 2003;22:329–35.
59. Hadzic N, Pagliuca A, Rela M, et al. Correction of the hyper-IgM syndrome after liver and bone marrow transplantation. N Engl J Med 2000;342:320–4.
60. Jasinska A, Kalwak K, Trelinska J, et al. Successful haploidentical PBSCT with subsequent T-cell addbacks in a boy with HyperIgM syndrome presenting as severe congenital neutropenia. Pediatr Transplant 2013;17:E37–40.
61. Kang EM, Marciano BE, DeRavin S, et al. Chronic granulomatous disease: overview and hematopoietic stem cell transplantation. J Allergy Clin Immunol 2011; 127:1319–26 [quiz: 1327–8].
62. Seger RA, Gungor T, Belohradsky BH, et al. Treatment of chronic granulomatous disease with myeloablative conditioning and an unmodified hemopoietic

allograft: a survey of the European experience, 1985-2000. Blood 2002;100: 4344–50.
63. Horwitz ME, Barrett AJ, Brown MR, et al. Treatment of chronic granulomatous disease with nonmyeloablative conditioning and a T-cell-depleted hematopoietic allograft. N Engl J Med 2001;344:881–8.
64. Gungor T, Teira P, Slatter M, et al. Reduced-intensity conditioning and HLA-matched haemopoietic stem-cell transplantation in patients with chronic granulomatous disease: a prospective multicentre study. Lancet 2014;383:436–48.
65. Nakano T, Boku E, Yoshioka A, et al. A case of McLeod phenotype chronic granulomatous disease who received unrelated cord blood transplantation. J Pediatr Hematol Oncol 1999;12:264.
66. Cole T, McKendrick F, Titman P, et al. Health related quality of life and emotional health in children with chronic granulomatous disease: a comparison of those managed conservatively with those that have undergone haematopoietic stem cell transplant. J Clin Immunol 2013;33:8–13.
67. Kuhns DB, Alvord WG, Heller T, et al. Residual NADPH oxidase and survival in chronic granulomatous disease. N Engl J Med 2010;363:2600–10.
68. Bonfim CM, de Medeiros CR, Bitencourt MA, et al. HLA-matched related donor hematopoietic cell transplantation in 43 patients with Fanconi anemia conditioned with 60 mg/kg of cyclophosphamide. Biol Blood Marrow Transplant 2007;13:1455–60.
69. Pasquini R, Carreras J, Pasquini MC, et al. HLA-matched sibling hematopoietic stem cell transplantation for Fanconi anemia: comparison of irradiation and nonirradiation containing conditioning regimens. Biol Blood Marrow Transplant 2008;14:1141–7.
70. Albert MH, Gennery AR, Greil J, et al. Successful SCT for Nijmegen breakage syndrome. Bone Marrow Transplant 2010;45:622–6.
71. Gruhn B, Seidel J, Zintl F, et al. Successful bone marrow transplantation in a patient with DNA ligase IV deficiency and bone marrow failure. Orphanet J Rare Dis 2007;2:5.
72. Buck D, Moshous D, de Chasseval R, et al. Severe combined immunodeficiency and microcephaly in siblings with hypomorphic mutations in DNA ligase IV. Eur J Immunol 2006;36:224–35.
73. Cagdas D, Ozgur TT, Asal GT, et al. Two SCID cases with cernunnos-XLF deficiency successfully treated by hematopoietic stem cell transplantation. Pediatr Transplant 2012;16:E167–171.
74. Faraci M, Lanino E, Micalizzi C, et al. Unrelated hematopoietic stem cell transplantation for Cernunnos-XLF deficiency. Pediatr Transplant 2009;13: 785–9.
75. Gadalla SM, Sales-Bonfim C, Carreras J, et al. Outcomes of allogeneic hematopoietic cell transplantation in patients with dyskeratosis congenita. Biol Blood Marrow Transplant 2013;19:1238–43.
76. Ayas M, Nassar A, Hamidieh AA, et al. Reduced intensity conditioning is effective for hematopoietic SCT in dyskeratosis congenita-related BM failure. Bone Marrow Transplant 2013;48:1168–72.
77. Henter JI, Horne A, Arico M, et al. HLH-2004: Diagnostic and therapeutic guidelines for hemophagocytic lymphohistiocytosis. Pediatr Blood Cancer 2007;48: 124–31.
78. Stephan JL, Donadieu J, Ledeist F, et al. Treatment of familial hemophagocytic lymphohistiocytosis with antithymocyte globulins, steroids, and cyclosporin A. Blood 1993;82:2319–23.

79. Ouachee-Chardin M, Elie C, de Saint Basile G, et al. Hematopoietic stem cell transplantation in hemophagocytic lymphohistiocytosis: a single-center report of 48 patients. Pediatrics 2006;117:e743–750.
80. Marsh RA, Vaughn G, Kim MO, et al. Reduced-intensity conditioning significantly improves survival of patients with hemophagocytic lymphohistiocytosis undergoing allogeneic hematopoietic cell transplantation. Blood 2010;116:5824–31.
81. Booth C, Gilmour KC, Veys P, et al. X-linked lymphoproliferative disease due to SAP/SH2D1A deficiency: a multicenter study on the manifestations, management and outcome of the disease. Blood 2011;117:53–62.
82. Marsh RA, Rao K, Satwani P, et al. Allogeneic hematopoietic cell transplantation for XIAP deficiency: an international survey reveals poor outcomes. Blood 2013; 121:877–83.
83. Pachlopnik Schmid J, Moshous D, Boddaert N, et al. Hematopoietic stem cell transplantation in Griscelli syndrome type 2: a single-center report on 10 patients. Blood 2009;114:211–8.
84. Tardieu M, Lacroix C, Neven B, et al. Progressive neurologic dysfunctions 20 years after allogeneic bone marrow transplantation for Chediak-Higashi syndrome. Blood 2005;106:40–2.
85. Barzaghi F, Passerini L, Bacchetta R. Immune dysregulation, polyendocrinopathy, enteropathy, x-linked syndrome: a paradigm of immunodeficiency with autoimmunity. Front Immunol 2012;3:211.
86. Rao A, Kamani N, Filipovich A, et al. Successful bone marrow transplantation for IPEX syndrome after reduced-intensity conditioning. Blood 2007;109:383–5.
87. Nademi Z, Slatter M, Gambineri E, et al. Single centre experience of haematopoietic SCT for patients with immunodysregulation, polyendocrinopathy, enteropathy, X-linked syndrome. Bone Marrow Transplant 2014;49:310–2.
88. Zhang Q, Davis JC, Lamborn IT, et al. Combined immunodeficiency associated with DOCK8 mutations. N Engl J Med 2009;361:2046–55.
89. McDonald DR, Massaad MJ, Johnston A, et al. Successful engraftment of donor marrow after allogeneic hematopoietic cell transplantation in autosomal-recessive hyper-IgE syndrome caused by dedicator of cytokinesis 8 deficiency. J Allergy Clin Immunol 2010;126:1304–5.e3.
90. Bittner TC, Pannicke U, Renner ED, et al. Successful long-term correction of autosomal recessive hyper-IgE syndrome due to DOCK8 deficiency by hematopoietic stem cell transplantation. Klin Padiatr 2010;222:351–5.
91. Ghosh S, Schuster FR, Adams O, et al. Haploidentical stem cell transplantation in DOCK8 deficiency - successful control of pre-existing severe viremia with a TCRass/CD19-depleted graft and antiviral treatment. Clin Immunol 2014;152: 111–4.
92. Al-Mousa H, Hawwari A, Alsum Z. In DOCK8 deficiency donor cell engraftment post-genoidentical hematopoietic stem cell transplantation is possible without conditioning. J Allergy Clin Immunol 2013;131:1244–5.
93. Boztug H, Karitnig-Weiss C, Ausserer B, et al. Clinical and immunological correction of DOCK8 deficiency by allogeneic hematopoietic stem cell transplantation following a reduced toxicity conditioning regimen. Pediatr Hematol Oncol 2012;29:585–94.
94. Barlogis V, Galambrun C, Chambost H, et al. Successful allogeneic hematopoietic stem cell transplantation for DOCK8 deficiency. J Allergy Clin Immunol 2011;128:420–2.e2.
95. Metin A, Tavil B, Azik F, et al. Successful bone marrow transplantation for DOCK8 deficient hyper IgE syndrome. Pediatr Transplant 2012;16:398–9.

Hematopoietic Stem Cell Transplantation for Patients with Sickle Cell Disease

Progress and Future Directions

Courtney D. Fitzhugh, MD[a], Allistair A. Abraham, MD[b], John F. Tisdale, MD[a], Matthew M. Hsieh, MD[a,*]

KEYWORDS

- Sickle cell disease • Matched sibling donor • Cord blood (CB) donor
- Haploidentical donor • Matched unrelated donor

KEY POINTS

- Progenitor cells (bone marrow, cord blood [CB], or peripheral blood stem cell) from matched sibling/related donors offer the best results of transplantation.
- Although there are insufficient data in sickle cell disease (SCD), fully matched unrelated marrow is likely the next best option. This donor source is rare for patients with SCD.
- No study directly compared fully with less well-matched unrelated CB transplants. The combined data showed 50% disease-free survival, 20% acute graft-versus-host disease (GVHD), and 15% mortality.
- The data from haploidentical (or mismatched related) transplants have 43% disease-free survival, 9% acute GVHD, and 9% mortality. The institutional expertise dictates whether haploidentical or unrelated CB is better suited; both should be performed in the context of clinical trials.
- Mismatched unrelated marrow (7/8 or less) in SCD is disappointing. This donor source should be studied only in the context of innovative clinical trials.

INTRODUCTION

The first reported bone marrow (BM) transplant (BMT) for sickle cell disease (SCD) was published in 1984 in a child who had developed acute myeloid leukemia (AML).[1] She was cured of both and remains alive almost 3 decades later. This proof-of-principle report paved the way for a series of pilot studies also showing that transplantation from HLA-matched sibling donors (MSD) could cure SCD.[2–5] Later, the multicenter

[a] 9000 Rockville Pike, Building 10/9N112, Bethesda, MD 20892, USA; [b] Division of Blood and Marrow Transplantation, Children's National Health System, George Washington University School of Medicine and Health Sciences, 111 Michigan Avenue, North West, Washington, DC 20010, USA

* Corresponding author.

E-mail address: matthewhs@mail.nih.gov

Hematol Oncol Clin N Am 28 (2014) 1171–1185
http://dx.doi.org/10.1016/j.hoc.2014.08.014
0889-8588/14/$ – see front matter Published by Elsevier Inc.

trial published by Walters and colleagues[6] in 1996 was instrumental in validating transplant as a bona fide treatment. In this landmark trial, 22 children with very symptomatic SCD underwent MSD marrow transplantation; overall and disease-free survival (DFS) estimates at 4 years were 91% and 73%, respectively. Since then, the procedure has become safer and more effective. This success is shown by the 95% DFS in 44 patients undergoing refined transplant procedures after January, 2000, as described by the French group.[7]

Traditionally, myeloablative conditioning was used in SCD transplants to maximize engraftment. Therefore, patients older than 16 years with significant sequelae of SCD, including considerable organ dysfunction, were often excluded. Less intense preparative regimens have made curative approaches available to adults. Increased rates of stable mixed chimerism are accepted as part of these less intense regimens, because the red cell compartment is replaced with normal donor red cells, and symptoms of SCD resolve with time. The largest report to date of such nonmyeloablative (NMA) transplantation was recently described,[8] in which 30 adults safely underwent matched sibling transplant, with an 87% DFS.

Over the last 2 decades, there has been significant progress in transplantation using alternative sources such as umbilical cord blood (CB) units, haploidentical donors, and unrelated donors to make this curative procedure more accessible to those who are eligible.

INDICATIONS FOR TRANSPLANTATION

Indications for transplant are either directed to patients requiring lifelong transfusion because of an increased risk of recurrent or primary stroke (stroke and increased transcranial Doppler velocity), a significant impact on quality of life (recurrent vaso-occlusive crises, priapism, acute chest syndrome, osteonecrosis of multiple joints, and symptomatic silent infarct), difficulty maintaining transfusion therapy because of the lack compatible units (red cell alloimmunization), or an association with increased mortality (tricuspid regurgitant jet velocity line [TRV] >2.5 m/sec, sickle-related liver injury, iron overload, and sickle nephropathy). These indications are summarized in **Table 1**.

Table 1
Indications for allogeneic HSCT in SCD

Established Indications	Potential Indications for Consideration
1. Clinically overt stroke 2. Increased transcranial Doppler velocity (>200 m/s) 3. Frequent vaso-occlusive crises (≥2 hospital admissions requiring parenteral narcotics while on a therapeutic dose of hydroxyurea) 4. Recurrent priapism requiring medical therapy 5. Acute chest syndrome (≥1 episode while on a therapeutic dose of hydroxyurea) 6. Red cell alloimmunization (typically in MSD transplant) 7. Osteonecrosis of ≥2 joints (typically in MSD transplant)	1. Silent infarct with severe anemia or neurocognitive dysfunction 2. TRV >2.5 m/s 3. Sickle-related liver injury or iron overload (typically in NMA transplant) 4. Renal insufficiency (requiring dialysis, nephrotic syndrome, or biopsy proven sickle nephropathy; typically in NMA transplant)

PATIENT EVALUATION OVERVIEW

SCD-related complications are important to identify before transplant. Not only do they drive the decision for transplant, but they also serve as a baseline for peritransplant and posttransplant care. Thus in addition to standard transplant-related blood (including renal/liver parameters and transfusion-related infectious pathogens), lung, and cardiac testing, evaluations for SCD-related end-organ injury should include the following:

- Brain MRI/MRA to establish the presence and extent of infarcts and vascular abnormalities
- Neurocognitive testing
- Echocardiographic estimate of pulmonary pressure (TRV)
- 6-minute walk test
- Consider right heart catheterization for suspected pulmonary hypertension
- Quantitative iron assessment, including ferritin, liver biopsy (if possible) to assess the extent of inflammation, fibrosis, and quantitative iron, or cardiac or liver magnetic resonance imaging for T2* measurements
- Creatinine clearance estimation by nuclear glomerular filtration rate (typically in children)
- Twenty-four hour urine collection for creatinine clearance and protein for adults: because patients with SCD often have serum creatinine levels of 0.6 mg/dL or less, higher levels may indicate subtle or overt renal injury
- Red cell phenotyping of the recipients and donors; the transfusion medicine department should be given ample time to store blood for patients who require difficult to match packed red blood cell units; patients should be screened for donor-directed antibodies to minor red blood cell antigens, because of the risk of pure red cell aplasia after transplant, particularly in the NMA setting[8]
- HLA-antibody testing of the recipients considering alternative donor transplantation; if donor-specific antibodies are detected, another donor may need to be identified because of the increased risk of graft rejection[9–11]

HLA-MATCHED HEMATOPOIETIC STEM CELL TRANSPLANTATION

HLA-Matched Sibling Donor

Myeloablative

The first transplant for SCD used BM from a MSD for AML.[1] The preparative regimen consisted of cyclophosphamide 120 mg/kg over 2 days and fractionated total body irradiation (TBI) of 11.5 Gy. Graft-versus-host disease (GVHD) prophylaxis was a short course of methotrexate (MTX) and 28 days of methylprednisolone. The patient was cured of both diseases. At about the same time, thalassemia major had been reported to be cured by MSD BMT, and myeloablation was achieved using the nonradiation-containing regimen of busulfan (Bu) and cyclophosphamide (Cy).[12,13] In the late 1980s and early 1990s, a few case series of patients with SCD undergoing myeloablative BuCy MSD BMT were reported, prompted by the successful outcomes using this approach in patients with thalassemia. The multicenter study published by Walters and colleagues[6] in 1996 showed that the myeloablative BuCy approach could reproducibly achieve good outcomes (73% DFS) in severe SCD. With better supportive care and in a larger cohort of patients, the addition of rabbit antithymocyte globulin (ATG) reduced the graft rejection rate from 23% (without ATG) to 3% (with ATG), as reported by Bernaudin and colleagues[7] in 2007. Many studies have now published the MSD BuCy + ATG regimen, and overall survival and DFS ranges from 90% to 100% and 77% to 100%, respectively (**Table 2**).

Table 2
Summary of transplant studies to date

References	Donor Source	Conditioning Regimen	HLA Match	Number of Patients (Age Range [y])[a]	DFS (%) (Number of Patients)[a]	Acute GVHD (Grade 2–4) (%)[a]	Chronic GVHD (Extensive) (%)[a]	Number of Deaths (%)[a]
7,14–16,22,39,47–49	Matched sibling[b]	Myeloablative	8/8 or 10/10	334 (1.2–27)	87 (290)	17	3	5
8,50–53	Matched sibling[c]	RTC and NMA	8/8 or 10/10	65 (1.8–65)	92 (60)	5	0	2
19,22,52,54–57	Related cord	Mostly myeloablative	Mostly 6/6	89 (1.8–20)	90 (80)	8	0	9
34,58–62	Unrelated cord	RTC and myeloablative	Mostly 4/6 and 5/6	41 (1–22)	49 (20)	20	7	15
38,39,63	Haploidentical	Mixed	Haploidentical	23 (4.2–42)	43 (10)	9	9	9

Abbreviation: RTC, reduced toxicity conditioning.

[a] DFS is an average of the total number of patients from all studies who were alive and without disease. The median follow-up time may be different across studies. Many references include patients with SCD and thalassemia, matched sibling and CB sources. Rates of GVHD and death were estimated, with the assumption that rates were the same for hemoglobin disorder type or graft source.

[b] Studies published after 2000.

[c] Studies published after 2005.

A few important points of this standard approach should be highlighted. Intravenous Bu has largely replaced the oral route of administration to reduce the incidence of sinusoidal obstructive syndrome. Bu is usually given as a 0.8 mg/kg/dose for 16 doses over 4 days (or 3.2 mg/kg once daily dosing), targeting steady state concentrations of 600 to 700 ng/mL or area under the curve of 900 to 1100 μmol/min/L.[14,15] Cy (50 mg/kg/dose) is given daily for 4 days. Equine ATG (30 mg/kg/dose for 3 days within the 4 days before transplant) or rabbit ATG (10–20 mg/kg divided over 4 days, typically days −6 to −3) is included. GVHD prophylaxis includes cyclosporine for 180 days after transplant and a short course of MTX. Central nervous system (CNS) protective measures include maintaining a platelet count greater than 50,000/uL, hemoglobin 9 to 11 g/dL, magnesium greater than 1.6 g/dL, aggressive antihypertensive management, and seizure prophylaxis while receiving Bu and calcineurin inhibition.[7]

- Myeloablative transplants from MSD are mostly performed in children and young adults.
- Excellent DFS has been achieved through improvements in supportive care, conditioning regimen, and CNS protective measures in this standard transplant approach.
- Although the rates of graft rejection (5%) and mortality (5%) have reduced recently, further optimization to decrease the rate of GVHD can make this standard regimen even more successful.

HLA-Matched Sibling

Reduced toxicity and nonmyeloablative

Because outcomes have been excellent with the myeloablative approach, investigators have attempted to offer transplant to previously excluded adult patients with SCD by using reduced toxicity (RTC) or NMA conditioning. Part of the premise is that achieving complete donor chimerism is not necessary, because many patients have been reported to have SCD symptom resolution with a stable mixed chimeric state, an expected scenario with RTC and NMA regimens.[16] In addition, patients undergoing transplant may benefit from less intense conditioning, potentially leading to decreased problems with fertility and other transplant-related organ dysfunction. However, earlier RTC and NMA experiences used transplant regimens from hematologic malignant transplants, and their results showed excessive GVHD leading to death in 1 series, and graft rejection in another.[17,18] These initial discouraging results prompted redesign of the conditioning regimen in SCD.

One such regimen was tested in 30 adult patients undergoing MSD peripheral blood stem cell transplants, conditioned with alemtuzumab, low-dose TBI (300 cGy), and sirolimus.[8] In this approach, alemtuzumab was chosen for in vivo T-cell depletion to prevent GVHD and rejection, TBI was increased to 300 cGy over the traditional 200 cGy to increase myelosuppression, and sirolimus was used for tolerance induction. Twenty-six of the 30 patients retained their graft, resulting in normalization of their hemoglobin level, and the approach was well tolerated without any GVHD. One patient died of intracranial hemorrhage after graft rejection. Although no patient achieved 100% donor chimerism in both T cells and myeloid cells, sirolimus was discontinued in 15 of 26 engrafted patients. Promising studies of HLA-matched RTC/NMA transplant for SCD are summarized in **Table 2**. Alemtuzumab was commonly included in several recent studies, and may contribute to the almost absent GVHD, mortality, and rejection rates. High CD34 cell counts may help overcome the host versus graft barrier. The relatively small numbers and mixed chimeric state do warrant larger trials with extended follow-up. Longer follow-up would also allow exploration regarding whether RTC/NMA regimens are associated with less infertility and organ toxicity, compared with myeloablative transplants.

- Although the collective experience of RTC/NMA transplants is less robust than myeloablative transplants, their results have dramatically improved recently.
- RTC/NMA transplantation is gaining acceptance as a standard option for older adults or those with organ damage.
- As with MSD myeloablative transplants, T-cell depletion is an essential component of the RTC/NMA conditioning regimen.

Related Umbilical Cord Blood Transplantation

The largest CB transplant (CBT) study was reported by the Eurocord and European Blood and Marrow Transplantation group in 2013.[19] Of 160 patients with SCD who underwent HLA-identical CBT or BMT, 30 received CBT. The 6-year DFS was 90% after CBT and 92% after BMT. Of all patients transplanted, those who received a CBT had significantly longer time to neutrophil and platelet engraftment compared with those who underwent BMT ($P<.005$). However, no patients who received CBT developed grade IV acute GVHD compared with 8 (2%) who received BM cells, and none of the CBT recipients experienced chronic extensive GVHD compared with 5% of the patients who received BMT.

Studies have shown that MTX affected outcome in patients with SCD and thalassemia major who undergo related CBT.[19,20] Patients who did not versus patients who did receive MTX had DFS of 90% versus 60%, respectively ($P<.001$). Patients who received thiotepa also did better, although thiotepa did not influence outcome in multivariate analysis. The total nucleated cell (TNC) dose infused did not affect outcome in patients who received CBT, although median TNC count was adequate at 3.9×10^7 cells/kg.

Recent studies have reported a more robust neutrophil (17 vs 25 days, $P = .013$) and platelet (29 vs 48 days, $P = .009$) recovery in patients who received CB along with BM compared with CB alone.[21] All 13 patients who received CB coinfused with BM remained engrafted, with a median follow-up greater than 5 years, with no acute grade 2 or greater GVHD or chronic GVHD. A second study showed long-term engraftment in all patients who received hydroxyurea before Bu, Cy, and ATG.[22] Therefore, CB and BM coinfusion as well as hydroxyurea treatment before conditioning seem to be viable options to explore further in young patients with HLA-MSD.

- Related CBT with mostly 6/6 matched units resulted in similar overall survival and DFS but lower incidence of chronic GVHD, compared with HLA-MSD BMT (see **Table 2**).
- Specific pretransplant and peritransplant treatment used (eg, hydroxyurea or MTX) affects CBT outcome.
- Coinfusion of CB and BM may shorten duration of BM recovery and improve CBT outcome.

ALTERNATIVE DONOR TRANSPLANTATION

Donor Availability

Although MSD transplants are safer, there remains the inherent problem of donor availability. The likelihood of 2 siblings being HLA identical is only 25%, and some siblings have SCD, further limiting the chance of having a suitable donor. Therefore, the field has moved to investigate alternative donor sources. Improved outcomes for malignancy and immunodeficiency have already been described with matched unrelated donor (MUD), umbilical CB, and haploidentical transplantation techniques in the last 2 decades.[23–26]

In 1 report from 2003 that evaluated searches performed by the National Marrow Donor Program, the chance of finding a potential 6/6 HLA MUD for a patient with SCD was approximately 60%.[27] In the same report, the chances of finding a 5/6 or 6/6 HLA-matched CB donor were approximately 62% and 30%, respectively. However, this matching was performed at the serologic level for HLA-A and HLA-B and at the potential allelic level for HLA-DRB1. A recent study with detailed matching reported that the chances of finding a potential allelic 8/8 HLA-A, HLA-B, HLA-C, and HLA-DRB1 MUD were only 19%.[28] Combining 5/6 and 6/6 HLA-matched cords (HLA-A, HLA-B antigen; DRB1 potential allele) with higher cell doses as needed for hemoglobin disorders (TNC count of $\geq 5 \times 10^7$ cells/kg) could increase the alternative donor option. When this factor was examined, the probability of a potential 8/8 MUD, 5/6 or 6/6 unrelated cord in SCD improved the chances, but they remained relatively low, at 45%.[28]

Matched Unrelated Donor Transplantation

Because of the low chance of finding appropriate donors, MUD marrow transplants have not been performed in enough patients with SCD. One report from Germany included 2 children who received fully matched MUD marrow transplant successfully.[29] Another report included 2 patients with 7/8 MUD and 4 patients with 4 to 5/6 matched unrelated CB units. Only 3 patients engrafted; 4 died of transplant-related complications, and the 2 patients who remained living had return of SCD.[30] The SCURT (Sickle Cell Unrelated Transplant) trial (BMT CTN 0601, NCT00745420) combined 8/8 MUD and myeloablative conditioning in children. The study has been open since 2008, and recently reached target accrual. Another study, STRIDE (Sickle Cell Transplantation to Prevent Disease Exacerbation, NCT01565616), has initiated accrual and will also evaluate 8/8 MUD marrow and myeloablative conditioning, but in adults aged 16 to 40 years. These study results will provide useful information about this donor option for patients with SCD. In thalassemia major, earlier reports of MUD marrow transplants from 10/10 matched donors showed that patients with Pesaro class 3 (higher severity) had a DFS of 55%, lower than 80% in less severe patients.[31,32] A recent large study of mostly Pesaro class 2 patients, which allowed 1 allele HLA-mismatched donors, showed DFS rate of 96%, with 8% acute GVHD.[33] Having more class 2 patients, using reduced doses of Cy, and using more current supportive care contributed to the better results reported in this recent cohort.

- DFS in MUD transplants for thalassemia major has improved recently, and the data from corresponding studies (SCURT and STRIDE) for SCD will be available soon.
- It may be reasonable to extrapolate the good DFS rate in 8/8 MUD transplants from thalassemia to SCD, but such donors are rare for patients with SCD.
- There are insufficient data in less than 8/8 MUD transplants; priority should be given to other donor options.

Unrelated Umbilical Cord Blood Transplantation

In contrast to the results in the related setting, unrelated CBT has been less successful. The largest study included 16 patients with SCD.[34] Nine of them received myeloablative regimens, whereas 7 underwent RTC. Although the overall survival was 94%, DFS was only 50%. The incidence of GVHD in the entire cohort of patients with SCD and thalassemia was reported as 22% acute grade 2 to 4 GVHD and 3% chronic extensive GVHD. There were additional reports that included small numbers of patients, and the results combined 6/6 with lower HLA matches. Some reports showed favorable results, but others had high rates of GVHD, with low rates of engraftment (see **Table 2**). Therefore, unrelated CBT for patients with SCD, even among recent reports, remains suboptimal and needs improvement.

There are additional considerations in unrelated CBT. Because TNC count is important, this source is better suited for children. Fully matched unrelated cord blood units are also rare for patients with SCD. Delayed platelet engraftment is typical with CBT and may lead to excessive morbidity because of the potential risk of bleeding in patients with red cell alloimmunization who require difficult to match red blood cell units or CNS vasculopathy, with the risk of intracranial hemorrhage in the setting of prolonged thrombocytopenia.

- Unrelated CBT has about 50% DFS, 20% acute GVHD, and 15% mortality (see **Table 2**).
- Further studies exploring fully versus less well-matched CB, better chemotherapy combinations, or improvement in GVHD prophylaxis are indicated to enhance outcome for unrelated CBT in patients with SCD.

Haploidentical Donor Transplantation

Because fully matched CB units are rare, and haploidentical donors are more accessible, a novel approach of using posttransplant administration of Cy in haploidentical transplantation was first explored in preclinical models, and later tested in the hematologic malignant setting.[35–37] Posttransplant Cy, when given a few days after donor cell infusion, was shown to preferentially target and remove proliferating T cells, which include alloreactive donor cells that lead to GVHD and host cells that mediate graft rejection. The largest study to date was reported by the Johns Hopkins group in 2012, in which 14 patients, mostly adults, were transplanted.[38] Although the rate of graft rejection was expectedly high in the setting of haploidentical donors, the sickle phenotype was completely reversed in 7 of the 14 patients. In addition, 1 other patient showed a mixture of donor and recipient erythroid cells with severe anemia and sickle hemoglobin (HbS) increased more than would be expected in a patient with sickle cell trait. Six of the patients with complete donor chimerism have stopped immunosuppressive therapy, consisting most recently of sirolimus and a short course of mycophenolate. None of the patients developed acute or chronic GVHD, and all of the patients are living. In contrast, a pediatric study involving 8 patients using ex vivo T-cell depletion reported an overall survival of 75% and DFS of 38%.[39] Two patients developed grade 2 acute GVHD, and 2 patients died of chronic extensive GVHD.

- Similar to unrelated CBT, haploidentical transplantation has 43% DFS, 9% acute GVHD, and 9% mortality (see **Table 2**).
- Posttransplant Cy has dramatically improved the safety of haploidentical transplantation by lowering GVHD rate and transplant-related mortality.
- The addition of sirolimus in haploidentical transplants in recent reports is credited to the tolerance induction achieved in patients.

TIMING AND PREPARATION FOR TRANSPLANTATION

Overall and SCD-free survival rates approaching 90% have prompted physicians to reconsider the methods and timing of treatment. The concept of transplantation earlier in the disease course was already being considered in the 1980s, as reported by investigators in Belgium.[40] In this study, 50 transplanted patients belonged to 1 of 2 groups: permanent residents of a European country who had already developed a severe sickle cell phenotype before transplant, or visiting patients who were transplanted earlier in the disease, because of a desire to return to their country of origin. The combined rate of nonengraftment, mixed chimerism, and death was significantly higher in the more diseased group (25% vs 7%, $P<.001$). Although transplanting patients earlier in their disease course was controversial in the 1980s, current understanding of the devastating nature of SCD has led providers to accept early transplant in less severe patients, such as those with an increased transcranial Doppler velocity.

In general, transplantation can proceed when patient's medical condition has stabilized, or sufficient time for recovery has elapsed to meet inclusion criteria (eg, Karnofsky score, pulmonary function). Fertility potential after transplantation should be discussed, and sufficient time allowed for consultation with fertility specialists for testing and cryopreservation of oocytes or spermatocytes. For patients undergoing NMA transplantation, preconditioning with hydroxyurea for at least several weeks may be important to reduce recipient hematopoiesis to improve transplant outcome. Preconditioning is less of a concern for patients undergoing myeloablative transplants. All patients should undergo simple or exchange red cell transfusions to target HbS of 30% within 1 week of starting the conditioning regimen to minimize sickle-related complications during the transplant.

NOVEL THERAPIES AND THEIR INTEGRATION IN TRANSPLANTATION

Based on the combined studies thus far, active research is most necessary for unrelated CB and haploidentical transplantation to improve outcome. Although the data in unrelated CBT have remained the same recently, results from the Hopkins group in haploidentical transplant showed no GVHD or mortality, giving enthusiasm for that donor source. The major obstacle with both approaches remains graft failure, and there are efforts to optimize the transplant regimens.

In the haploidentical transplants, reduction of donor-specific HLA antibodies is actively being investigated to improve engraftment.[41] Their desensitization methods of plasmapheresis, intravenous immunoglobulin, tacrolimus, and mycophenolate mofetil, starting 1 to 2 weeks before transplant conditioning, seems to be promising.[42] Other strategies include rituximab and bortezomib.[43] Another ongoing study is evaluating whether tolerance induction using alemtuzumab and sirolimus as a backbone with escalating doses of posttransplant Cy may decrease the risk of graft rejection in the haploidentical setting (NCT00977691).

Double cord transplantation is also being studied in hemoglobin disorders. The currently open trial (NCT00920972), which evaluates alemtuzumab, fludarabine, and melphalan conditioning, has strata dedicated to single and double cord transplants.

A limiting factor for CBT is cord size/cell dose. A study published from the Eurocord Registry, the Center for International Blood and Marrow Transplant Research, and the New York Blood Center[34] describing outcomes of unrelated cord transplants for hemoglobin disorders recommended a TNC count of at least 5×10^7 cells/kg for single cord transplants to maximize engraftment. Such high cell doses can restrict cord options for patients, especially for adults. In the last few years, many approaches have expanded hematopoietic stem cells (HSCs) in the basic science laboratory and translated to clinical practice. The most impressive report to date[44] described 31 adults with hematologic malignancy who received unrelated double umbilical cord transplants. In this trial, 1 cord was cocultured ex vivo with mesenchymal stromal cells before infusion, resulting in a 12-fold increase in TNC count and a 30-fold increase in CD34+ cell content. Neutrophil engraftment rate by day 42 improved in patients who received the expanded cord as part of their transplant (96%), compared with 2 separate control cohorts receiving unmanipulated double cords (83% and 78%). Although the expanded cord contributed to hematopoiesis early on, the predominant donor-derived chimerism was from the unmanipulated unit in most of the patients at 1 year. This finding questions whether expanded units, despite having increased numerical cell doses, behave functionally similar to unmanipulated grafts of similar size and are capable of lifelong engraftment. Preliminary data in transplants for malignancy have supported the NiCord trial[45] for SCD (NCT01590628), which is evaluating the use of double cord transplantation after myeloablative conditioning, when one of the cord units is expanded ex vivo with cytokines and nicotinamide. The study is estimated to complete in 2015.

GENE THERAPY

Autologous transplantation for hemoglobin disorders has only been considered in gene therapy trials. Clinical trials using lentiviral vectors to correct autologous HSCs have begun in France (NCT02151526) and New York City (Memorial Sloan Kettering Cancer Center, NCT01639690) for patients with thalassemia. Patients typically received close to myeloablative doses of Bu to enhance the engraftment of genetically modified cells. Patients achieving transfusion independence have been reported.[46] A gene therapy trial for SCD is expected to begin enrollment soon.

SUMMARY

Substantial progress in allogeneic hematopoietic stem cell transplantation has been made (**Fig. 1**). These transplant studies can be summarized into the following key points, and applied to children and adults (**Fig. 2**).

- Marrow, peripheral blood-derived, or CB progenitor cells from matched sibling/related donors offer the best results of transplantation.

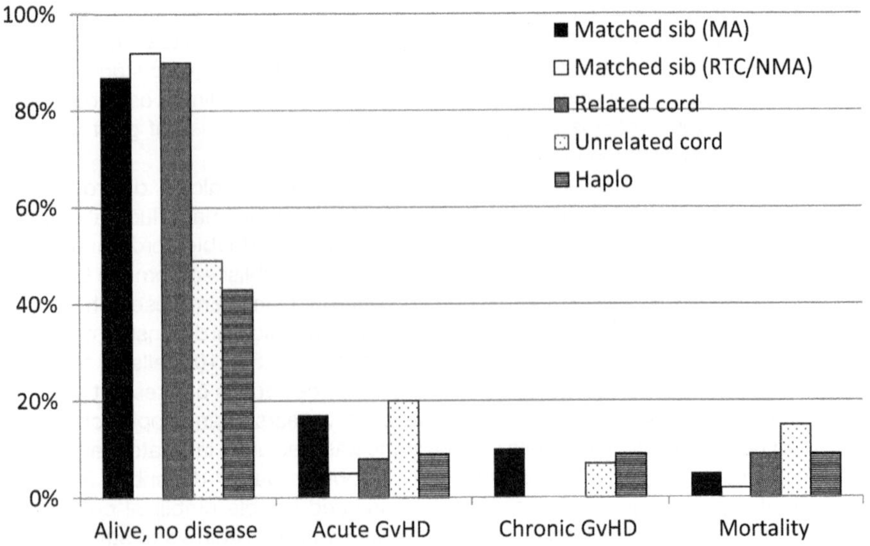

Fig. 1. Summary of allogeneic HSCT for SCD. Data for MUD transplantation are not available. Acute GVHD includes grade 2 to 4, and chronic GVHD includes only extensive.

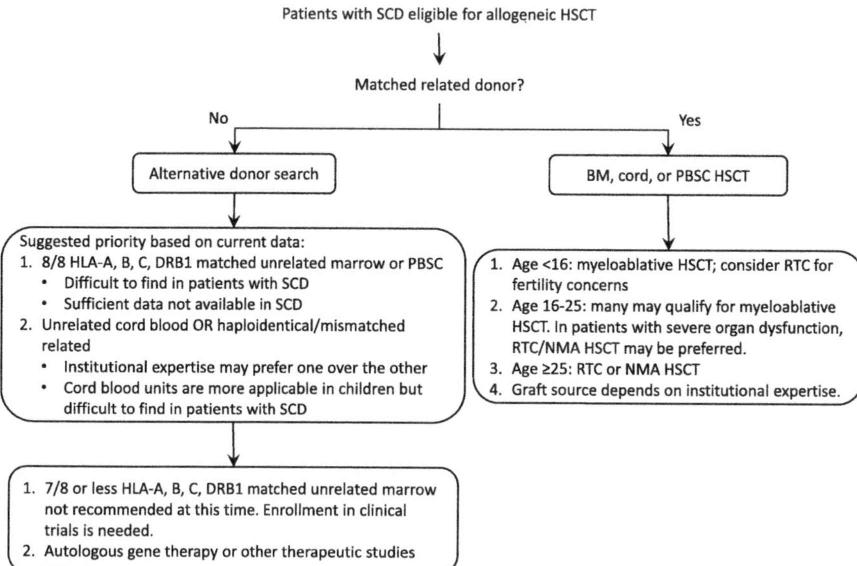

Fig. 2. Suggested priority in decision making among transplant options.

- Fully matched unrelated marrow (8/8 or 10/10 allelic match) is likely the next best option, as described in patients with thalassemia from 2 reasonably sized studies in different populations.[32,33] There are insufficient data in SCD thus far, but the results from the SCURT trial (NCT00745420) should be available soon. This donor source is rare for patients with SCD.
- Although fully matched unrelated CB units seem to be the next reasonable option, no study directly compared fully with less well-matched units.
- Haploidentical (or mismatched related) donors have emerged as a reasonable alternative. The data from a recent series showed better survival and lower GVHD rates.[38]
- At this time, unrelated CB units are not clearly more preferable than haploidentical donors. The institutional expertise dictates which source is better suited, and transplantation in the context of clinical trials is preferable.
- Mismatched unrelated marrow (7/8 or less) in SCD to date is disappointing. This donor source should be studied only in the context of innovative clinical trials.

REFERENCES

1. Johnson FL, Look AT, Gockerman J, et al. Bone-marrow transplantation in a patient with sickle-cell anemia. N Engl J Med 1984;311(12):780–3.
2. Vermylen C, Fernandez Robles E, Ninane J, et al. Bone marrow transplantation in five children with sickle cell anaemia. Lancet 1988;1(8600):1427–8.
3. Vermylen C, Cornu G. Bone marrow transplantation for sickle cell disease. The European experience. Am J Pediatr Hematol Oncol 1994;16(1):18–21.
4. Ferster A, De Valck C, Azzi N, et al. Bone marrow transplantation for severe sickle cell anaemia. Br J Haematol 1992;80(1):102–5.
5. Johnson FL, Mentzer WC, Kalinyak KA, et al. Bone marrow transplantation for sickle cell disease. The United States experience. Am J Pediatr Hematol Oncol 1994;16(1):22–6.

6. Walters MC, Patience M, Leisenring W, et al. Bone marrow transplantation for sickle cell disease. N Engl J Med 1996;335(6):369–76.
7. Bernaudin F, Socie G, Kuentz M, et al. Long-term results of related myeloablative stem-cell transplantation to cure sickle cell disease. Blood 2007;110(7):2749–56.
8. Hsieh MM, Fitzhugh CD, Weitzel R, et al. Nonmyeloablative HLA-matched sibling allogeneic hematopoietic stem cell transplantation for severe sickle cell phenotype. JAMA 2014;312(1):48–56.
9. Brand A, Doxiadis IN, Roelen DL. On the role of HLA antibodies in hematopoietic stem cell transplantation. Tissue Antigens 2013;81(1):1–11.
10. Ciurea SO, Thall PF, Wang X, et al. Donor-specific anti-HLA Abs and graft failure in matched unrelated donor hematopoietic stem cell transplantation. Blood 2011;118(22):5957–64.
11. Takanashi M, Atsuta Y, Fujiwara K, et al. The impact of anti-HLA antibodies on unrelated cord blood transplantations. Blood 2010;116(15):2839–46.
12. Thomas ED, Buckner CD, Sanders JE, et al. Marrow transplantation for thalassaemia. Lancet 1982;2(8292):227–9.
13. Lucarelli G, Galimberti M, Polchi P, et al. Marrow transplantation in patients with advanced thalassemia. N Engl J Med 1987;316(17):1050–5.
14. McPherson ME, Hutcherson D, Olson E, et al. Safety and efficacy of targeted busulfan therapy in children undergoing myeloablative matched sibling donor BMT for sickle cell disease. Bone Marrow Transplant 2011;46(1):27–33.
15. Maheshwari S, Kassim A, Yeh RF, et al. Targeted busulfan therapy with a steady-state concentration of 600-700 ng/mL in patients with sickle cell disease receiving HLA-identical sibling bone marrow transplant. Bone Marrow Transplant 2014;49(3):366–9.
16. Walters MC, Patience M, Leisenring W, et al. Stable mixed hematopoietic chimerism after bone marrow transplantation for sickle cell anemia. Biol Blood Marrow Transplant 2001;7(12):665–73.
17. Iannone R, Casella JF, Fuchs EJ, et al. Results of minimally toxic nonmyeloablative transplantation in patients with sickle cell anemia and beta-thalassemia. Biol Blood Marrow Transplant 2003;9(8):519–28.
18. van Besien K, Bartholomew A, Stock W, et al. Fludarabine-based conditioning for allogeneic transplantation in adults with sickle cell disease. Bone Marrow Transplant 2000;26(4):445–9.
19. Locatelli F, Kabbara N, Ruggeri A, et al. Outcome of patients with hemoglobinopathies given either cord blood or bone marrow transplantation from an HLA-identical sibling. Blood 2013;122(6):1072–8.
20. Locatelli F, Rocha V, Reed W, et al. Related umbilical cord blood transplantation in patients with thalassemia and sickle cell disease. Blood 2003;101(6):2137–43.
21. Soni S, Boulad F, Cowan MJ, et al. Combined umbilical cord blood and bone marrow from HLA-identical sibling donors for hematopoietic stem cell transplantation in children with hemoglobinopathies. Pediatr Blood Cancer 2014;61:1690–4.
22. Dedeken L, Le PQ, Azzi N, et al. Haematopoietic stem cell transplantation for severe sickle cell disease in childhood: a single centre experience of 50 patients. Br J Haematol 2014;165(3):402–8.
23. Gooley TA, Chien JW, Pergam SA, et al. Reduced mortality after allogeneic hematopoietic-cell transplantation. N Engl J Med 2010;363(22):2091–101.
24. Hahn T, McCarthy PL Jr, Hassebroek A, et al. Significant improvement in survival after allogeneic hematopoietic cell transplantation during a period of

significantly increased use, older recipient age, and use of unrelated donors. J Clin Oncol 2013;31(19):2437–49.
25. Ballen KK, Gluckman E, Broxmeyer HE. Umbilical cord blood transplantation: the first 25 years and beyond. Blood 2013;122(4):491–8.
26. Cavazzana-Calvo M, Andre-Schmutz I, Fischer A. Haematopoietic stem cell transplantation for SCID patients: where do we stand? Br J Haematol 2013; 160(2):146–52.
27. Krishnamurti L, Abel S, Maiers M, et al. Availability of unrelated donors for hematopoietic stem cell transplantation for hemoglobinopathies. Bone Marrow Transplant 2003;31(7):547–50.
28. Justus D, Perez E, Dioguardi J, et al. Allogeneic donor availability for hematopoietic stem cell transplantation in patients with sickle cell disease. World Cord Blood Congress IV and Innovative Therapies for Sickle Cell Disease. Monaco, October 24–27, 2013.
29. Mynarek M, Bettoni da Cunha Riehm C, Brinkmann F, et al. Normalized transcranial Doppler velocities, stroke prevention and improved pulmonary function after stem cell transplantation in children with sickle cell anemia. Klin Padiatr 2013; 225(3):127–32.
30. Kharbanda S, Smith AR, Hutchinson SK, et al. Unrelated donor allogeneic hematopoietic stem cell transplantation for patients with hemoglobinopathies using a reduced-intensity conditioning regimen and third-party mesenchymal stromal cells. Biol Blood Marrow Transplant 2014;20(4):581–6.
31. La Nasa G, Giardini C, Argiolu F, et al. Unrelated donor bone marrow transplantation for thalassemia: the effect of extended haplotypes. Blood 2002;99(12): 4350–6.
32. La Nasa G, Argiolu F, Giardini C, et al. Unrelated bone marrow transplantation for beta-thalassemia patients: the experience of the Italian Bone Marrow Transplant Group. Ann N Y Acad Sci 2005;1054:186–95.
33. Li C, Wu X, Feng X, et al. A novel conditioning regimen improves outcomes in beta-thalassemia major patients using unrelated donor peripheral blood stem cell transplantation. Blood 2012;120(19):3875–81.
34. Ruggeri A, Eapen M, Scaravadou A, et al. Umbilical cord blood transplantation for children with thalassemia and sickle cell disease. Biol Blood Marrow Transplant 2011;17(9):1375–82.
35. Luznik L, Engstrom LW, Iannone R, et al. Posttransplantation cyclophosphamide facilitates engraftment of major histocompatibility complex-identical allogeneic marrow in mice conditioned with low-dose total body irradiation. Biol Blood Marrow Transplant 2002;8(3):131–8.
36. Luznik L, O'Donnell PV, Symons HJ, et al. HLA-haploidentical bone marrow transplantation for hematologic malignancies using nonmyeloablative conditioning and high-dose, posttransplantation cyclophosphamide. Biol Blood Marrow Transplant 2008;14(6):641–50.
37. Munchel AT, Kasamon YL, Fuchs EJ. Treatment of hematological malignancies with nonmyeloablative, HLA-haploidentical bone marrow transplantation and high dose, post-transplantation cyclophosphamide. Best Pract Res Clin Haematol 2011;24(3):359–68.
38. Bolanos-Meade J, Fuchs EJ, Luznik L, et al. HLA-haploidentical bone marrow transplantation with posttransplant cyclophosphamide expands the donor pool for patients with sickle cell disease. Blood 2012;120(22):4285–91.
39. Dallas MH, Triplett B, Shook DR, et al. Long-term outcome and evaluation of organ function in pediatric patients undergoing haploidentical and matched

related hematopoietic cell transplantation for sickle cell disease. Biol Blood Marrow Transplant 2013;19(5):820–30.
40. Vermylen C, Cornu G, Ferster A, et al. Haematopoietic stem cell transplantation for sickle cell anaemia: the first 50 patients transplanted in Belgium. Bone Marrow Transplant 1998;22(1):1–6.
41. Ciurea SO, de Lima M, Cano P, et al. High risk of graft failure in patients with anti-HLA antibodies undergoing haploidentical stem-cell transplantation. Transplantation 2009;88(8):1019–24.
42. Gladstone DE, Zachary AA, Fuchs EJ, et al. Partially mismatched transplantation and human leukocyte antigen donor-specific antibodies. Biol Blood Marrow Transplant 2013;19(4):647–52.
43. Yoshihara S, Taniguchi K, Ogawa H, et al. The role of HLA antibodies in allogeneic SCT: is the 'type-and-screen' strategy necessary not only for blood type but also for HLA? Bone Marrow Transplant 2012;47(12):1499–506.
44. de Lima M, McNiece I, Robinson SN, et al. Cord-blood engraftment with ex vivo mesenchymal-cell coculture. N Engl J Med 2012;367(24):2305–15.
45. Horwitz ME, Chao NJ, Rizzieri DA, et al. Umbilical cord blood expansion with nicotinamide provides long-term multilineage engraftment. J Clin Invest 2014; 124:3121–8.
46. Cavazzana-Calvo M, Payen E, Negre O, et al. Transfusion independence and HMGA2 activation after gene therapy of human beta-thalassaemia. Nature 2010;467(7313):318–22.
47. Panepinto JA, Walters MC, Carreras J, et al. Matched-related donor transplantation for sickle cell disease: report from the Center for International Blood and Transplant Research. Br J Haematol 2007;137(5):479–85.
48. Majumdar S, Robertson Z, Robinson A, et al. Outcome of hematopoietic cell transplantation in children with sickle cell disease, a single center's experience. Bone Marrow Transplant 2010;45(5):895–900.
49. Soni S, Gross TG, Rangarajan H, et al. Outcomes of matched sibling donor hematopoietic stem cell transplantation for severe sickle cell disease with myeloablative conditioning and intermediate-dose of rabbit anti-thymocyte globulin. Pediatr Blood Cancer 2014;61:1685–9.
50. Horwitz ME, Spasojevic I, Morris A, et al. Fludarabine-based nonmyeloablative stem cell transplantation for sickle cell disease with and without renal failure: clinical outcome and pharmacokinetics. Biol Blood Marrow Transplant 2007; 13(12):1422–6.
51. Krishnamurti L, Kharbanda S, Biernacki MA, et al. Stable long-term donor engraftment following reduced-intensity hematopoietic cell transplantation for sickle cell disease. Biol Blood Marrow Transplant 2008;14(11):1270–8.
52. Matthes-Martin S, Lawitschka A, Fritsch G, et al. Stem cell transplantation after reduced-intensity conditioning for sickle cell disease. Eur J Haematol 2013; 90(4):308–12.
53. Bhatia M, Jin Z, Baker C, et al. Reduced toxicity, myeloablative conditioning with BU, fludarabine, alemtuzumab and SCT from sibling donors in children with sickle cell disease. Bone Marrow Transplant 2014;49:913–20.
54. Brichard B, Vermylen C, Ninane J, et al. Persistence of fetal hemoglobin production after successful transplantation of cord blood stem cells in a patient with sickle cell anemia. J Pediatr 1996;128(2):241–3.
55. Miniero R, Rocha V, Saracco P, et al. Cord blood transplantation (CBT) in hemoglobinopathies. Eurocord. Bone Marrow Transplant 1998;22(Suppl 1): S78–79.

56. Gore L, Lane PA, Quinones RR, et al. Successful cord blood transplantation for sickle cell anemia from a sibling who is human leukocyte antigen-identical: implications for comprehensive care. J Pediatr Hematol Oncol 2000;22(5):437–40.
57. Walters MC, Quirolo L, Trachtenberg ET, et al. Sibling donor cord blood transplantation for thalassemia major: experience of the Sibling Donor Cord Blood Program. Ann N Y Acad Sci 2005;1054:206–13.
58. Mazur M, Kurtzberg J, Halperin E, et al. Transplantation of a child with sickle cell anemia with an unrelated cord blood unit after reduced intensity conditioning. J Pediatr Hematol Oncol 2006;28(12):840–4.
59. Adamkiewicz TV, Szabolcs P, Haight A, et al. Unrelated cord blood transplantation in children with sickle cell disease: review of four-center experience. Pediatr Transplant 2007;11(6):641–4.
60. Sauter C, Rausen AR, Barker JN. Successful unrelated donor cord blood transplantation for adult sickle cell disease and Hodgkin lymphoma. Bone Marrow Transplant 2010;45(7):1252.
61. Kamani NR, Walters MC, Carter S, et al. Unrelated donor cord blood transplantation for children with severe sickle cell disease: results of one cohort from the phase II study from the Blood and Marrow Transplant Clinical Trials Network (BMT CTN). Biol Blood Marrow Transplant 2012;18(8):1265–72.
62. Radhakrishnan K, Bhatia M, Geyer MB, et al. Busulfan, fludarabine, and alemtuzumab conditioning and unrelated cord blood transplantation in children with sickle cell disease. Biol Blood Marrow Transplant 2013;19(4):676–7.
63. Raj A, Bertolone S, Cheerva A. Successful treatment of refractory autoimmune hemolytic anemia with monthly rituximab following nonmyeloablative stem cell transplantation for sickle cell disease. J Pediatr Hematol Oncol 2004;26(5):312–4.

Allogeneic Stem Cell Transplantation for Thalassemia Major

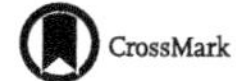

Vikram Mathews, MD, DM[a,*], Alok Srivastava, MD, FRACP, FRCPA[a], Mammen Chandy, MD, FRACP, FRCPA[b]

KEYWORDS

- Thalassemia major • Allogeneic stem cell transplant • Conditioning regimens
- Treosulfan • Sinusoidal obstruction syndrome • Peripheral blood stem cell graft
- Cord blood stem cells • Haploidentical transplants

KEY POINTS

- Allogeneic stem cell transplant remains the only curative option for patients with thalassemia major.
- Current risk stratification strategies have limitations and fail to recognize a very high risk subset of patients in whom a conventional conditioning regimen is associated with an unacceptable risk of treatment related mortality, especially in countries where pre-transplant medical therapy is sub-optimal.
- A number of novel conditioning regimen have been evaluated in an effort to improve the transplant outcomes in high risk patients. In the absence of controlled clinical trials to compare these it is difficult to make strong recommendation for one or the other of these approaches. A treosulfan based conditioning regimen has shown promise in high risk cases.
- Bone marrow is the preferable source of stem cells. While there is data to suggest a potential role for peripheral blood stem cells in reducing the risk of graft rejection in high risk cases this cannot be considered a recommendation based on the available data.
- Results from matched unrelated donor stem cell transplant have improved with the use of high resolution leukocyte antigen (HLA) typing and can be considered in low risk patients with a fully matched donor. There is a potential role for related cord blood transplants and if done should be in a center which has facilities with considerable experience in this procedure. It should preferably be done only in low risk cases. Unrelated cord blood transplants and haploidentical transplants should preferably be done only in the setting of a clinical trial.

[a] Department of Haematology, Christian Medical College, Ida Scudder Road, Vellore, TN 632004, India; [b] Department of Haematology and Bone Marrow Transplant, Tata Medical Center, Rajarhat, Kolkata 700020, India

* Corresponding author.

E-mail address: vikram@cmcvellore.ac.in

Hematol Oncol Clin N Am 28 (2014) 1187–1200

http://dx.doi.org/10.1016/j.hoc.2014.08.009 hemonc.theclinics.com

INTRODUCTION

Allogeneic stem cell transplantation (SCT) remains the only curative option for patients with β-thalassemia major.[1] The correction of this disorder by an allogeneic stem cell transplant was first described by Thomas and colleagues.[2] A conditioning regimen of busulfan and cyclophosphamide was subsequently established for SCT in this condition.[3] This myeloablative therapy forms the basis for the current conditioning regimens in this condition. Reduced-intensity conditioning regimens have been attempted, with some success, although the increased risk of rejection with this approach has limited its widespread acceptance.[1] To date more than 3000 transplants have been reported worldwide for this condition.[1] The current risk stratification of patients with β-thalassemia major undergoing a myeloablative allogeneic SCT classifies them into 3 risk groups (Pesaro classes I, II, and III), based on liver size (>2 cm), presence of liver fibrosis, and inadequate iron chelation.[4,5] Recent advances have attempted to improve on the risk stratification to better identify subsets that are likely to do poorly and need alternative/improved strategies to reduce rejection and treatment-related mortality (TRM) among patients in class III.[6–8] There has been some progress in developing new protocols; preliminary studies have shown the ability of such regimens to reduce TRM and rejection. Of special interest is the role of intravenous busulfan[9] and treosulfan[10,11] in conditioning regimens and efforts to reduce the risk of sinusoidal obstruction syndrome (SOS). The development of new conditioning regimens has, in general, been empiric with the evaluation of a variety of drugs and doses and schedules with no controlled studies to validate the claims of superiority of one rather than another. Of recent interest is the role of matched unrelated donor (MUD) stem cell transplants, cord blood stem cell transplants, and haploidentical stem cell transplants. Their potential lies in expanding the number of recipients for this curative strategy. Although there have been significant challenges and concerns with these alternate donor sources there have also been steady improvements in clinical outcome with these approaches that has put them on the threshold of being considering as standard of care. The role of splenectomy before allogeneic SCT is unclear, although there are theoretic benefits. There are limited data on optimal posttransplant chelation therapy, immune reconstitution, and long-term care after transplantation. In the absence of controlled clinical trials to address issues such as optimal conditioning regimen, graft source, use of alternate donors, and graft-versus-host disease (GVHD) prophylaxis clinicians have to rely on expert and consensus opinions, which have significant limitations. This article addresses some of these issues and the advances in each of these areas.

PRETRANSPLANT RISK STRATIFICATION AND AGE AT TRANSPLANTATION

The conventional risk stratification of patients with β-thalassemia major undergoing a myeloablative allogeneic SCT classifies them into 3 risk groups (Pesaro classes I, II, and III) based on liver size (>2 cm), presence of liver fibrosis, and inadequate iron chelation (adequate chelation was defined as initiation of chelation by 18 months from date of first transfusion and chelation with deferoxamine administered subcutaneously over 8–10 hours/d for at least 5 days a week).[4,5] Patients with none of these risk factors are classified as class I, those with 1 or 2 of these risk factors are class II, whereas those patients who have all 3 adverse risk factors are classified as class III. Patients in class I and II are considered to be low risk and have excellent long-term outcomes following an allogeneic SCT. In contrast, class III patients are considered high risk and have inferior outcomes following SCT. The authors further showed the ability of this classification to discriminate the thalassemia-free survival (TFS) and overall survival (OS) between these groups. In that initial report, age up to 15 years did not affect TFS.

This risk stratification has not been validated in different populations, especially in a group of patients with inadequate medical care before an allogeneic SCT (as commonly seen in developing countries where such transplants are increasingly done). When applied to such a population with inadequate medical therapy before transplantation there was skewing in the distribution of patients, with most being class III, and there was also significant heterogeneity in clinical outcomes among this class III subset that could not be recognized by the existing risk stratification strategy. We had previously reported on the limitations of this classification in our population and, based on statistical analysis, had further subdivided class III patients into a high-risk subset (class III HR) based on age greater than or equal to 7 years and liver size greater than or equal to 5 cm (**Fig. 1**).[6] We had proposed that this high-risk subset would need innovative strategies for improving outcomes following an allogeneic SCT, in view of their dismal outcomes with the conventional busulfan plus cyclophosphamide conditioning regimens. A subsequent registry-based analysis Center for International Blood and Marrow Transplant Research (CIBMTR) showed a similar adverse effect of age greater than or equal to 7 years and hepatomegaly on clinical outcomes after transplantation. In contrast with this, the European Society for Blood and Bone Marrow Transplantation (EBMT) registry analysis showed that the adverse effect of age occurred at a threshold of 14 years.[1] This difference in the threshold age predicting poor clinical outcome is probably directly related to adequacy of medical care before transplantation in Europe in contrast with our series and the CIBMTR series in which a significant proportion of cases (>60%) were

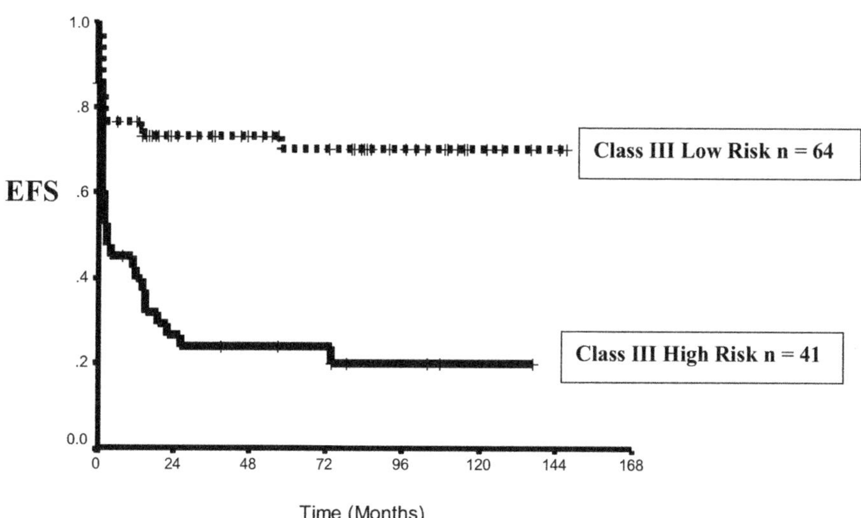

Fig. 1. Comparison of 5-year event-free survival (EFS) of class III transplants in the high-risk group (class III HR; n = 41) and the rest of transplants in class III (class III low risk; n = 64). (*From* Mathews V, George B, Deotare U, et al. A new stratification strategy that identifies a subset of class III patients with an adverse prognosis among children with beta thalassemia major undergoing a matched related allogeneic stem cell transplantation. Biol Blood Marrow Transplant 2007;13:892; with permission.)

from developing countries. Based on the available data, it is reasonable to retain the Pesaro risk stratification strategy, recognizing its limitations and its inability to identify a very-high-risk subset.

Patients should ideally receive an allogeneic SCT within the first 2 to 3 years of life before significant iron-related organ damage has set in.[1] There are very limited data for allogeneic SCT in adults (>18 years), although the TRM has consistently been reported to be more than 25%[12] and is probably best avoided.

CONDITIONING REGIMENS

The Pesaro group initially reported the adverse outcome in class III patients conditioned with a similar regimen as used for class I and II, with a TFS of 53% among class III patients versus 85% for the rest.[13] They also noted a nonrejection mortality of 39% in this group. To improve on the outcome and reduce non–transplant-related mortality they reduced the dose of cyclophosphamide to 160 mg/kg from 200 mg/kg. This small change reduced TRM but resulted in an increase in rejection rate from 7% to 30%.[14] The same group in March 1997 developed a conditioning regimen that started on day -45 with azathioprine and hydroxyurea, fludarabine from day -17 to -13, and busulfan 14 mg/kg with cyclophosphamide 160 mg/kg. With this new regimen, this group reported an 85% event-free survival (EFS) and a rejection rate of 8%.[15]

Class III and, more specifically, the class III HR subset have a high risk of graft rejection and regimen-related toxicity (RRT), especially SOS leading to multiorgan failure and death. These complications are related to the high degree of alloimmunization and iron overload–related end-organ damage in this cohort. The poor clinical outcome in this subset of older patients with very poor pretransplant medical therapy, as reported previously, is not reflected in the Western literature because of the use of adequate blood transfusion and chelation support before transplantation. However, when such a population is transplanted, even in a developed country with expertise in such transplants, the rejection rate is as high as 34%.[16]

The introduction of intravenous busulfan into conditioning regimens had the promise of more uniform pharmacokinetics and reduced toxicity (reviewed by Ciurea and Andersson[17]). A recent study of 57 patients with thalassemia major conditioned with intravenous busulfan along with oral defibrotide for SOS prophylaxis had a low incidence of SOS, with only 1 of 63 patients fulfilling the criteria for SOS.[18] However, there are too few data on clinical outcomes comparing oral versus intravenous busulfan to state conclusively that the latter is superior with regard to TFS and OS.

Treosulfan (dihydroxybusulfan), has recently attracted a lot of attention as an agent to replace busulfan in view of its favorable toxicity profile.[19] It is structurally similar to busulfan. Unlike busulfan it is water soluble and easy to reconstitute and administer intravenously. It also has a linear pharmacokinetic profile with good systemic exposure and very low intraindividual and interindividual pharmacokinetic variability.[20,21] In phase I studies even at cumulative doses of 56 gm/m^2 (a dose not usually reached when used as an agent in conditioning regimens) there was no dose-limiting hepatic, renal, neurologic, or cardiac toxicity.[22] Hepatic SOS is a common problem with conventional busulfan-based myeloablative regimens with an incidence ranging from 5% to 40%.[18] Use of a busulfan-based conditioning regimen was associated with an increased incidence of SOS on a multivariate analysis in a prospective study.[23] The link between pretransplant iron overload and SOS is similarly well recognized.[24] Although targeted busulfan levels and prophylaxis with defibrotide have significantly reduced this complication in patients with thalassemia major,[16,18] it is still a significant complication among class III HR patients. In the absence of such interventions, the cumulative incidence of SOS in the very-high-risk subset (class III HR) of patients has been reported to be as high as 78% and, in 24% of such cases, it led to multiorgan failure and death.[11] Treosulfan was hence especially attractive in the context of an allogeneic SCT for high-risk β-thalassemia major because of its reported low hepatic toxicity profile and consistent pharmacokinetic profile, which are both significant problems with conventional busulfan in this population.[6,25,26] However, it is also important to recognize that the pharmacokinetic profile of treosulfan-based regimens, both in patients with thalassemia major and when it is combined with other high-dose chemotherapeutic agents as part of the conditioning regimen, have not been studied extensively.

The first report on the use of treosulfan being used as part of the conditioning regimen for thalassemia was by Bernado and colleagues[27] in a small series of 20 patients, of whom 45% were class III and 18 received matched unrelated stem cell transplants. Only 2 patients in this series developed transient liver enzyme increase. In addition, the conditioning consisted of thiotepa and fludarabine, was well tolerated, and 17 cases had complete chimerism. The same group recently reported on their expanded experience with this reduced toxicity myeloablative regimen.[10] In this expanded series of 60 cases with thalassemia major the median age was 7 years, although only 7% of the 48 children were class III and the remaining 12 patients were adults. Forty (67%) of the patients received an unrelated donor transplant and in 47 (79%) the stem cell source was bone marrow. The regimen as previously reported was well tolerated with low (<10%) graft failure and a TFS of 84%.

A small series reported a comparable outcome between a similar treosulfan-based (n = 28) and a historical busulfan-based regimen (n = 12).[28] However, the median age in the busulfan group was 7 years versus 9.6 years in the treosulfan group, and the treosulfan group had 75% class III patients of whom 52.4% were class III HR as defined previously. In the busulfan arm 58% were class III and the number that fulfilled the criteria of class III HR is not available. The age and risk group of the patients in the treosulfan arm who died because of RRT (n = 4) and those who had a graft rejection (n = 2) are not available. As reported previously, the outcome of class III HR can be significantly different from class III as a whole.[6] Interpreting these data and comparing the 2 groups without this information must be done with caution, especially because of the small numbers in both groups. The inferior outcome in the treosulfan arm is likely to be related to the biology of class III HR rather than the conditioning regimen.

Our group recently reported our experience showing a clear advantage of a treosulfan-based regimen on the clinical outcome of class III as a whole and the subset of class III HR was recently reported.[11] A significant reduction in nonrelapse mortality and RRT, especially SOS, was shown in the class III HR compared with a historical control arm that had used a conventional busulfan-based conditioning regimen.[11]

However, in this very-high-risk group there was a significantly increased risk of mixed chimerism, which could be overcome with the use of a peripheral blood stem cell graft (PBSC). The use of this regimen with a PBSC graft translated to a significantly superior OS and EFS in the class III HR subset without a significant increased risk of GVHD.[11]

More recently, Anurathapan and colleagues[29] reported a novel approach of administration of 1 or 2 courses of immune-suppressive therapy with a combination of fludarabine and dexamethasone 1 to 2 months before the start of conditioning and followed this up with a reduced toxicity myeloablative conditioning regimen consisting of fludarabine, intravenous busulfan, and antithymocyte globulin with promising results in a small series of 18 patients with class III HR thalassemia major. **Table 1** summarizes the data on attempts to improve the clinical outcome.

Table 1
Major reported clinical studies that have attempted to improve the outcome of patients with class III thalassemia major

Study, Year	N	Median Age (y)/(Range)	Proportion in Class III (%)	Proportion in Class III HR[a] (%)	Major Defining Feature of Change in Protocol	TRM (%)	Graft Rejection (%)	EFS (%)	OS (%)
Lucarelli et al,[13] 1996[b]	115	11 (3–16)	100	NA	Reduction in cumulative cyclophosphamide from 200 mg/kg to 160 mg/kg	24	35	49	74
Sodani et al,[15] 2004	33	11 (5–16)	100	NA	Reduction in cyclophosphamide dose to ≤160 mg/kg. Addition of azathioprine and fludarabine and intensification of immunosuppression. Suppression of erythropoiesis by hypertransfusion, chelation, and hydroxyurea starting from day -45	6	6	85	93
Gaziev et al,[9] 2010	71	9 (1.6–27)	57.3	NA	Intravenous busulfan, dose adjustments with therapeutic drug monitoring	7	5	87	91
Chiesa et al,[16] 2010	53	8 (1–17)	47	NA	Intravenous busulfan, dose adjustments with therapeutic drug monitoring	4	15	79	96

Chiesa et al,[16] 2010[c]	25	NA	100	NA	Intravenous busulfan, dose adjustments with therapeutic drug monitoring	4	34	66	96
Bernardo et al,[10] 2012	60	7 (1–37)	27[d]	NA	Treosulfan-based conditioning regimen	7	9	84	93
Choudhary et al,[28] 2013	28	9.6 (2–18)	75	39	Treosulfan-based conditioning regimen	21	7	71	79
Anurathapan et al,[29] 2013	18	14 (10–18)	100	NA	Preconditioning immunosuppression therapy with fludarabine and dexamethasone; 1 or 2 courses 1 to 2 mo before transplantation. Conditioning regimen of fludarabine with intravenous busulfan	5	0	89	89
Mathews et al,[11] 2013	50	11 (2–21)	100	48	Treosulfan-based conditioning regimen with PBSC graft in 74%	12	8	79	87
Mathews et al,[11] 2013[e]	24	12 (3–21)	100	100	Treosulfan-based conditioning regimen with PBSC graft in 74%	13	8	78	87

Abbreviation: NA, not available.
[a] As defined previously.[6]
[b] Only patients less than 17 years of age are included in this table.
[c] Subset of high-risk cases from same article.
[d] Includes all adult cases as well (assumed to be class III).
[e] Subset of high-risk cases from same article.

The caveat to interpretation and comparison of clinical outcomes to compare different conditioning regimens is that the proportion of class III patients varies and the subset of patients who would fulfill the criteria for class III HR is often not available. These variables, especially the proportion in class III HR, significantly affect the clinical outcome and make such comparisons difficult.

BONE MARROW VERSUS PERIPHERAL BLOOD STEM CELL GRAFTS

Bone marrow has been the preferred choice of stem cells to reduce the risk of GVHD in this nonmalignant condition, although the incidence of both acute and chronic GVHD in this predominantly pediatric population is low.[26,30] PBSC have been reported to be associated with faster engraftment and lower requirement of blood product support in the peritransplant period[11,31,32] and have also been associated with a low incidence of graft rejection.[8,11] However, the risk of chronic GVHD is increased.[11,31,32] Our experience of using a PBSC graft with a treosulfan-based regimen to overcome early mixed chimerism and potential graft failure remains to be validated in larger studies. Larger prospective studies are required to confirm the benefit of PBSC compared with bone marrow in thalassemia major.

ALTERNATE DONOR SOURCES

Matched Unrelated Stem Cell Transplants

Only 25% to 30% of patients with thalassemia major have a human leukocyte antigen (HLA)–matched sibling donor, which limits the utility of an allogeneic SCT. Use of an MUD SCT has the potential to overcome this. The initial results with this approach were dismal, with a 55% graft rejection.[33] Since then there has been significant interval improvement in MUD SCT, with high-resolution molecular typing becoming standard in donor selection and outcome in malignant disorders with MUD being comparable with that of HLA-matched sibling transplants. More recent data suggest that OS of 79% can be achieved with this approach with TFS of 66% and a 25% chance of TRM.[34] The study also suggested that an extended haplotype match was associated with a superior outcome. The overall data suggest that MUD SCT should only be considered in centers that have reasonable experience with this approach and preferably in low-risk patients. High-resolution HLA typing with a full (10 of 10) match is the preferred donor and in addition they should ideally not have HLA-DP1 mismatches in the direction favoring graft rejection.[35]

Cord Blood Transplants

Cord blood transplants over the last decade have been the most rapidly growing source of stem cells for allogeneic SCT. However, for patients with thalassemia major, there are limited data. Using cord blood stem cells for allogeneic SCT in thalassemia major must be considered under 2 headings, which are distinctly different in terms of comparison of clinical outcome:

1. Related cord blood transplant: when an HLA-matched or partly mismatched sibling is the source of stem cells.
2. Unrelated cord blood transplant: when an unrelated cord blood product is procured from a cord blood bank as part of donor search for an allogeneic SCT. There could be varying degrees of HLA mismatch.

Using related cord blood, the Eurocord Transplant Group reported a 2-year probability of EFS of 79% in 33 patients with thalassemia. There was a 21% (7 rejections) risk of rejection of the graft, in spite of none of the patients being class III; 20 (61%) of the patients were class I.[36] A few smaller series have reported lower rejection rates but the numbers are small.[37,38] A large recently reported Eurocord and EBMT analysis showed comparative clinical outcomes with bone marrow and a fully HLA-matched related cord.[39] However, of the 96 related HLA cord blood transplants in this recent report, only 2 patients were class III and the rest (96%) were class I (61%) or II (35%). In spite of this statistically significantly higher proportion of class I cases in the related cord blood arm the graft rejections were higher at 10.4%. These data cannot and be extrapolated to populations in which most patients are class III; we would err on waiting for 2 years and do a regular bone marrow harvest and stem cell transplant from the same donor without this increased risk of graft rejection. The proposed reduction in acute GVHD from approximately 20% to 10% with the related cord blood transplant must be tempered by the fact that only 2% of patients in the bone marrow arm developed grade 4 GVHD.[39] There is a theoretically reduced risk of GVHD and, more importantly, less donor discomfort with a related donor cord blood transplant.

Unrelated cord blood transplant increases the potential pool of donors for patients with thalassemia major. However, the published data are limited. In a recent review of 6 studies a total of 19 patients were reported.[40] After combining data from 3 different registries, Rugeeri and colleagues[41] reported in 2011 that the cumulative graft failure rate was an unacceptable 52%. At this time, an unrelated cord blood transplant cannot be recommended outside the setting of a clinical trial.

Haploidentical Stem Cell Transplants

There is a lot of interest in haploidentical stem cell transplants worldwide over the last few years. Novel conditioning and GVHD prophylaxis regimens have resulted in dramatic improvements in clinical outcome even without T-cell depletion of the graft. However, there are very limited data in thalassemia major. In one small series (n = 22) using T-cell depletion grafts the graft rejection rate was 27% and the TFS about 67%. More recently the use of grafts with depletion of CD3$\alpha\beta$ T cells looks promising with a few successful reports.[42] Haploidentical SCT cannot be recommended at this time outside the setting of a clinical trial.

STEM CELL DOSE AND IMMUNE RECONSTITUTION AFTER TRANSPLANTATION AND ITS IMPACT ON CLINICAL OUTCOMES

At our center we prospectively evaluated bone marrow graft cellular subsets and patterns of immune reconstitution in a cohort of 63 consecutive patients with thalassemia major who underwent an HLA-matched sibling allogeneic SCT.[30] Data from this analysis suggest that, in this cohort of patients, increasing the stem cell dose reduces the risk of posttransplant bacterial and fungal infections. We hypothesize that faster immunologic recovery occurs with higher CD34 cell doses and, consequently, diminishes the risk of bacterial and fungal infections, as observed in a previous report.[43] However, we were not able to show a correlation in speed of recovery of any specific cellular subset in relation to the stem cell dose. We also noted that patients in the highest quartile of the stem cell dose did not have an increased risk of acute or chronic GVHD (data not shown). Although the number of events is few and the cohort studied small, it would still be reasonable in future, based on the available data, to target a CD34 cell dose of 79 $\times$ 10^6/kg to 9 $\times$ 10^6/kg. At these doses, our data suggest that there should be a significant reduction in posttransplant infection without an increased risk of GVHD.[30] We also noted an association with the day 28 natural killer cell count recovery and graft rejection. Patients who achieved less than the median level on day 28 after transplantation were significantly more likely to have secondary graft rejection.[30]

ROLE OF PRETRANSPLANT SPLENECTOMY

Massive splenomegaly in patients with β-thalassemia major is often a reflection of inadequate medical care and/or advanced disease and is often seen in class III patients.[44] It is associated with increased blood transfusion requirement.[45] Splenectomy is conventionally indicated when the transfusion requirement exceeds 220 mL of packed red blood cells per kilogram per year.[46] Splenectomy is also indicated if there is significant abdominal discomfort, splenic infarction, or symptomatic hypersplenism.[45]

Presence of splenomegaly before an SCT raises the theoretic concern of sequestration of infused stem cells, which can potentially have an adverse impact on engraftment. Splenectomy before an SCT could alter engraftment kinetics, which in turn could have an impact on graft tolerance and development of GVHD.[47] Splenectomy before an allogeneic SCT has the potential of reducing peritransplant transfusion requirement and hastening engraftment.[48]

Splenectomy in patients with β-thalassemia major is also considered a surrogate marker of high-risk disease, because it is often performed in older patients or in those who have had inadequate medical care. Splenectomy is reported to be associated with increased risk of pulmonary hypertension,[49] progressive restrictive pulmonary disease,[49] and alteration in hemostatic parameters that favor thrombosis.[50–52] It has also been reported to be associated with an increased risk of infections.[53] All the factors discussed earlier could contribute to an adverse outcome following an allogeneic SCT.

In a retrospective analysis done at our center we evaluated the impact of pretransplant splenectomy on clinical outcomes.[54] Our analysis suggests that, although pretransplant splenectomy among patients with thalassemia major was associated with faster engraftment and reduced transfusion support, it did not translate to an improved TFS or OS because of the higher RRT and peritransplant infection-related deaths in the splenectomized group. On multivariate analysis splenectomy was not an independent adverse factor and its perceived adverse effect on survival was probably caused by its association with other adverse features such as older age group and inadequate medical therapy before transplant. We could not show any significant beneficial effect that would warrant considering this procedure routinely before transplantation.[54,55]

POSTTRANSPLANT CARE AND MANAGEMENT OF IRON OVERLOAD

The iron overload state continues to require attention after transplantation. After a successful transplantation, provided the patient is stable and the hemoglobin is more than 100 g/L, the preferred method of iron removal is phlebotomy. It can be repeated once in 14 days and a volume of 6 mL/kg can be removed in 1 sitting.[56] If the hemoglobin level is not adequate or if phlebotomy is not possible, then the patient should be started on chelation therapy. It should be continued (maybe for years) until the ferritin level is less than 100 ng/mL. The optimal pharmacologic agents and chelation regimen after transplantation remain to be defined. In addition to chelation, these patients need close attention to immunization, endocrine dysfunction, and organ dysfunction secondary to iron overload.

SUMMARY

Significant progress has been made in the understanding of allogeneic stem cell transplant with regard to risk stratification, optimal conditioning regimens, and alternative stem cell sources, and this has translated to improved clinical outcomes for patients. However, there are limitations to the advances that can readily be translated to the larger worldwide community, and the major constraint is the cost of therapy; as a result, an allogeneic SCT is an option that is available only to a small fraction of patients. Efforts to further improve conditioning regimens with low toxicity profiles and reduced requirement of supportive care along with effective strategies to increase the donor pool are critical to increase access to this therapy to most patients.

REFERENCES

1. Angelucci E, Matthes-Martin S, Baronciani D, et al. Hematopoietic stem cell transplantation in thalassemia major and sickle cell disease: indications and management recommendations from an international expert panel. Haematologica 2014; 99:811–20.
2. Thomas ED, Buckner CD, Sanders JE, et al. Marrow transplantation for thalassaemia. Lancet 1982;2:227–9.
3. Lucarelli G, Polchi P, Galimberti M, et al. Marrow transplantation for thalassaemia following busulphan and cyclophosphamide. Lancet 1985;1:1355–7.
4. Lucarelli G, Galimberti M, Polchi P, et al. Bone marrow transplantation in patients with thalassemia. N Engl J Med 1990;322:417–21.
5. Lucarelli G, Galimberti M, Polchi P, et al. Bone marrow transplantation in adult thalassemia. Blood 1992;80:1603–7.
6. Mathews V, George B, Deotare U, et al. A new stratification strategy that identifies a subset of class III patients with an adverse prognosis among children with beta thalassemia major undergoing a matched related allogeneic stem cell transplantation. Biol Blood Marrow Transplant 2007;13:889–94.
7. Sabloff M, Chandy M, Wang Z, et al. HLA-matched sibling bone marrow transplantation for beta-thalassemia major. Blood 2010;117:1745–50.
8. Li C, Wu X, Feng X, et al. A novel conditioning regimen improves outcomes in beta-thalassemia major patients using unrelated donor peripheral blood stem cell transplantation. Blood 2012;120:3875–81.
9. Gaziev J, Nguyen L, Puozzo C, et al. Novel pharmacokinetic behavior of intravenous busulfan in children with thalassemia undergoing hematopoietic stem cell transplantation: a prospective evaluation of pharmacokinetic and pharmacodynamic profile with therapeutic drug monitoring. Blood 2010;115: 4597–604.
10. Bernardo ME, Piras E, Vacca A, et al. Allogeneic hematopoietic stem cell transplantation in thalassemia major: results of a reduced-toxicity conditioning regimen based on the use of treosulfan. Blood 2012;120:473–6.
11. Mathews V, George B, Viswabandya A, et al. Improved clinical outcomes of high risk beta thalassemia major patients undergoing a HLA matched related allogeneic stem cell transplant with a treosulfan based conditioning regimen and peripheral blood stem cell grafts. PLoS One 2013;8:e61637.
12. Gaziev J, Sodani P, Polchi P, et al. Bone marrow transplantation in adults with thalassemia: treatment and long-term follow-up. Ann N Y Acad Sci 2005;1054: 196–205.
13. Lucarelli G, Clift RA, Galimberti M, et al. Marrow transplantation for patients with thalassemia: results in class 3 patients. Blood 1996;87:2082–8.
14. Lucarelli G, Andreani M, Angelucci E. The cure of thalassemia by bone marrow transplantation. Blood Rev 2002;16:81–5.

15. Sodani P, Gaziev D, Polchi P, et al. New approach for bone marrow transplantation in patients with class 3 thalassemia aged younger than 17 years. Blood 2004;104:1201–3.
16. Chiesa R, Cappelli B, Crocchiolo R, et al. Unpredictability of intravenous busulfan pharmacokinetics in children undergoing hematopoietic stem cell transplantation for advanced beta thalassemia: limited toxicity with a dose-adjustment policy. Biol Blood Marrow Transplant 2010;16:622–8.
17. Ciurea SO, Andersson BS. Busulfan in hematopoietic stem cell transplantation. Biol Blood Marrow Transplant 2009;15:523–36.
18. Cappelli B, Chiesa R, Evangelio C, et al. Absence of VOD in paediatric thalassemic HSCT recipients using defibrotide prophylaxis and intravenous Busulphan. Br J Haematol 2009;147(4):554–60.
19. Danylesko I, Shimoni A, Nagler A. Treosulfan-based conditioning before hematopoietic SCT: more than a BU look-alike. Bone Marrow Transplant 2012;47:5–14.
20. Hilger RA, Harstrick A, Eberhardt W, et al. Clinical pharmacokinetics of intravenous treosulfan in patients with advanced solid tumors. Cancer Chemother Pharmacol 1998;42:99–104.
21. Glowka FK, Karazniewicz-Lada M, Grund G, et al. Pharmacokinetics of high-dose i.v. treosulfan in children undergoing treosulfan-based preparative regimen for allogeneic haematopoietic SCT. Bone Marrow Transplant 2008;42(Suppl 2):S67–70.
22. Scheulen ME, Hilger RA, Oberhoff C, et al. Clinical phase I dose escalation and pharmacokinetic study of high-dose chemotherapy with treosulfan and autologous peripheral blood stem cell transplantation in patients with advanced malignancies. Clin Cancer Res 2000;6:4209–16.
23. Cesaro S, Pillon M, Talenti E, et al. A prospective survey on incidence, risk factors and therapy of hepatic veno-occlusive disease in children after hematopoietic stem cell transplantation. Haematologica 2005;90:1396–404.
24. de Witte T. The role of iron in patients after bone marrow transplantation. Blood Rev 2008;22(Suppl 2):S22–8.
25. Srivastava A, Poonkuzhali B, Shaji RV, et al. Glutathione S-transferase M1 polymorphism: a risk factor for hepatic venoocclusive disease in bone marrow transplantation. Blood 2004;104:1574–7.
26. Chandy M, Balasubramanian P, Ramachandran SV, et al. Randomized trial of two different conditioning regimens for bone marrow transplantation in thalassemia–the role of busulfan pharmacokinetics in determining outcome. Bone Marrow Transplant 2005;36:839–45.
27. Bernardo ME, Zecca M, Piras E, et al. Treosulfan-based conditioning regimen for allogeneic haematopoietic stem cell transplantation in patients with thalassaemia major. Br J Haematol 2008;143:548–51.
28. Choudhary D, Sharma SK, Gupta N, et al. Treosulfan-thiotepa-fludarabine-based conditioning regimen for allogeneic transplantation in patients with thalassemia major: a single-center experience from north India. Biol Blood Marrow Transplant 2013;19:492–5.
29. Anurathapan U, Pakakasama S, Rujkijyanont P, et al. Pretransplant immunosuppression followed by reduced-toxicity conditioning and stem cell transplantation in high-risk thalassemia: a safe approach to disease control. Biol Blood Marrow Transplant 2013;19:1259–62.
30. Rajasekar R, Mathews V, Lakshmi KM, et al. Cellular immune reconstitution and its impact on clinical outcome in children with beta thalassemia major undergoing a

matched related myeloablative allogeneic bone marrow transplant. Biol Blood Marrow Transplant 2009;15:597–609.
31. Iravani M, Tavakoli E, Babaie MH, et al. Comparison of peripheral blood stem cell transplant with bone marrow transplant in class 3 thalassemic patients. Exp Clin Transplant 2010;8:66–73.
32. Ghavamzadeh A, Iravani M, Ashouri A, et al. Peripheral blood versus bone marrow as a source of hematopoietic stem cells for allogeneic transplantation in children with class I and II beta thalassemia major. Biol Blood Marrow Transplant 2008;14:301–8.
33. Gaziev D, Galimberti M, Lucarelli G, et al. Bone marrow transplantation from alternative donors for thalassemia: HLA-phenotypically identical relative and HLA-nonidentical sibling or parent transplants. Bone Marrow Transplant 2000;25:815–21.
34. La Nasa G, Giardini C, Argiolu F, et al. Unrelated donor bone marrow transplantation for thalassemia: the effect of extended haplotypes. Blood 2002;99:4350–6.
35. Fleischhauer K, Locatelli F, Zecca M, et al. Graft rejection after unrelated donor hematopoietic stem cell transplantation for thalassemia is associated with nonpermissive HLA-DPB1 disparity in host-versus-graft direction. Blood 2006;107:2984–92.
36. Locatelli F, Rocha V, Reed W, et al. Related umbilical cord blood transplantation in patients with thalassemia and sickle cell disease. Blood 2003;101:2137–43.
37. Lisini D, Zecca M, Giorgiani G, et al. Donor/recipient mixed chimerism does not predict graft failure in children with beta-thalassemia given an allogeneic cord blood transplant from an HLA-identical sibling. Haematologica 2008;93:1859–67.
38. Walters MC, Quirolo L, Trachtenberg ET, et al. Sibling donor cord blood transplantation for thalassemia major: Experience of the Sibling Donor Cord Blood Program. Ann N Y Acad Sci 2005;1054:206–13.
39. Locatelli F, Kabbara N, Ruggeri A, et al. Outcome of patients with hemoglobinopathies given either cord blood or bone marrow transplantation from an HLA-identical sibling. Blood 2013;122:1072–8.
40. Pinto FO, Roberts I. Cord blood stem cell transplantation for haemoglobinopathies. Br J Haematol 2008;141:309–24.
41. Ruggeri A, Eapen M, Scaravadou A, et al. Umbilical cord blood transplantation for children with thalassemia and sickle cell disease. Biol Blood Marrow Transplant 2011;17:1375–82.
42. Bertaina A, Merli P, Rutella S, et al. HLA-haploidentical stem cell transplantation after removal of alphabeta+ T and B-cells in children with non-malignant disorders. Blood 2014;124(5):822–6.
43. Bittencourt H, Rocha V, Chevret S, et al. Association of CD34 cell dose with hematopoietic recovery, infections, and other outcomes after HLA-identical sibling bone marrow transplantation. Blood 2002;99:2726–33.
44. Rund D, Rachmilewitz E. Beta-thalassemia. N Engl J Med 2005;353:1135–46.
45. Panigrahi I, Marwaha RK. Common queries in thalassemia care. Indian Pediatr 2006;43:513–8.
46. Cohen A, Markenson AL, Schwartz E. Transfusion requirements and splenectomy in thalassemia major. J Pediatr 1980;97:100–2.
47. Shatry AM, Jones M, Levy RB. The effect of the spleen on compartmental levels and distribution of donor progenitor cells after syngeneic and allogeneic bone marrow transplants. Stem Cells Dev 2004;13:51–62.
48. Li Z, Gooley T, Applebaum FR, et al. Splenectomy and hemopoietic stem cell transplantation for myelofibrosis. Blood 2001;97:2180–1.

49. Phrommintikul A, Sukonthasarn A, Kanjanavanit R, et al. Splenectomy: a strong risk factor for pulmonary hypertension in patients with thalassaemia. Heart 2006; 92:1467–72.
50. Tripatara A, Jetsrisuparb A, Teeratakulpisarn J, et al. Hemostatic alterations in splenectomized and non-splenectomized patients with beta-thalassemia/ hemoglobin E disease. Thromb Res 2007;120(6):805–10.
51. Pattanapanyasat K, Gonwong S, Chaichompoo P, et al. Activated platelet-derived microparticles in thalassaemia. Br J Haematol 2007;136:462–71.
52. Singer ST, Kuypers FA, Styles L, et al. Pulmonary hypertension in thalassemia: association with platelet activation and hypercoagulable state. Am J Hematol 2006;81:670–5.
53. Robin M, Guardiola P, Devergie A, et al. A 10-year median follow-up study after allogeneic stem cell transplantation for chronic myeloid leukemia in chronic phase from HLA-identical sibling donors. Leukemia 2005;19:1613–20.
54. Mathews V, George B, Lakshmi KM, et al. Impact of pretransplant splenectomy on patients with beta-thalassemia major undergoing a matched-related allogeneic stem cell transplantation. Pediatr Transplant 2009;13:171–6.
55. Bhatia M, Cairo MS. Splenectomy or no splenectomy prior to allogeneic stem-cell transplantation in patients with severe thalassemia: this is the question. Pediatr Transplant 2009;13:143–5.
56. Angelucci E, Muretto P, Lucarelli G, et al. Phlebotomy to reduce iron overload in patients cured of thalassemia by bone marrow transplantation. Italian Co-operative Group for Phlebotomy Treatment of Transplanted Thalassemia Patients. Blood 1997;90:994–8.

Referral to Transplant Center for Hematopoietic Cell Transplantation

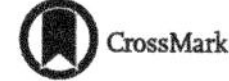

Navneet S. Majhail, MD, MS[a], Madan Jagasia, MBBS, MS[b,*]

KEYWORDS

- Hematopoietic cell transplantation • Transplant center • Referral • Patient
- Referring physician • Payors

KEY POINTS

- Transplant center referrals are a complex, multistep process that involves patients, physicians, and payors.
- Timely referral of the patient requires education of the referring physician.
- Transplant indications continue to evolve with improved transplant outcome and emergence of better nontransplant therapies.
- Care of transplant patients after discharge from the transplant center needs to be considered during initial referral along with other factors.

INTRODUCTION

Hematopoietic cell transplantation (HCT) is a complex and highly specialized medical procedure limited to institutions that can dedicate the required resources, personnel, and infrastructure toward a transplant program.[1–3] It is offered by approximately 170 to 180 transplant centers in the United States. Many states have only one institution that conducts this procedure and some states do not have an active transplant program. Most HCT programs are located in academic tertiary care medical centers. Hence, patients who may be candidates for transplantation frequently have to be referred by their treating hematologist and/or oncologist to a transplant center. The transplant referral process is multistep with many variables that are often not systematically studied. These factors can be classified as physician-, patient-, and payor-based. This article reviews the process of referral to a transplant center and discusses perspectives that patients, referring physicians, and payors may consider when

Financial Disclosure: None of the authors has a financial conflict of interest to disclose.
[a] Blood & Marrow Transplant Program, Cleveland Clinic Taussig Cancer Institute, 9500 Euclid Avenue, Cleveland, OH 44195, USA; [b] Division of Hematology-Oncology, Vanderbilt University Medical Center, 3973 TVC, Nashville, TN 37232, USA
* Corresponding author.
E-mail address: madan.jagasia@vanderbilt.edu

Hematol Oncol Clin N Am 28 (2014) 1201–1213
http://dx.doi.org/10.1016/j.hoc.2014.08.007 **hemonc.theclinics.com**
0889-8588/14/$ – see front matter

determining which center to select for transplantation. This article is written from the viewpoint of the US health care system. Although referral practices for HCT vary considerably among countries because of the differences in health care system organization and delivery, the general principles discussed in this review are still relevant.

CARE MODELS FOR TRANSPLANT CENTER REFERRAL

The mechanism for referral usually depends on where a patient receives therapy for his or her underlying disease and can occur under one of the following scenarios:

- For most patients, the transplant referral is initiated by a hematologist-oncologist practicing at a site other than the transplant center (eg, community or another academic institution). Patients are often referred to a transplant center that is located within the same geographic region. This may be a geographic feature, but more often than not, referring physicians in the "catchment" area of a tertiary center have an established working relationship with hematologists and transplant physicians at the tertiary center.
- Most transplant centers have a robust hematologic malignancy program and thus some patients receive a within-institution referral. They are treated by a hematologist-oncologist who practices at the same institution but is often not a member of the transplant team. Patients are referred to the transplant program within that institution if they are potential candidates for transplantation.
- Some institutions are organized in a manner such that the same physician provides primary management of the underlying disease and then takes care of the transplant portion of the treatment. There is no formal referral in this case. However, personnel who constitute the rest of the transplant team are frequently different, even within the same institution, and some element of transition of care does occur for the patient.
- Health care payors often determine the transplant center of choice based on "in-network" and "out of network" privileges.
- Finally, the patient may self-refer himself or herself to a transplant center or may do so at the behest of a caregiver or family member.

Most of the transplant referrals are initiated by physicians. Pidala and colleagues[4] conducted a survey of practice variation in physician referrals for allogeneic stem cell transplantation (SCT). Despite recent advances in SCT, and the abundance of data showing improved outcomes for older age, there was a significant bias against referring older patients for SCT (age 60 vs age 30; odds ratio, 8.3; 95% confidence interval, 5.9–11.7; *P*<.0001). Thus, continued education of the referring physician regarding the evolving outcomes of SCT remains an important unmet need. As nontransplant options, albeit noncurative, increase, the role of SCT needs to be continually reassessed. As expected, lack of health care coverage was a deterrent to referral (no coverage vs coverage; odds ratio, 6.9; 95% confidence interval, 5.2–9.1). With the implementation of the Affordable Care Act, it is likely that more patients who currently do not have health care coverage can access life-saving procedures like SCT.

Payors often determine the choice of the transplant center based on "in-network" and "out of network" status of the transplant centers. The "in-network" centers are often in geographic proximity of the patient and maintain excellent outcomes, but on multiple occasions patients have to travel significant distances to go to an "in-network" center. These "forced" referrals are often disruptive to patients and their caregivers.

Some patients are self-referred and "shop-around" for transplant centers with specific expertise in the underlying disease or in search of specific clinical trials. In these instances, it is important to ensure that interim therapy is not compromised while a determination of the transplant center is being made.

TIMING OF TRANSPLANT REFERRAL

Among transplant recipients, HCT earlier in the disease course is associated with better outcomes compared with transplantation for late-stage relapsed or active disease.[5,6] Hence, for patients in whom HCT may be potentially considered as a part of the overall treatment plan, it is critical that referral to a transplantation center occurs sooner in the disease course. The logistics of organizing a transplant can take time (eg, identifying a donor, arranging caregivers, additional treatment, and financial clearance), and hence early consultation is appropriate even though some patients may not need a transplant. **Box 1** summarizes the general guidelines

Box 1
National Marrow Donor Program and American Society for Blood and Marrow Transplantation guidelines for recommended timing for transplant consultation for adults with hematologic malignancies (complete guidelines are available at www.bethematchclinical.org)

Acute myeloid leukemia

- Early after initial diagnosis, all patients including
  - First complete remission, except favorable-risk leukemia
  - Antecedent hematologic disease (eg, myelodysplastic syndrome)
  - Treatment-related leukemia
  - Primary induction failure or relapse
  - Presence of minimal residual disease after initial or subsequent therapy, if not evaluated previously

Acute lymphoblastic leukemia

- Early after initial diagnosis, all patients including
  - First complete remission
  - Primary induction failure or relapse
  - Presence of minimal residual disease after initial or subsequent therapy, if not evaluated previously

Myelodysplastic syndromes

- Any intermediate or high International Prognostic Scoring System score myelodysplastic syndrome
- Any myelodysplastic syndrome with poor prognostic features, including
  - Treatment-related myelodysplastic syndrome
  - Refractory cytopenia
  - Adverse cytogenetics
  - Transfusion dependence

Chronic myeloid leukemia

- Inadequate hematologic or cytogenetic response after trial of tyrosine kinase inhibitor
- Disease progression
- Intolerance to tyrosine kinase inhibitor

- Accelerated phase
- Blast crisis

Chronic lymphocytic leukemia

- High-risk cytogenetics or molecular features (eg, del[11q] or del[17p], unmutated Ig VH)
- Short initial remission
- Poor initial response
- Fludarabine resistant
- Richter transformation

Follicular non-Hodgkin lymphoma

- Poor response to initial treatment
- Initial remission duration of less than 12 months
- First relapse
- Transformation to diffuse large B-cell lymphoma

Diffuse large B-cell lymphoma

- At first or subsequent relapse
- First complete remission with high or high-intermediate International Prognostic Index risk
- No complete remission with initial treatment
- Second or subsequent remission

Mantle cell lymphoma

- After initiation of therapy

Other high-risk lymphomas

- After initiation of therapy

Hodgkin lymphoma

- Primary induction failure or relapse
- Second or subsequent remission

Multiple myeloma

- All patients after initiation of primary therapy
- At first progression

Severe aplastic anemia

- At diagnosis

Courtesy of National Marrow Donor Program and American Society for Blood and Marrow Transplantation, Arlington Heights, IL; with permission.

for the appropriate timing to refer patients to a transplant center that have been developed by the National Marrow Donor Program and the American Society for Blood and Marrow Transplantation. These guidelines need to be continually reassessed as nontransplant therapy changes. The referring physician may have a bias toward "late" transplantation especially in diseases where there are several second- or third-line therapy options, even though they may be noncurative. The absence of prospective randomized controlled trials regarding the benefit of transplant over nontransplant therapy in most disease indications makes decision making complex and contentious. The risk-benefit assessments of early transplant versus nontransplant options are best done in collaboration with the transplant physician. The patient should ideally receive an unbiased balanced opinion of the outcome of early transplant versus delaying the transplant for a subsequent progression. These decisions are often taken in the context of team meetings and should ideally also be attended by nontransplant physicians.

TRANSPLANT CENTER CONSIDERATIONS

This section describes some general processes that a transplant center follows when it receives a patient referral (**Fig. 1**). The first step is a consultation with a transplant physician, where patient suitability for transplantation is assessed based on an evaluation of disease status and comorbidities. Patients may be sent back to their referring physician if additional therapy is warranted before transplantation. Some centers also do a detailed psychosocial assessment at this time through an interview with a social worker or another transplant provider. The patient's health insurance provider is contacted by the transplant center to assess benefits for transplantation and to obtain clearance for transplant-related care. For patients who need an allogeneic HCT, an evaluation of donor options begins at this stage with typing of related donors. If related donors are not available, a search for an unrelated donor or umbilical cord blood units is initiated.

Before transplantation, the patient usually returns for a pretransplant work-up. During this phase, evaluations are conducted for disease status, infectious disease markers, organ function, and psychosocial status. The time between initial consultation and pretransplant assessment depends on whether the patient needs additional therapy before transplantation, and in patients being considered for allogeneic HCT, the time to identify a suitable donor. For patients whose disease status is optimal and who are being considered for autologous or related donor transplantation, the time between initial and pretransplant assessment can be as short as 2 to 4 weeks. This interval is longer for patients who need an unrelated donor for transplantation.[7]

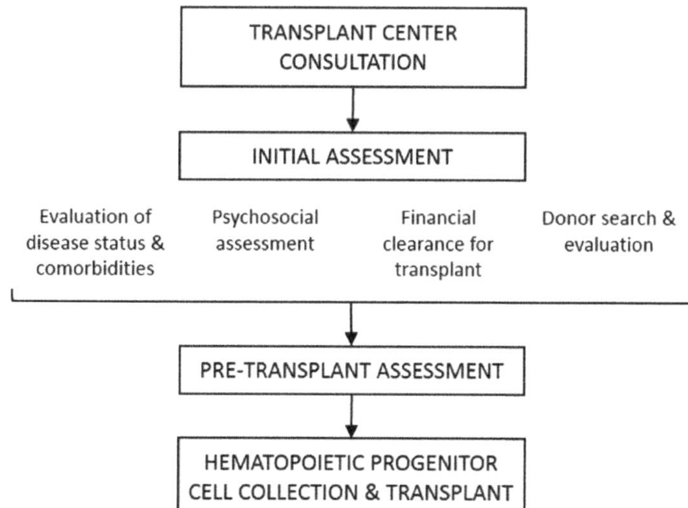

Fig. 1. Process for evaluation of a patient who has been referred to a transplant center.

ISSUES TO CONSIDER WHEN CHOOSING A TRANSPLANT CENTER

Perspectives that patients, referring physicians, and payors consider when choosing a transplant center vary (**Box 2**). In our experience, most patients go to a transplant center that is recommended by their hematologist-oncologist, provided that the procedure at that center is covered by their health insurance. For referring physicians, the most important factor for referring a patient to a particular transplant center is their relationship with that center, largely based on experience and outcomes for previously transplanted patients. Some common issues to consider are discussed next.

Transplant Center Outcomes

Patients like to know a center's experience and outcomes for other patients with the same diagnosis. Similarly, referring physicians and payors consider outcomes an important factor when determining where to send patients for transplantation. In the United States, the Center for International Blood and Marrow Transplant Research performs a center outcomes analysis annually for all centers that perform allogeneic HCT. Results show the observed 1-year survival for related and unrelated donor

Box 2
Transplant center characteristics considered by patients, referring physicians, and payors in selecting a center

Patients

- Referring physician recommendation
- Health insurance coverage for care at the transplant center
- Transplant center outcomes and experience
- Type and breadth of patient support services
- Distance of primary residence from the transplant center
- Options for temporary housing near the transplant center
- Financial issues (eg, out-of-pocket costs)

Referring physicians

- Relationship with transplant center
- Transplant center outcomes
- Transplant center reputation and experience
- Health insurance coverage for care at the transplant center
- Center communication with referring physician
- Patient convenience
- Type and breadth of patient support services
- Patient financial issues

Payors

- Transplant center outcomes
- Presence of a quality management program
- Accreditation (eg, by Foundation for Accreditation of Cellular Therapy)
- Type and breadth of patient support services
- Costs of transplant

HCT at each center and compare it with the expected survival for patients transplanted at that center. The findings are publically reported and are available at the Web site bloodcell.transplant.hrsa.gov.

Transplant Center Accreditation

Programs that are accredited by the Foundation for Accreditation of Cellular Therapy or its Europe equivalent, the Joint Accreditation Committee of the International Society for Cellular Therapy-European Society for Blood and Marrow Transplantation (ISCT-EBMT), have demonstrated that they meet a minimum but rigorous set of standards for providing high-quality care to HCT recipients. Other organizations (eg, National Marrow Donor Program) also require transplant centers to meet certain standards before they can use their services.

Financial Considerations

HCT is an expensive procedure and whether their health insurance covers transplantation in a particular center is an important consideration for patients and their physicians. Patients may also consider out-of-pocket costs, such as the expenses associated with relocation and temporary housing. Payors may restrict transplant coverage for their health plan enrollees to selected centers within a geographic area. In making such decisions, they generally focus on value where they balance the center outcomes and quality of care with the overall costs for transplantation. Many transplant centers have financial counselors that interact with patients before transplant to explain the various nuances of their health care coverage policy.

Geographic Location

Location of the transplant center is an important determinant of where patients will receive a transplant. Most patients prefer to stay close to their home. Most physicians refer their patients to the nearest transplant center. With the way most health insurance plans are organized, most payors recommend a transplant center that is close to the patient's place of residence. At times, the payors are "in network" with a select group of transplant centers designated as "center of excellence" and patients may be forced to seek care further away from home. Most patients stay in the vicinity of the transplant center for the first 3 to 4 months after an allogeneic HCT. The follow-up after discharge from the transplant center is significantly influenced by the distance from the patient's home to the transplant center. Recent data have suggested that distance from the transplant center may influence outcome. In a recent study by Abou-Nassar and colleagues,[8] patients with long driving time had worse overall survival 1 year after HCT compared with patients living closer to the transplant center, independent of other patient-, disease-, and transplant-related variables. The optimal health care delivery model for patients after the initial departure from the transplant center continues to evolve. **Fig. 2** shows the various models that are commonly used in follow-up of patients. At some centers, there is a dedicated long-term follow-up program with a focus on graft-versus-host disease (GVHD) management and survivorship. At many centers, patients return frequently for longitudinal follow-up. At other centers, patients are followed by "proxy" along with their local referring physicians and in some cases, primary practice physicians. Many academic centers do not have a dedicated long-term follow-up unit, and patients are reintegrated into hematology clinics without a focus on GVHD, late effects, and survivorship issues. The interplay of distance from the transplant center and the various models of health care delivery probably influence outcome but have not been well studied. In a recent study by Ragon and colleagues,[9] distance from the transplant center did not influence outcome contrary to the previous

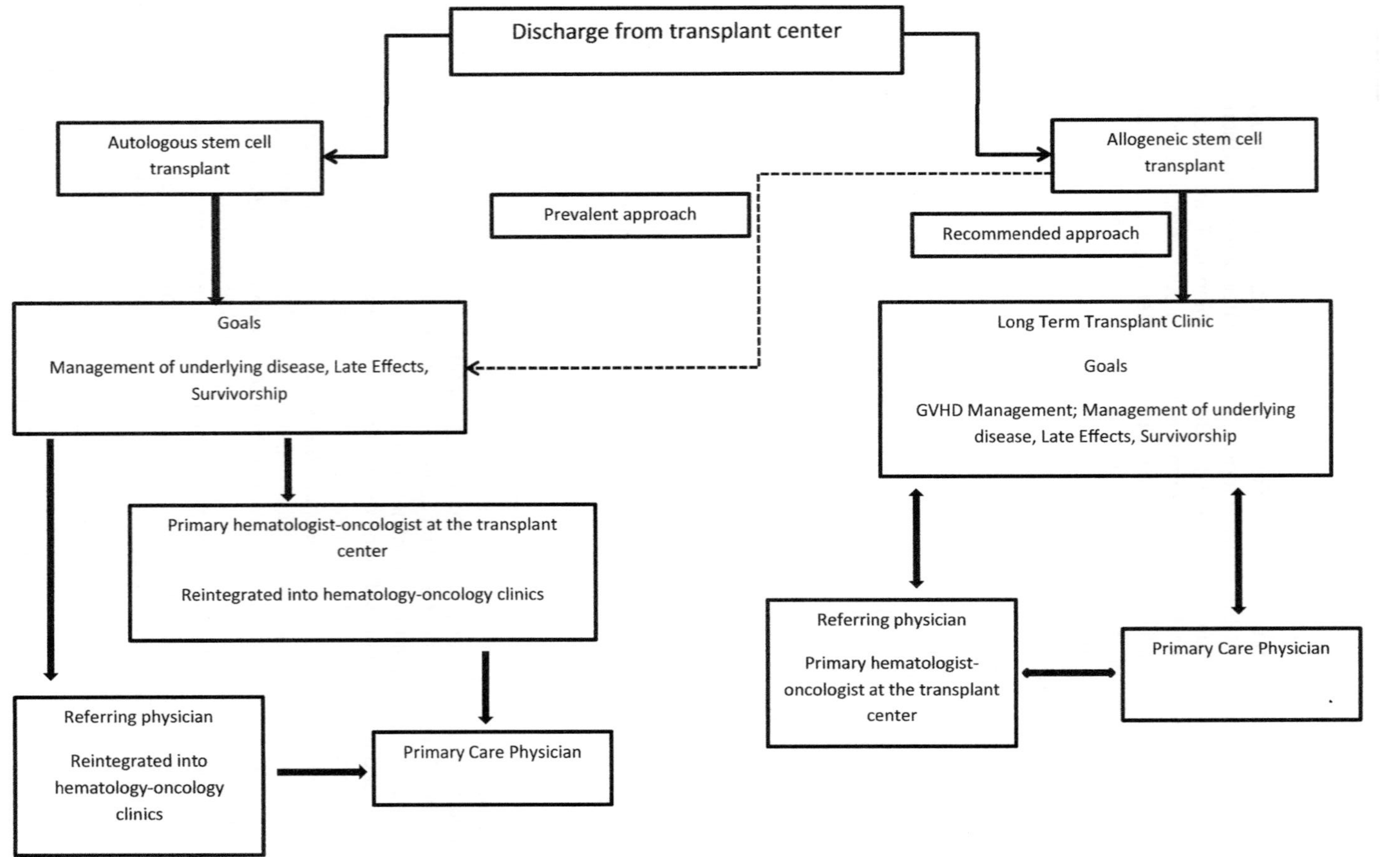

Fig. 2. Models of care after discharge from the transplant center. GVHD, graft-versus-host disease.

report, but patients were followed in a longitudinal long-term transplant model with focus on multidisciplinary care.

Care After Discharge from the Transplant Center

Although, accreditation agencies focus on volume of the transplant center along with stringent standards for the first 100 days after transplant, many important outcome determinants require close attention to the processes that affect outcome after patient departure from the transplant center. As the early transplant-related mortality improves, chronic GVHD management, late effects, and survivorship issues need more attention.

The optimal model of health care delivery to the transplant patients after discharge from the transplant center is not known. Follow-up care after autologous transplant often mimics the care of the nontransplant patient. Many patients return to the transplant center for "day 100" and annual disease reassessment. Interim disease reassessment and maintenance chemotherapy (multiple myeloma) is often coordinated by referring physicians. Even in this seemingly uncomplicated group of patients, unique posttransplant complications can occur. Referring physicians need to be educated to identify these clinical scenarios and reach out to the transplant center.

The care of the allogeneic transplant recipient is complex and requires continued interaction with the transplant center. There are multiple models that are currently prevalent in the country. At many centers, the care of these patients is transitioned to the hematologist-oncologist at the transplant center. These patients are reintegrated into general hematology clinics. At other centers, patients are referred back to their community hematologist-oncologist and continue to receive guidance from the transplant center.

It is becoming increasingly evident that chronic GVHD along with non-GVHD late effects remains an important challenge after allogeneic transplantation and impacts long-term survival of the transplant recipient.[10–12] Many transplant centers have formed long-term follow-up clinics with focus on GVHD, survivorship, or both. These programs should ideally be staffed by physicians with expertise in these areas. Given the breadth of clinical problems that these patients encounter, midlevel providers and program coordinators are often needed to orchestrate multidisciplinary care. If the patient is able to follow longitudinally at the transplant center, the care is delivered on site at the transplant center. If a patient is not in geographic proximity to the transplant center, the long-term follow-up clinic coordinates the care with the referring hematologist-oncologist, or often the primary care provider. As health care informatics evolves, patients have ever-increasing access to their records through World Wide Web portals that access their electronic medical records. Electronic communication with the health care provider is becoming increasingly prevalent and should allow seamless communication between the long-term follow-up clinic provider and the patient. These advances in informatics need to be leveraged to allow for complex interdisciplinary care of the patient.

It is important to establish minimal standards of care in the long-term follow-up clinic. Implementation of these standards in a uniform manner will likely improve outcomes. The transplant community has published many guidelines and consensus documents for chronic GVHD, vaccinations, and late effects.[13–26] Until these guidelines are operationalized in clinics, it is unlikely to impact patient outcome.

Care after discharge from the transplant center may not be an important factor that decides the initial referral but probably has a high impact on outcome of the patient, especially after allogeneic transplant. The patient, referring physician, and payor all need to consider this at the time of the initial referral.

Patient Support Services

Although not a critical determinant for where a patient is referred for transplantation, patients and their caregivers usually appreciate availability of patient support services at a transplant center (eg, resources for psychosocial support, nutrition, physical therapy, education, and financial support).

Psychosocial Support

Although the goal of transplant is curative in most diseases, it is often complicated by significant early and late morbidity. This involves not only the patient, but influences the patient's social support system. Most transplant centers have social workers as part of their team. It is important for the patient to undergo psychosocial evaluation before transplant, but more importantly the resources need to be available in the post-transplant period. Psychologists and psychiatrists, who are familiar with transplant issues, are invaluable in taking care of the transplant recipient with psychiatric comorbidities, substance abuse issues, and complex family dynamics. The role of the caregivers cannot be underestimated. Resources are often also needed to support the caregivers.[27–29]

Financial Counseling

Transplant is a complex and expensive procedure. Despite health care coverage, patients and families experience out-of-pocket costs. These costs can be significant and vary based on duration of stay in the vicinity of the transplant center. Most programs have a financial counselor who can interact with the patient and educate them. Many transplant centers have in-house charity programs to offset cost of food, accommodation, and travel based on means-testing.

Role of the Nutritionist and Pharmacist

Transplant patients are often malnourished in the pretransplant setting and remain at a high risk of rapid weight loss with onset of chemotherapy toxicity and GVHD. As the incidence of obesity increases, the role of the nutritionist becomes challenging. Drug interactions, monitoring of drug levels, coordinating preparative regimen chemotherapy orders, and counseling patients on compliance with medications requires the presence of a pharmacist dedicated to the transplant team.

Rehabilitation and Physical Therapy

Many transplant patients get deconditioned during transplant and require referral for physical therapy. The role of pre-emptive physical therapy remains to be validated. At some programs, physical therapists assess transplant patients during initial evaluation and recommend an exercise program.

The use of the previously mentioned resources in the care of the transplant patient may not influence outcome, but are often made available to the transplant patient and their family to provide a holistic approach to transplant and at the same time maintain team efficiency.

SUMMARY

HCT has undergone tremendous advances in the last two decades. The patient can benefit from these only if they are referred to a transplant center in a timely manner. The complex interplay of the patient, the referring physician, the payor, and the transplant center make the referral process challenging. These need to be comprehensively studied and streamlined to deliver optimal care in an effective and efficient manner.

Table 1
Information resources about transplant centers in the United States

Organization	Web Site
CW Bill Young Transplantation Program	bloodcell.transplant.hrsa.gov
National Marrow Donor Program	bethematch.org
Foundation for the Accreditation of Cellular Therapy	www.factwebsite.org
BMT InfoNet	bmtinfonet.org

Both payors and accreditation agencies should attempt to elevate the standards of care that affect the patient after discharge from the transplant center because it impacts transplant outcome. The high cost of transplant procedure and the anticipated increase in transplant patients in a more restrictive financial health care climate underscores the importance of studying the transplant center referral process in a scientific manner to allow patients to access these services at the right time.

INFORMATION RESOURCES

Resources that can assist patients and referring providers in learning more about transplant centers in the United States are listed in **Table 1**.

REFERENCES

1. Majhail NS, Murphy EA, Omondi NA, et al. Allogeneic transplant physician and center capacity in the United States. Biol Blood Marrow Transplant 2011;17: 956–61.
2. Majhail NS, Murphy EA, Denzen EM, et al. The National Marrow Donor Program's Symposium on hematopoietic cell transplantation in 2020: a health care resource and infrastructure assessment. Biol Blood Marrow Transplant 2012;18:172–82.
3. Denzen EM, Majhail NS, Stickney Ferguson S, et al. Hematopoietic cell transplantation in 2020: summary of year 2 recommendations of the National Marrow Donor Program's System Capacity Initiative. Biol Blood Marrow Transplant 2013;19:4–11.
4. Pidala J, Craig BM, Lee SJ, et al. Practice variation in physician referral for allogeneic hematopoietic cell transplantation. Bone Marrow Transplant 2013;48: 63–7.
5. Pasquini MC, Wang Z. Current use and outcome of hematopoietic stem cell transplantation: CIBMTR summary slides. 2013. Available at: http://www.cibmtr.org/referencecenter/slidesreports/summaryslides/pages/index.aspx.
6. Armand P, Gibson CJ, Cutler C, et al. A disease risk index for patients undergoing allogeneic stem cell transplantation. Blood 2012;120:905–13.
7. Majhail NS, Lazarus HM. Many are called but few are chosen: under-utilization of unrelated donor transplantation. Biol Blood Marrow Transplant 2013;19:1414–5.
8. Abou-Nassar KE, Kim HT, Blossom J, et al. The impact of geographic proximity to transplant center on outcomes after allogeneic hematopoietic stem cell transplantation. Biol Blood Marrow Transplant 2012;18:708–15.
9. Ragon BK, Clifton C, Chen H, et al. Geographic distance is not associated with inferior outcome when using long-term transplant clinic strategy. Biol Blood Marrow Transplant 2014;20:53–7.
10. Wingard JR, Majhail NS, Brazauskas R, et al. Long-term survival and late deaths after allogeneic hematopoietic cell transplantation. J Clin Oncol 2011;29:2230–9.

11. Majhail NS, Rizzo JD. Surviving the cure: long term followup of hematopoietic cell transplant recipients. Bone Marrow Transplant 2013;48:1145–51.
12. Majhail NS. Secondary cancers following allogeneic haematopoietic cell transplantation in adults. Br J Haematol 2011;154:301–10.
13. Majhail NS, Rizzo JD, Lee SJ, et al. Recommended screening and preventive practices for long-term survivors after hematopoietic cell transplantation. Bone Marrow Transplant 2012;47:337–41.
14. Majhail NS, Rizzo JD, Lee SJ, et al. Recommended screening and preventive practices for long-term survivors after hematopoietic cell transplantation. Biol Blood Marrow Transplant 2012;18:348–71.
15. Savani BN, Griffith ML, Jagasia S, et al. How I treat late effects in adults after allogeneic stem cell transplantation. Blood 2011;117:3002–9.
16. Tomblyn M, Chiller T, Einsele H, et al. Guidelines for preventing infectious complications among hematopoietic cell transplantation recipients: a global perspective. Biol Blood Marrow Transplant 2009;15:1143–238.
17. Greinix HT, Loddenkemper C, Pavletic SZ, et al. Diagnosis and staging of chronic graft-versus-host disease in the clinical practice. Biol Blood Marrow Transplant 2011;17:167–75.
18. Wolff D, Schleuning M, von Harsdorf S, et al. Consensus Conference on Clinical Practice in Chronic GVHD: second-line treatment of chronic graft-versus-host disease. Biol Blood Marrow Transplant 2011;17:1–17.
19. Wolff D, Gerbitz A, Ayuk F, et al. Consensus conference on clinical practice in chronic graft-versus-host disease (GVHD): first-line and topical treatment of chronic GVHD. Biol Blood Marrow Transplant 2010;16:1611–28.
20. Pavletic SZ, Lee SJ, Socie G, et al. Chronic graft-versus-host disease: implications of the National Institutes of Health consensus development project on criteria for clinical trials. Bone Marrow Transplant 2006;38:645–51.
21. Martin PJ, Weisdorf D, Przepiorka D, et al. National Institutes of Health consensus development project on criteria for clinical trials in chronic graft-versus-host disease: VI. Design of Clinical Trials Working Group report. Biol Blood Marrow Transplant 2006;12:491–505.
22. Couriel D, Carpenter PA, Cutler C, et al. Ancillary therapy and supportive care of chronic graft-versus-host disease: National Institutes of Health consensus development project on criteria for clinical trials in chronic graft-versus-host disease: V. Ancillary Therapy and Supportive Care Working Group report. Biol Blood Marrow Transplant 2006;12:375–96.
23. Pavletic SZ, Martin P, Lee SJ, et al. Measuring therapeutic response in chronic graft-versus-host disease: National Institutes of Health consensus development project on criteria for clinical trials in chronic graft-versus-host disease: IV. Response Criteria Working Group report. Biol Blood Marrow Transplant 2006; 12:252–66.
24. Schultz KR, Miklos DB, Fowler D, et al. Toward biomarkers for chronic graft-versus-host disease: National Institutes of Health consensus development project on criteria for clinical trials in chronic graft-versus-host disease: III. Biomarker Working Group report. Biol Blood Marrow Transplant 2006;12:126–37.
25. Shulman HM, Kleiner D, Lee SJ, et al. Histopathologic diagnosis of chronic graft-versus-host disease: National Institutes of Health consensus development project on criteria for clinical trials in chronic graft-versus-host disease: II. Pathology Working Group report. Biol Blood Marrow Transplant 2006;12:31–47.
26. Filipovich AH, Weisdorf D, Pavletic S, et al. National Institutes of Health consensus development project on criteria for clinical trials in chronic graft-

versus-host disease: I. Diagnosis and Staging Working Group report. Biol Blood Marrow Transplant 2005;11:945–56.
27. Wulff-Burchfield EM, Jagasia M, Savani BN. Long-term follow-up of informal caregivers after allo-SCT: a systematic review. Bone Marrow Transplant 2013;48: 469–73.
28. Wulff-Burchfield EM. Caregivers of long-term survivors. In: Savani BN, editor. Blood and marrow transplantation long term management: prevention and complications. Hoboken (NJ): Wiley-Blackwell; 2013. p. 340.
29. Stokes K. Prevalent psychosocial adjustment issues and solutions: lifestyle and social challenges. In: Savani BN, editor. Blood and marrow transplantation long term management: prevention and complications. Hoboken (NJ): Wiley-Blackwell; 2013. p. 368.

Index

Note: Page numbers of article titles are in **boldface** type.

Hematol Oncol Clin N Am 28 (2014) 1215–1226
http://dx.doi.org/10.1016/S0889-8588(14)00138-5

B

F

H

I

L

M

R

S

T

Printed and bound by CPI Group (UK) Ltd, Croydon, CR0 4YY

03/10/2024

01040491-0007